EVERYDAY ETHICS
Resolving Dilemmas in Nursing Home Life

EVERYDAY ETHICS
Resolving Dilemmas in
Nursing Home Life

Rosalie A. Kane
Arthur L. Caplan

Editors

SPRINGER PUBLISHING COMPANY
New York

mR

Springer Publishing Company, Inc.
536 Broadway
New York, NY 10012

91 92 93 94 / 5 4 3 2

ISBN: 0-8261-6640-7

Printed in the United States of America

This book is gratefully dedicated to the memory of Joan Knowlton, who lived at Hopkins Health Care Center in Hopkins, Minnesota, for 24 years. She was a leader in the struggle to protect the rights of nursing home residents and an example of how a person with a nursing home address can live a life connected to the outside. Until her death in December 1988, she was a member of the advisory group for the study on which this work is based.

CONTENTS

Preface   xi

Acknowledgments   xv

PART I. INTRODUCTION: THE PROBLEM

Chapter 1   Everyday Life in Nursing Homes: "The Way Things
             Are" .... Rosalie A. Kane   3

Chapter 2   Life in an Institution: A Sociological and
             Anthropological View............ Steven S. Foldes   21

Chapter 3   The Morality of the Mundane: Ethical Issues
             Arising in the Daily Lives of Nursing Home
             Residents..................... Arthur L. Caplan   37

PART II. CASES AND COMMENTARIES

Chapter 4   About the Cases ....
             .... Rosalie A. Kane and Arthur L. Caplan   53

Chapter 5   Good Citizen, Bad Citizen......................
              Case Commentary.................. Ruth Macklin   58

Chapter 6   The Chair and Other Public Space ....
              Case Commentary............. Margaret P. Battin   71

Chapter 7   If You Let Them They'd Stay in Bed All Morning:
              The Tyranny of Regulation in Nursing Home Life
              Case Commentary............. James F. Childress   79

Chapter 8   Intimate Strangers: Roommates in Nursing Homes
              Case Commentary: Accommodating Room and
              Roommate Preferences ....
              .... Steven H. Miles and Greg A. Sachs   90

Chapter 9   Till Death Us Do Part: Married Life in Nursing
              Homes ....
              Case Commentary.............. Rosemarie Tong   100

Chapter 10   Thought for Food: Nursing Home Meals ....
              Case Commentary: Something to Chew On........
              ....Mary Ellen Waithe   109

Chapter 11   Phone Privileges ....
              Case Commentary....... Laurence B. McCullough   125

Chapter 12   Guardian Angles ....
              Case Commentary...............Robert Schwartz   137

Chapter 13   Leaving Homes: Residents on Their Own
              Recognizance ....
              Case Commentary.............Reinhard Priester   155

Chapter 14   Let My Persons Go! Restraints of the Trade........
              Case Commentary...............Andrew Jameton   165

Chapter 15   Bathing: On the Boundaries of Health Treatment...
              Case Commentary.............Mila Ann Aroskar   178

Chapter 16   Caring on Demand: How Responsive Is Responsive
              Enough?.......................................
              Case Commentary....................Sara T. Fry   190

Chapter 17   Beyond the Call of Duty: A Nurse's Aide Uses Her
              Judgment.....................................
              Case Commentary..............Diane K. Kjervik   199

Chapter 18   Death of a Resident. . . . .
             Case Commentary: Care of the Dying and the
             Newly Dead . . . . Terrie Wetle   209

Chapter 19   Dressing For "Success" . . . .
             Case Commentary. . . . . Martin Benjamin   223

Chapter 20   Tips and Favors . . . .
             Case Commentary: Private Contracts Between
             Residents and Staff . . . . David J. Mayo   235

Chapter 21   Finding a Home . . . .
             Case Commentary. . . . . Harry R. Moody   245

Chapter 22   Letter of the Law: Eviction from Homes . . . .
             Case Commentary. . . . . Loren E. Lomasky   258

PART III: TOWARD SOLUTIONS

Chapter 23   Building an Effective Caregiving Staff:
             Transforming the Nursing Services. . . . .
             Mila Ann Aroskar, Ene Kristi Urv-Wong, and
             Rosalie A. Kane   271

Chapter 24   Developing Systems That Promote Autonomy:
             Policy Considerations. . . . . Iris C. Freeman   291

Chapter 25   Avenues to Appropriate Autonomy: What Next?. . . .
             Rosalie A. Kane, Arthur L. Caplan, Iris C. Freeman,
             Mila Ann Aroskar, and Ene Kristi Urv-Wong.   306

Contributors   319

PREFACE

This book had its genesis in an idea and a study. The idea was that it is possible and necessary to describe in considerable detail the kind of personal autonomy that is wanted and wanting in America's nursing homes. Part of this idea was that a multidisciplinary group of philosophers and ethicists, as well as social scientists and practitioners, should take on the task of identifying and thinking about the everyday problems that affect residents of nursing homes.

THE STUDY

The University of Minnesota, in collaboration with the Minnesota Alliance for Health Care Consumers, was awarded a grant from The Retirement Research Foundation to conduct a 2-year study of autonomy in the everyday lives of nursing home residents. The following premises underlay our initial efforts:

> Personal autonomy is a complex phenomenon in nursing homes because of the nature of the nursing home as a social setting, the

public policies that govern these institutions, the heterogeneity of the residents, and the multiplicity of purposes and prognoses that residents bring to a nursing home setting.

Matters of life in nursing homes are as worthy of attention as are the more widely discussed matters of dying and death in nursing homes. Issues concerning the right to have treatment withheld or discontinued, the do-not-resuscitate and do-not-intubate controversies, and other questions concerned with the use of life-prolonging technology at the end of life are, of course, important. But complicated ethical issues are raised in the course of ordinary nursing home life. These have far-reaching ramifications for the quality of life of those who live in nursing homes.

To try to enhance personal autonomy for physically impaired nursing home residents is to grapple with a paradox: The more physically impaired the nursing home resident, the more he or she must depend on help from others to carry out his or her autonomous designs. Those who depend on help in order to be autonomous are in an ambiguous position. Staff members who strive to promote both increased physical independence and autonomy of nursing home residents are often uncertain about how to act in specific cases.

Facilitating appropriate autonomy involves a dual challenge: first, to define what is appropriate; and second, to identify the barriers interfering with what is appropriate. Thus, we faced two related but distinct tasks: finding out what is right to do and finding out how to do what is right.

The barriers to appropriate autonomy, however appropriate autonomy is further specified, are likely to be multiple and complex. Removing them will involve changes in public law and regulation, educational strategies, and organizational strategies. Perhaps, too, more money or different ways of using money will be needed to improve chances for autonomy among nursing home residents.

Our study had three general components: empirical, ethical, and strategic. The empirical side involved detailed interviews with large numbers of nursing home residents and nurses' assistants, as well as the review and analysis of nursing home complaint records. In this book we do not present these findings in detail, but we do draw on them heavily to illustrate our points.

For the ethical component, we created 18 "cases," derived directly from our own data. These cases are complex, as is the nursing home. They may illustrate the predicament of more than one resident and perhaps of several staff members as well. Each case was presented to a philosopher or other ethicist, who, in turn, prepared a commentary on how to approach the ethical issues raised by the case. In October 1988 we held a meeting in Minneapolis during which researchers, ethicists-commentators, practitioners, and policymakers from Minnesota came together. The revised case studies were tempered in the crucible of that lively meeting.

The third part of the study was a policy analysis of the factors that facilitate and impede the kind of autonomy the case commentators deemed appropriate.

ORGANIZATION OF THE BOOK

Part I sets the stage for presentation and analysis of case material. In Chapter 1, Rosalie Kane describes everyday life for those who live and work in nursing homes, borrowing generously from the words of those we interviewed as well as from other sources. In Chapter 2, anthropologist Steven Foldes suggests that the case material is partly explained by the role the nursing home plays in our society. Then, in Chapter 3, Arthur Caplan lays out ethical considerations pertaining to "the morality of the mundane"—that is, the ordinary events that befall denizens of the nursing home.

Part II, the heart of the book, contains cases and commentaries on the cases. Although identifying information about nursing homes, residents, and staff is disguised, and although we have combined the stories of several people into a single "case," all of the incidents and reactions were reported to us. True stories all, they should ring true to nursing home life. For many of the philosophers and ethicists who wrote the case commentaries, it was a new experience to apply paradigms and principles to homely topics such as how one decides who rooms with whom in a nursing home, what the extent of the staff's obligations are to help an immobile resident remain continent, or who has the right to sit in a particular dayroom chair.

In Part III we reach for more general, or systemic, solutions. In Chapter 23, Aroskar, Urv-Wong, and Kane discuss approaches to organizing the all- important nursing service as a force for resident empowerment. In Chapter 24, Iris Freeman describes both external and internal approaches to promoting autonomy; in so doing, she gives attention to the thorny subject of nursing home regulations, which may have either an enabling or a chilling effect on resident autonomy. In the last chapter, the study team presents a list of issues for future work on autonomy in long-term-care contexts.

Despite the varied styles of the contributors, we have strived for an even tone and a coherent ordering of materials. It should be possible for an interested person to read the book from beginning to end. It should also be possible for instructors to use the material for courses in long-term care and in ethics. To that end, each case is self-contained and presents a set of questions for further study. Because we hope this book will be useful for long-term-care practitioners and their students, and for philosophers and their students, we have tried to protect each group as much as possible from the jargon of the other.

ROSALIE A. KANE
ARTHUR L. CAPLAN

ACKNOWLEDGMENTS

An enterprise such as we describe above necessarily accrues many debts of gratitude along the way. The study itself had four major investigators. These were the editors and Mila Ann Aroskar, RN, EdD, of the University of Minnesota School of Public Health, and Iris C. Freeman, executive director of the Minnesota Alliance for Health Care Consumers. An interdisciplinary team that included a social work researcher, a social work advocate, a nurse, and a philosopher made for a lively mix. As editors, we are exceedingly grateful to our primary colleagues in this work. As well, we thank Ene Kristi Urv-Wong, then a research associate, who managed the project from the beginning; and Meribeth Arndt of the Minnesota Alliance for Health Care Consumers, who conducted a retrospective review of nursing home ombudsman records.

Knowing that Minnesota does not necessarily represent the country, we replicated our work in four communities. We thank Susan O. Mercer of the University of Arkansas, School of Social Work, and her assistant, Maybian Sloane, who did related studies in Little Rock, Arkansas, and Sante Fe, New Mexico; Rose Dobrof, of Hunter College's Brookdale Center on Aging, and her assistant the Twaha Bukenya, who did related studies in New York City; and Elyse Salend, of the University of California's Division of Geriatric Medicine, and her assistant, Anna Rahman, who did related studies in Los Angeles.

In Minnesota, our data collectors—all graduate students at the University of Minnesota at the time—were Nancy Oxton, Julie Portesan (who also assisted with analysis), Julie Scher, and Debora Smith. In latter stages, Jody M. Schueneman served as the project's research assistant. We are grateful to them all.

Pretesting of resident interview formats was enabled by nursing home residents Joan Knowlton and Ben Miller. Pretesting of nurse's aides questionnaires was made possible by administrator Rachel Rustad, who arranged for us to visit her facility, Stevens Square Home, and talk to her staff.

Over the 2-year period this study has enjoyed the energetic and thoughtful advice of an advisory group that represents many important areas of leadership in the state. Members included Sue Bannick, MD, Hennepin County Medical Center; Inez Bonk, chair, Family Council, Minnesota Veterans Home; Barbara Ann Brown, RN, MS, St. Paul Ramsey Medical Center; Barbara J. Blumer, JD, Broeker, Geer, Fletcher & LaFond, Ltd.; Rick E. Carter and his representative, Dean Newman, Care Providers of Minnesota; Steven S. Foldes, PhD, Minnesota Department of Health; George K. Gordon, EdD, University of Minnesota; Kenneth Hepburn, PhD, Veterans Administration Medical Center; Joan E. Knowlton, Residents' Council, Hopkins Care Center; Gayle M. Kvenvold and her representative, Darrell Schreve, Minnesota Association of Homes for the Aging; Margaret A. McManus, MSW, Minnesota Nursing Home Social Workers Association; Ben Miller, Residents' Council, Baptist Residence; Jean Klein Orsello, Minnesota Board on Aging; Pamela J. Parker, Minnesota Department of Human Services; James J. Pattee, MD, University of Minnesota; Paul O. Sand, National Conference of Christians and Jews, Inc.; Susan Schaffer, RN, JD, Broeker, Geer, Fletcher & LaFond, Ltd.; Clarice Seufert, Minnesota Department of Health; Michael Tripple, Minnesota Department of Health; Evelyn Van Allen, Minnesota Network for Institutional Ethics Committees. Particular thanks are due to the Minnesota Association of Homes for the Aging and Care Providers of Minnesota for their endorsement of this study with their members.

This study would have been impossible without the generous support and intellectual leadership of the Retirement Research Foundation. Vice-President Brian Hofland, who served as project officer, was an unfailing source of help.

Ann Mulally has typed many pounds of material in the course of this research including the earliest version of the manuscript itself. In later phases, Pat Thomas, with assistance from Ann Mulally and Leticia Fernandez, labored prodigiously to produce the final manuscript and the disks for typesetting. We thank them all for their cheerful competence.

Last and never least, we are deeply grateful to the nursing home residents and staff members, in particular the nurses' assistants, who shared their lives and work with us.

R. A. K.
A. L. C.

PART I

INTRODUCTION: THE PROBLEM

Chapter 1

EVERYDAY LIFE IN NURSING HOMES: "The Way Things Are"

Rosalie A. Kane

BACKGROUND

During youth and middle age, few contemplate the prospect of someday taking up residence in a nursing home. When the subject painfully intrudes, typically because a relative or friend needs the care or protection a nursing home affords, we react with a mingling of fear (because it could happen to anyone), anxiety (because the sounds, smells, and sights of nursing homes may be upsettingly foreign), sadness (because our friend's life seems somehow diminished by her new address), and guilty relief (because we are thankful to be "on the outside").

If it has been our unhappy lot to make the arrangements for a relative, perhaps a parent, to enter a nursing home, the predominant emotion may be guilt, regardless of the valid reasons that made it impossible to save our parent from this fate. Even if our exposure to nursing homes is more perfunctory, perhaps limited to an occasional visit or an organized event such as Christmas caroling in a neighborhood facility, we are likely to react to the experience with superstitious dread. Many middle-aged people say to their own children, "I pray I never get like that," or more directively, "Don't ever let me get that way."

Most people, therefore, ignore nursing homes unless they absolutely cannot, and then they tend to be shocked, dismayed, and ultimately resigned to what they find. But the nursing home is and in some form will continue to be a dominant theme in the lives of disabled adults, particularly the elderly. At present, 5% of people over age 65 live in nursing homes, and those surviving to 65 have at least a 25% chance of living in a nursing home before they die. With odds of admission so high, the nursing home directly and indirectly affects millions of American lives. The current mixture of avoidance and resignation (that is, avoiding the issue as long as possible and then resigning oneself to presumably inevitable conditions) is the worst possible recipe for identifying and, as much as possible, changing the conditions that make nursing homes dreaded places to live.

Novels sometimes describe nursing home proprietors who are genuinely evil (Hassler, 1979; Sarton, 1973). But when nursing home residents themselves write true or thinly veiled fictional accounts of life in nursing homes, their stories have few villains. Carobeth Laird (1979) a nursing home resident for many years while in her 80s, calls her memoir *Limbo* and refers to herself as a "nursing home survivor." She begins her book this way:

> If you expect a tale of horror, of filth and overt cruelty, read no further. . . .
> It is instead an account of one person's efforts to hold onto sanity and identity in an atmosphere which was, by its very nature, dehumanizing. It dwells of necessity upon those trivialities of daily routine which loom so large in the lives of the helpless and isolated. (p. 1)

Similarly, Janet Tulloch (1975), an extremely physically disabled woman who entered a nursing home at age 40 when her parents died, prefaces her book this way: "Millions of words have been written about the horrors of living in nursing homes and other institutions. However, indifference and insensitivity are more devastating crimes than intentional cruelty and premeditated assault" (p. 15). In the early 1980s, California newspaper readers were regularly confronted with the struggle of an elderly inmate in a state prison for women who steadfastly refused parole lest she be sent to a nursing home. Ms. Lang was a longtime prisoner who, in her 70s, was released to a quiet life in the community, complete with pet cat. Five years later a fall catapulted her into a nursing home. Unable to tolerate the shared room and the confused environment, she committed a technical parole violation and returned to prison where she had a room of her own. There her physical condition declined further, and in her 80s she annually and gallantly held forth against the parole board, which questioned whether a prison could or should care for the frail elderly. She protested that she still could work at folding laundry and that, except for a little help getting in and out of bed, she was managing on her own. With its usual sympathetic appreciation for an individual underdog, the public responded, and Ms. Lang was released to someone who volunteered to give her a home. But with its usual failure to extend its sympathy beyond the dramatic single case, public reaction did not extend to the similar predicaments of thousands of other nursing home residents who had committed no crime and therefore had no recourse to prison as an alternative.

However atypical this case may be, the plain fact that Ms. Lang, a woman who had experienced both settings, preferred a prison to a nursing home is a severe indictment of our national provisions for the frail elderly. Her stance is consistent with the eloquent testimony of Laird (1979) and Tulloch (1975) and other nursing home survivors. The complaints of these and other chroniclers of life in nursing homes rarely deal with issues of technical medical treatment or life-and-death decisions. Rather, they deal with the nagging indignities and losses of ordinary life. Given that national attention must turn to ways of developing better living environments for the frail elderly, providing a detailed record of these everyday issues can energize and direct that effort.

As a backdrop to later chapters that explore personal autonomy for nursing home residents using cases and case commentaries, this chapter examines the American nursing home as an environment for living. As we began to study this topic, we assumed that appropriate personal autonomy would be as difficult to define as it is theoretically desirable. Moreover, even if agreement could be achieved about situations and conditions under which personal autonomy ought to be protected, we knew that putting these principles into operation would be extraordinarily difficult. In fact, infringements of personal autonomy are so commonplace and efforts to protect agreed-upon areas of autonomy so unsuccessful that many observers have come to accept rather severe limits in personal autonomy as the "way things are."

This chapter depicts "the way things are" under several headings: the residents, the staff, the home itself, the typical programs, and the public policies governing nursing homes. These components in interaction— residents, staff, place, programs, and policies—define everyday life in nursing homes. Although not all of the features are mutable, some could be altered in the service of greater personal autonomy for nursing home residents.

THE RESIDENTS

Nursing Home Residents Are Heterogeneous

The first fact about nursing home residents is heterogeneity. Although homes may and do specialize somewhat, the usual nursing home is multipurpose. It houses short-stay and long-stay residents. It houses those who have come to die and those who have come to attempt a life with a nursing home address. It houses some who have come to convalesce after surgery or to receive rehabilitation after a stroke or a hip fracture (this latter group often returns home). Depending on the purpose for entering a nursing home, the expected length of stay, and the prognosis, residents will have different priorities and wishes for how they spend their time.

Statistics about nursing home length of stay underscore the multipurpose use of the nursing home. Although the public and nursing home residents themselves may view admission to a facility as the last move on the way to death, the facts differ. Using data from the 1977 National Nursing Home Survey, Keeler, Kane and Solomon (1981) showed that 50% of all nursing home admissions resulted in discharge within 3 months; more than half of those persons were alive at the time of discharge. Of those discharged alive, about half went to hospitals and half went home. Those who went to hospitals later either went back to a nursing home or to a lesser level of care in the community. Considering all nursing home residents, the average length of stay was about 1 year, but this masks the fact that some residents had very long nursing home stays indeed—measured in decades rather than years—whereas others had remarkably short stays. Thus, even though some residents may be making their long-term home in a nursing home, the setting itself is marked by flux. Every week new residents must be accommodated, and perhaps current residents must be discommoded in the process.

Preliminary findings from the most recent (1985) National Nursing Home Survey (Sekscenski, 1987) describe a large probability sample of nursing home dischargees during the course of a year; 72% were discharged alive and 28% dead. The median length of stay was 82 days for live dischargees and 163 days for those who died. However, about 7% of those discharged alive in 1985 and 20% of those discharged dead had stayed in the nursing home more than 3 years; 11% of those who died had lengths of stay of more than 5 years. Thirty percent of those discharged alive went directly to a residence in the community; the rest went to hospitals or other health facilities. Again these data confirm diverse patterns of nursing home use.

Heterogeneity is not confined to disabilities and lengths of stay. As others point out (see Macklin, this volume), the nursing home is an accidental community. Its residents are even less likely to be similar than tenants of housing developments on the outside. Unsurprisingly, nursing home residents differ in interests, tastes, cultural background, social class, educational status, former occupations, and income.

Nursing home residents even represent a wide age spectrum. True, the average age of a nursing home resident is about 84, and most nursing home residents are over 65. The 1985 National Nursing Home Survey showed that the proportion of residents over age 85 had increased since the 1977 survey. Extrapolating to all residents, the 1985 survey suggests that 45% of elderly residents are over 85, 39% are between 75 and 84, and 16% are between 65 and 84 (Hing, 1987). But younger adults are also found in nursing homes. Some of the younger residents are physically disabled, whereas others are chronically mentally ill—the products of the deinstitutionalization movement of the mid-1960s in the state mental hospitals. Moreover, the 35-year age span from 65 to 100 + is too broad to be conveniently classified under the heading "old." After all, among those aged 65 to 100, we should expect as much diversity as in a group ranging in age from 20 to 55!

Nursing Home Residents Are Functionally Impaired

Functional impairment is a common denominator in the nursing home. Nursing home residents tend to need help with one or more basic activities of daily living such as dressing and grooming themselves, bathing, getting to the toilet, getting in and out of bed, and even eating. They may need to have objects fetched for them; someone else may need to do the reaching. They may need help in dialing a telephone or holding its receiver.

In fact, help with the basic functions of daily life that most people take for granted is translated into the job description of nurse's aides. They do "transfers" (i.e., help a person get in and out of bed), they give baths, and they "toilet" the residents. The routines of the morning are often known as "morning cares," to be contrasted with "evening cares." Those who need to be spoon-fed are colloquially known as "feeders," a term internalized by residents themselves. (More than one resident explained to our interviewers: "I'm a feeder.")

Functional disability among residents means a high degree of dependence on staff, and it means that the day is dominated by issues concerned with the mechanics of living. Serving as an object of care can be a demoralizing role. As one resident told us, "I'd just as well be dead. I'm clean, have clean food, and they wash me." Residents are aware that their care routines are not their own. In the words of another resident, "It's not like at home where if you get a little hungry, you go and get some coffee, or you lay down or move around." Or as another woman put it, "It feels awkward to have someone write down a description of how much you ate at meals."

According to the 1985 Nursing Home Survey (Hing, 1987), 91% of residents needed help with bathing, 75% with dressing, 63% with getting in and out of bed or a chair, and 40% with eating. Half experienced at least some bladder or bowel incontinence. These bleak statistics of dependency are, in part, created by nursing home policy. For instance, few nursing homes permit residents to bathe unassisted. Furthermore, need for assistance is a matter of degree. Assistance in eating, for example, could be limited to cutting food, it could involve watching to be sure the resident does not choke, or it could require literal spoon-feeding. Finally, nursing home staff, who provided the survey data, have a propensity to assume physical dependency. All of these caveats aside, functional dependency is still a central reality in the nursing home.

Residents who are functionally impaired will often need help from a staff member to put their wishes and choices into action. Some are literally unable to implement a decision about what to wear, where to sit, when and what to eat without help. Staff members have the power to refuse to take them where they want to go, or to take them to activities when they choose to stay in their rooms. In the nursing home, there is a paradox: Physically dependent people require help from others to execute their independent designs.

Sensory Impairments Are Common

Vision, hearing, and speech deficits are common in nursing homes. These sensory impairments affect the personal autonomy of nursing home residents in two ways. First, they create difficulties in communication. As already noted, physical disability forces many nursing home residents to depend on staff to carry out their wishes. Add sensory deficits, and residents will have trouble even conveying those wishes. It takes time, patience, and ingenuity (all scarce commodities) for a staff member to receive the message that such a resident is trying to convey. Second, sensory impairments greatly diminish opportunities for nursing home residents to fashion meaningful lives.

Cognitive Impairment Is Common

The 1985 National Nursing Home Survey reports that 63% of nursing home residents are demented or have memory impairments (Hing, 1987). Disorientation was defined as being unable to remember dates or time, identify familiar locations or people, recall important aspects of recent events, or make straightforward judgments.) The survey further reports that 47% of the residents had either senile dementia or organic brain damage. Even more than the functional data, these data must be interpreted carefully. They were supplied by staff members and thus are subject to the careless labeling of cognitive impairment that staff members often make. The diagnostic data may be based on a note in the record that itself was the result of an assumption rather than a serious workup. Moreover, cognitive impairment itself ranges widely among residents who share the label of "dementia," and cognitive abilities also wax and wane for particular residents. A resident may experience periods of lucidity interspersed with periods of confusion.

All that being said, undoubtedly considerable cognitive impairment is present in nursing homes with all of the problems for the exercise of personal autonomy that cognitive deficits introduce.

Nursing Home Residents Are Usually Female

A nursing home tends to be a woman's world. Most residents are female. Widows predominate, and women who have never married are overrepresented compared to their presence in the population. The 25% of male nursing home residents may find few programs slanted to their interests. On the other hand, women who enter nursing homes must surely notice that their world is strangely devoid of men.

Nursing Home Residents Are Often Poor

Money is power. Functionally disabled people of means have a better chance of implementing their wishes than do those who are poor. About half of all nursing home residents are supported by the Medicaid program, a state-run medical-care-financing program for the poor. To qualify for this coverage, residents must have virtually depleted their assets and have incomes that fall below the costs of their care. Medicaid allows a fixed monthly fund for personal spending, known as a "comfort allowance."

In most states, the comfort allowance does not exceed $40 a month. From that sum, nursing home residents on Medicaid must pay for cosmetics and toiletries, clothing, postage stamps and stationery, books, entertainment, transportation for nonmedical reasons, telephone bills (if they have a phone), any any other items they need or want. Clearly, residents financed by Medicaid must lower their sights. A pair of shoes could consume more than a month's allowance. For a resident to send gifts or even greeting cards to family members, she may need to forgo something for herself that could hardly be called a luxury. Some nursing home residents enter facilities with sufficient assets to pay the bills—at least in the short run—and have funds left over. Although half of nursing home residents are, by definition, poor, many are not. Most typically, however, even cognitively intact residents have no direct access to their own money. For convenience, arrangements are usually made with a family member or other third party to administer the resident's funds. If a resident needs to undertake a process to request access to her own resources, and if she sometimes has to accept no for an answer, the functional result is very much like poverty. To have lost control over a checkbook in 20th-century America is, by definition, a loss of autonomy.

Admission Is Often Involuntary and Traumatic

Entering a nursing home is often an emergency matter. It seldom involves the active participation of the resident. The vast majority of the residents who spoke to us did not pick out the nursing home. Most believed they were there as a result of a doctor's recommendation; the majority had been in a hospital immediately before admission to a nursing home, which compromised their ability to shop for a facility. Family members were often involved in the original selection, and when a resident was moved to a different home, he or she accounted for it by saying that a son or daughter wanted them somewhere else. Surprisingly often, our informants had already made a move to the community of an adult child, and, as strangers to the community, had little frame of reference to choose a facility. Sometimes plans to live with a relative went wrong; sometimes the resident's condition deteriorated and made these plans impractical.

Even residents making the decision from the community rather than a hospital used language like "I felt a little railroaded" or said that the description of the home did not match the reality. One resident, aged 83, had lived alone in Texas but was brought to the city where her son lived. The initial plan had been to add a room to her son's house. After a precipitating illness, she was admitted to a nursing home.

I expected to stay three weeks," she said, "and it became three months, and now it looks like forever. I have no place to go. My daughter who owned the house in Texas sold the house and all the furniture. I have nothing of my household with me. They were going to add a room to the house, but I guess now they won't. My grandson got divorced, and he is left with 6 kids to be raised by him and his parents. My son has that responsibility now. *When we are robbed of our independence, we lose our confidence.* (emphasis added)

The last words here are eloquent. The typical process by which older people move to nursing homes does tend to rob them of their confidence.

Residents may feel bereft, without even personal possessions to remind them of their former selves. For example, one 77-year-old woman, paralyzed with stroke, who had been in a nursing home for 4 years described it this way:

I lived in Florida until my husband died. We had no kids, so I came here [a different state]. My brother made the decisions. I was in another home for a year, but he decided this place was nicer and moved me here. I never saw either place or had any say about the decision. He sold my home and all my things and never asked me or told me what he was doing, and I don't know anything about the money from the sale. He never told me. I have not one thing but a snapshot of me and my husband to remind me or come with me from my former life with my husband.

Families Play Pivotal Roles

As was shown, family members play a major role in getting the resident to a nursing home in the first place. They also can be lifelines to former identities and to the community. Although inability of the family to give the necessary care is cited as the reason for admission, families nevertheless provide large amounts of hands-on practical care to relatives in nursing homes. They also offer companionship and help with business affairs. It is not unusual for a nursing home resident to be visited daily by an interested family member. As already stated, nursing home residents also have considerable financial dependence on family, even for the use of their own resources. Personal autonomy of nursing home residents, therefore, is facilitated and (sometimes impeded) by family members. Family members may give instructions to staff (for example, about the use of physical restraints) that oppose those of the resident.

Other residents have no family within a reasonable distance for interaction. In stark contrast to residents whose family members become fixtures in the home, these residents may have no visitors at all. Although the case examples in this book describe some conflict-ridden situations in which family members are imperfect spokespeople for the resident's interests, those without family have no natural advocates at all.

In summary, nursing home residents are heterogeneous in length of stay, prognosis, and purpose of the admission, as well as along social dimensions. They tend to be functionally impaired in a way that prevents carrying out some or all basic self-care activities without help. They may also have sensory impairment that limits communication, or cognitive impairment that limits decision-making capacities. They are most likely to be women and often poor; when not poor, they seldom have direct control over their finances. Admission to the facility often occurs in a crisis, and the resident often feels out of control. Possessions and properties are mysteriously gone. For some residents, family members are conspicuously and helpfully present, whereas others have no family involvement in their care. All of this adds up to a difficult test case for realization of personal autonomy.

THE STAFF

Perhaps appropriately, the nursing home is hardly a highly professional environment. Unlike a hospital, it is, after all, meant to be a place to live. On the other hand, residents and their families who have been convinced they should enter a nursing home because of the demands of a medical condition requiring "24-hour care" are often surprised to realize how little contact they have with doctors or even nurses after their admission.

Typically, a nursing home has an administrator and a director of nursing (DON) at the helm. Although there will nominally be a medical director, house physicians are unusual and the medical director's presence may not be felt. Ironically, despite the fact that most residents are Medicare beneficiaries who are entitled to regular physician visits, nursing home residents often complain that they lack chances to confer with a doctor.

Although nursing as a discipline dominates the nursing home, the ratio of registered nurses to residents is low, usually conforming to but not surpassing minimum requirements for federal certification. Residents may rarely see a registered nurse, particularly at night. Licensed practical nurses (LPNs) and certified nursing assistants (CNAs), the latter known as nurse's aides or nursing assistants, are the mainstay of care. A home will also have a social worker and activities director on staff (sometimes combined in the same person), a consultant dietician, a consultant pharmacist, and perhaps a physical therapist.

The paraprofessional labor pool, which forms the bulk of the work force is the group that most frequently comes into contact with the resident. Nurse's aides and even dietary aides have the greatest likelihood of influencing the daily life of residents.

This paraprofessional work force tends to be poorly paid, minimally trained, and overworked. The nursing home is largely nonunionized, and nurse's aides often barely exceed the minimum wage. A minimum amount of training is now mandated prior to employment, but most of the learning is on-the-job. And the job itself involves heavy labor and unpleasant routines. Especially on evening and night shifts, one aide may be assigned to 50 or even 100 residents. Nurse's aides may also be relatively uneducated and perhaps functionally illiterate in the English language. This is not universally true, however; the position also attracts college students and transitional people who may have more extensive educations. Some of the latter may be new immigrants who have health care backgrounds but do not share the language of the residents and lack formal credentials to practice their old jobs in the United States. They may perceive the position as temporary, a stepping-stone to a better-paying job in the hospital sector. Some nurse's aides plan to become licensed practical nurses. Overall, turnover tends to be high, because of nurse's aides moving from facility to facility or deciding to leave the industry entirely.

Some nurse's aides are highly motivated despite the pay and the working conditions. In our own studies we found that many are inspired by a desire to work with old people, and some impute almost religious significance to their work. Unfortunately, there are virtually no career ladders that would allow the most effective nurse's aides to progress markedly in either responsibility or earning capacity.

In some communities the nursing home staff almost entirely represents ethnic minority groups, whereas the majority of the residents are white and "Anglo." Sometimes staff members report that they are at the receiving end of racial slurs. When the prejudiced remarks result from the released inhibitions or changed personalities of persons with Alzheimer's disease, the staff member has little choice but to shrug them off. Nevertheless, they substantially reduce the quality of the working environment.

THE PLACE

The newly admitted nursing home resident may well find the environment a shock. In the first scene of *A Home Is Not a Home*, Janet Tulloch (1975) depicts two new residents at their first meal in the facility:

> Cecile was spreading vanilla ice cream on her sauerkraut. She had flattened the briny mound into a pale field. Very carefully, she scooped the ice cream from its styrofoam container, spreading it as glazed snow. Smiling with accomplishment, she traded spoon for fork and deposited the goo

in her waiting mouth. Her air of confidence seemed to say that her action was perfectly natural. Her companions at the table gave a collective gasp before accepting the act and continuing with their own less exotic meals. However the two newcomers did experience more than a flurry of emotion. . . . Both of them needed to sort all the events of that day to put them in perspective. (p. 19)

Decades of social activities do not prepare nursing home residents for the multiple instances of "ice cream mixed with sauerkraut" that they encounter upon admission.

These and other odd experiences occur partly because in most nursing homes the cognitively impaired and the cognitively intact are housed in close proximity. These close quarters mean that residents who are lucid may be frightened or annoyed by screams, moans, and other repetitive noises or by confused people invading their personal space. It means that programs are often cast to the lowest common denominator. From the viewpoint of the person with dementia, it may also mean that their mobility may be restricted to produce a somewhat normal environment for the others.

Living in a nursing home in all likelihood means living in a shared bedroom. Though most residents prefer a single room if they can afford the price difference, there are simply not enough single rooms to go around. Nursing home life means reducing one's space to a few square feet around a bed and to have no ultimate control over who occupies the next bed. Although staff may try to accommodate preferences, the mathematics of room arrangements interfere. Even those nobody wants to room with need partners. Residents may share their quarters with the dying, with the demented, or with a succession of roommates, none of whom they have chosen. Several cases in this volume deal with the ethical ramifications of room assignments (see Miles and Sachs, this volume, and Tong, this volume). The residents we interviewed told us many poignant stories about their difficulties with roommates.

The resident is not even guaranteed that she will remain in the same room throughout her stay. Residents may be moved either to make the logistics of room assignments work out or to meet the demands of caregiving and reimbursement categories. For example, only some beds will be certified for Medicare, so a resident whose condition temporarily merits Medicare coverage may be summarily moved to a room with a higher staffing level. Or some residents may be moved closer to the nurses' station so that they can be more closely or conveniently watched. If several women are admitted and vacancies happen to be in men's rooms, an adjustment will be made.

Quite often the more severely disabled residents are housed on upper floors, and deterioration is marked by moving upstairs. Such relocation can have severe symbolic as well as realistic effects on the resident. Our review of complaints to the ombudsman showed that residents returning from a brief hospitalization could be very upset to find that their old room had been reassigned and they were temporarily or permanently installed in another area of the home. Given these circumstances, the contract between a resident and a nursing home would be more accurately be described as an arrangement for a "space" rather than for a particular bed or room.

Privacy in a nursing home is at a premium. The dining room, which often doubles as an activity room, is a major congregating place. Small dayrooms may also be available. Communal televisions often have hard-to-reach controls and are perpetually playing. A resident with a double room may be hard-pressed to find a private place to sit with visitors. Typically, a single chair is available by each bed. Although enlightened homes encourage staff to knock on the doors, this is more generally done to announce entry rather than to request it.

Physical restraints are in wide use in nursing homes. These include restraining "geri-chairs" (similar to high chairs), waist and "possey" restraints that tie the resident to a chair, wrist restraints that are applied to residents at night, and side rails that prohibit residents from getting out of bed. (In our interviews one resident even told us about a leash like arrangement that she had observed being used for another resident and which she found demeaning.) Ethicists have given virtually no thought to physical restraints and their proper use. (See Jameton, this volume, for a beginning formulation.)

It is difficult to determine how often restraints are used, but the use is high (Evans & Strumpf, 1989). One statistic has it that physical restraints were in use for 30% of nursing home residents in a sample of New York State facilities (Zimmer, Watson, & Treat, 1984). By contrast, in many European countries physical restraints are not used at all, and alternative methods are found to promote safety.

Nursing home residents cannot bring much with them. First, space is severely limited. Storage space is insufficient even for a meaningful selection of personal clothes. Second, the safety of personal possessions is not guaranteed. Some losses occur because confused residents appropriate (and perhaps hide) others' things. Some loss is a result of theft on the part of staff. Because it is always possible to attribute disappearance of possessions to the first cause, it is easier for the second cause to go unchecked. A nursing home administrator who spent 9 days in the role of a wheelchair-bound resident suddenly began to view his "enlightened" policies designed to give residents a sense of personal possession (Bennett, 1980) as hollow gestures. For example, previously he had taken pride in the policy of printing residents' names on their wheelchairs, making cellophane tape available to put greeting cards on walls, encouragement of family photos, and respectful laundering of residents' clothes. After 9 days in a nursing home these efforts seemed "minuscule, just token expressions of good will. The magnitude of patients' personal property deprivation is great and almost total. . . . Irrespective of the patients' prior lifestyles, being bereft of their property makes them seem destitute" (p. 79).

This context of deprivation of possessions provides the background against which the case and comment by Battin (this volume) acquires its poignancy.

In summary, the nursing home typically affords little privacy, personal space, or opportunity to use public space. The policy of enforced roommates minimizes the chance for personal autonomy. Even though special units for senile dementia are becoming more common, in most nursing homes the interspersing of the confused and the lucid can create a world of the absurd for cognitively intact residents. And too often nursing home residents are literally tied or otherwise physically restrained, a crude and extreme form of behavior control.

THE PROGRAMS

The life of a nursing home is driven by routines. There are fixed times for baths, meals, medications, getting up, and going to bed. The major job of the staff is to make sure all of the routines are properly performed.

The major mechanism that guides the care of a particular resident is known as the care plan. Nursing homes are expected to have care plans that are carefully thought out and suitable to the needs of the resident. In some nursing homes residents are permitted to be involved in developing their care plans. (In Minnesota, for example, the Bill of Rights for Nursing Home Residents asserts that a resident or, if the resident is incapacitated, a resident's surrogate must be permitted to attend the meetings at which the care plan is developed or otherwise participate in forging the plan.) It is the care plan that puts the individualized touches on a resident's routines.

Unfortunately, many residents are unaware of how all-embracing a care plan can be. It may include details about what the resident may eat, whom she can see, whether she is permitted to stay up late enough to watch a favorite television show, whether she will have a bath or a shower, and whether this will be twice a week or daily and what time of day it will occur. Life by care plan means that all of the elements of daily life that one takes for granted on the outside need to be negotiated.

Nursing home programming may be geared to the lowest common denominator. Bingo is a staple, as are arts and crafts and decorating for every holiday. Birthday parties tend to be held monthly, adding an impersonal touch to recognition of the birthdays of everyone born that month. Religious observation may be relentlessly ecumenical, thus stripped of the symbols that people find important.

It is unfair to indict all nursing home programming with sweeping generalizations. Yet as one considers the domination of care plans and routines, the popularity of programs often associated with children, and the long empty spaces—particularly during the weekends, when there is little to do but anticipate the next meal—a single word comes to mind that best captures the average nursing home day: boring.

POLICIES GOVERNING NURSING HOMES

Nursing homes are shaped by outside forces. Perhaps the most prominent influence is regulation. The nursing home is a minutely regulated entity. Federal requirements—called Conditions of Participation—must be met before a nursing home may receive federal Medicare or Medicaid funds (the latter being a shared federal and state financing program that is administered by each state). With a strong emphasis on Medicaid, most nursing homes depend heavily on public financing programs, which may be supporting more than half of the residents at any given time.

Nursing home regulations emphasize safety above all. They also concentrate on the physical environment, the resident record system, and the dietary routines—in other words, the procedures thought necessary for a safe environment. A widely hailed report by the Institute of Medicine (1986) suggested some reshaping of the regulations to emphasize quality of life and civil rights in addition to health and safety. It also proposed changing the means of measuring compliance with regulations to emphasize outcomes as well as procedures. (For example, for restorative nursing programs, a procedural measure would be that bowel and bladder training programs are started for residents likely to benefit, and an outcome measure would be reduced levels of incontinence and use of urinary catheters.) Simple outcome measures that can be counted for the whole facility include bed sores, proportion of residents up and dressed, and proportion of residents needing to be fed. Harder to measure and count are outcomes reflective of emotional or social well-being—for example, proportion leaving the facility for short periods, proportion with visitors in a given week, proportion of residents who are depressed. Unusually high negative outcomes in any sphere—physical, psychological, social—do not automatically reflect poor care. For example, a nursing home may simply have admitted a sicker or more depressed group of residents. But a preponderance of negative outcomes, in the view of the Institute of Medicine committee, should trigger a careful examination of the reasons.

The panel also urged that information be gathered through interview with and observation of residents rather than relying on medical records and staff reports alone. Since 1986 the routine inspection process has included direct contact with a sample of residents. Many of the Institute of Medicine's findings were embodied in 1987 legislation, but the net effect has not been regulatory relief for nursing homes. They are still subject to a large number of rules that govern their activities. Furthermore, regulations are administered by hundreds of inspectors (called surveyors). The idiosyncratic judgments of one surveyor may be inconsistent with the views of the previous one. There is also a danger that surveyors will focus on eliminating potential hazards and achieving a level of cleanliness in a way that threatens residents' preferred activities and even their cherished possessions.

Nursing home regulation is surely necessary. The present state evolved as a response to scandals of the 1960s and early 1970s. However, at present the regulator, rightly or wrongly, is viewed as an irrational tyrant, and almost all of the deadening routines, rituals, and deprivations of the setting—again, rightly or wrongly—have been attributed to the exigencies of regulation. As we discuss later (see in particular Freeman, this volume, and Childress's case comment, this volume), meaningful personal autonomy is unlikely to occur unless we learn how to make regulations serve us rather than vice versa.

With some justice on their side, nursing homes also complain that parsimonious levels of state reimbursement militate against the niceties of individualized care. Certainly, enormous variation exists in state payment rates under Medicaid and in details of the reimbursement systems, which in turn create incentives for a facility's policies. (For example, if facilities are paid substantially more when a resident is functionally limited and presumed to need more nursing help, the facility has a financial disincentive to help the resident achieve more independence.) Undoubtedly, too, the public reimbursement rates in some states are artificially low. In almost all states, facilities can balance their books by charging higher prices to residents who are paying for care privately, thus hastening the moment when they have expended their funds and are eligible for Medicaid (see Lomasky, Chapter 22, this volume). Facilities also take a keen interest in admitting no more than a fixed proportion of residents soon likely to be on Medicaid as well as in seeking residents who are profitable to serve (see Moody, Chapter 21, this volume). Although they set the tone, the twin scapegoats of reimbursement systems and regulation cannot be held culpable for all of the elements of nursing home life described in this chapter. Many routines have been developed for the convenience of staff. Orthodoxies evolve, and routines harden into fixed policies.

LOOKING AHEAD

This chapter has been somber, deliberately so. Without detracting from the dedication and the fine, often thankless work of many nursing homes, we must acknowledge in plain language that nursing homes are not nice places to live. In many instances they also are not nice places to work. This book and the research project that gave it life are dedicated to the proposition that it is unnecessary and improper to accept these conditions as immutable. Rather, we need to give serious attention to livability in nursing homes and to the maintenance of personal identity. As a step in that direction, we have asked philosophers and other leaders in biomedical ethics to think through the rights and wrongs of homely subjects such as meals, telephone use, and toileting. Their thoughts form the large midsection of the book.

The points in this chapter about nursing home life can be summarized by a new version of "the three Rs." Three enemies of personal autonomy for nursing home residents are: routine, regulation, and restricted opportunity. It is a challenge to determine what can and should be done about them, but surely they should not be ignored.

REFERENCES

Bennett, C. (1980). *Nursing home life: What it is and what it could be.* New York: The Iresias Press.

Evans, L., & Strumpf, N. (1989). Tying down the elderly: A review of the literature on physical restraint. *Journal of the American Geriatrics Society, 37,* 65–74.

Hassler, J. (1979). *Simon's night.* New York: Ballantine.

Hing, E. (1987). Use of nursing homes by the elderly: Preliminary data from the 1985 National Nursing Home Survey. *Advance Data from Vital and Health Statistics,* No. 135. (DHHS Publication No. PHS

87-1275). Hyattsville, MD: National Center for Health Statistics, Public Health Service.

Institute of Medicine. (1986). *Improving quality in nursing homes.* Washington, DC: Academy Press.

Keeler, E., Kane, R., & Solomon, D. (1981). Short and long-term residents of nursing homes. *Medical Care, 19,* 363–370.

Laird, C. (1979). *Limbo.* Novato, CA: Chandler & Sharp.

Sarton, M. (1973). *As we are now.* New York: W. W. Norton.

Sekscenski, E. (1987). Discharges from nursing homes: Preliminary data from the 1985 National Nursing Home Survey. *Advance Data from Vital and Health Statistics,* No. 142. (DHHS Publication No. PHS 87-1250). Hyattsville, MD: National Center for Health Statistics, Public Health Service.

Tulloch, J. C. (1975). *A home is not a home (life within a nursing home).* New York: Seabury.

Zimmer, J., Watson, N., & Treat, A. (1984). Behavioral problems among patients in skilled nursing facilities. *American Journal of Public Health, 74,* 1118–1121.

Chapter 2

LIFE IN AN INSTITUTION:
A Sociological and Anthropological View

Steven S. Foldes

A person needs nothing worse over him than another person.
Yɪᴅᴅɪsʜ ᴘʀᴏᴠᴇʀʙ

Is a free, "normal" life possible in a nursing home? After all, people who live in nursing homes do so because, as a result of the debilities of illness or advancing age, they can no longer live as usual in their own homes and communities. In this context, the expectation of many families is that the nursing home will act as a guardian for its residents, an expectation that is often supported by regulations and liability case law. If continuing medical care also is needed, the nursing home is expected to provide it. But in addition, many residents and their families expect the nursing home to provide a homelike setting. To the administrator of a nursing home it appears self-evident that an institution must have rules to govern how people live together, especially with limited staff and resources available. If all residents were to exercise their wills freely, surely this could result only in daily chaos, with its attendant legal liability. This chapter considers the social context of the nursing home and the implications of this context for the autonomy of the residents.

It will come as no surprise to people who work in nursing homes, or to social scientists who study how people live together, that these frequently contradictory goals lead to many conflicts and dilemmas. The brief case studies in this book chronicle many of the most common problems of daily living in the nursing home context. They show that the conflicts frequently involve the most ordinary and mundane details of life: Schedules for communal meals, the organization of residents' wardrobes or possessions, use of the telephone or commonly held space, and leaving the premises for outings are examples of daily situations that can and do lead to conflicts. The case studies indicate that these conflicts sometimes take the form of overt disputes, but more often they simmer as unstated disappointments of residents' personal expectations.

To be sure, some of the problems are not particular to the nursing home. Sometimes the nursing home is merely the setting in which a conflict occurs, by virtue of the presence of the resident. For instance, when Mrs. Allison, a resident, wishes to call her children repeatedly in a way they find disagreeable, the nursing aides who must help her dial the phone are only tangentially involved in a family conflict, even if that conflict eventually draws in the staff (McCullough, this volume). Other problems, however, seem to arise from the nature of life in a nursing home. The ubiquitous problem of compatibility among "roommates" in the nursing home finds its origin in the economics and design common to this institution. The use of physical and chemical restraints, inconsistencies between residents' expectations and staff performance, and the simple facts of regimentation of daily life are all problems that emerge from the organization and management of daily life in the nursing home. As the case studies in Part II show, conflicts arise between residents or between residents and their families, which often involve the staff, and more directly between the residents and the staff or management.

THE GENESIS OF CONFLICTS

Families, in their many permutations throughout the world and over the course of human history, have always played a key role in the protection and care of those who are incapable of a more independent existence, primarily children and the aged and infirm. But in American society the demands of making a living, the need for mobility, and the cultural emphasis on youth conspire to make institutions necessary in assuming some of the familial burdens of care. When an old or infirm person requires more care than the family is able or willing to offer, whether that care is custodial or quasi-medical, the nursing home is available as an alternative. From the perspective of a resident's family, and often from the resident's perspective as well, the nursing home is expected to serve as a kind of extension of the nurturing function of the family. Even though it is clear that the nursing home is an impersonal setting by comparison with the family, it is the common hope and expectation that the staff will act in the family's stead to provide professional caring and appropriate protection.

This expectation underlies the reason for the existence, the very legitimacy, of nursing homes in American society. It justifies the enterprise morally and provides meaning and purpose to the activities of the people who manage it and work there. Whether the nursing home is viewed as a residential facility or as medical care facility, it is ideally understood as an establishment marked by beneficence toward its residents. But there is no place in this portrait for conflicts of the type revealed in this research project. Whether custodians or caregivers, the staff is expected to nurture, not fight with, residents. What is the origin, then, of the many daily conflicts and problems described in this book? Do conflicts and disappointments arise because caregivers are routinely insensitive to the dignity and indifferent to the autonomy of residents? Are conflicts the result of insufficient resources or a surfeit of regulations?

Answering these questions requires moving beyond the expressed justification for the nursing home to a cultural and sociological perspective. Through a cultural and sociological lens the nursing home can be seen as American society's predominant solution for dealing with those aged and disabled among us who are unfortunate enough to outlive their social and economic usefulness in a society notable for its lack of respect for the aged and infirm. Unlike some societies in which advanced age is accompanied by greater political and religious power and personal influence, American society has few places for the aged, especially as they become less able to live on their own. Most Americans do not wish to be confronted by the dependent aged and appear content with their invisibility in the nation's nursing homes.

Because the behavior of the aged and the infirm often diverges from the acceptable range of social and economic behavior in everyday life, the nursing home may be viewed as an institution that has as one of its purposes management of the behavior of the individuals who live there. Indeed, there is irony in the fact that, having distanced and isolated the aged and infirm, American society demands that they behave in ways that are sensible and orderly from our cultural perspective. In childhood, people are typically expected to become unique individuals even as they learn to assume defined social roles. In old age in the nursing home, however, people are expected to follow the opposite path; to homogenize their individual traits and eccentricities to a remarkable extent in order to fit into a bureaucratically defined behavioral norm. Lumped together with strangers who share little besides their ages and debilities, nursing home residents are expected to "socialize" with each other and not complain about it. This cultural expectation makes it possible for social workers and aides to exhort residents toward conformity with the institution and to rationalize many kinds of intrusions as necessary for the residents' own good.

The Nursing Home as Cultural Microcosm

However, lumping strangers together to socialize rarely leads to social tranquility. The cases in this book demonstrate some of the common complexities that emerge from the swirl of people and their expectations in these settings. For a wide variety of reasons, residents often do not like being in close daily proximity with each other, and their behavior and expectations frequently conflict with the institution's rules and the staff's tolerance. However, aside from the annoyances of daily living, which are well represented in these case studies, residents and staff alike bring to this setting differences in ethnic, class, and gender backgrounds. Nursing homes vary greatly in the extent to which they admit people of diverse backgrounds. Some nursing homes are fairly homogeneous ethnically or religiously, and others are highly diverse. Even those that are relatively homogeneous may host considerable diversity in the range of residents' disabilities, including cognitive impairment. Class and gender differences also may exist, particularly between residents and staff. Currently, most residents are female, white, and middle class, whereas aides tend to be from poor, minority backgrounds. These diverse groups have difficulty coexisting in American society at large, where considerable social distance separates them on a daily basis. In the nursing home, particularly in those homes with less religious or ethnic homogeneity, people from all backgrounds are brought into daily and often intimate contact. In this sense the nursing home may be seen as a microcosm of American society, much like the public schools, where the nation's underlying social cleavages and conflicts are magnified by more intense daily interaction.

Such heterogeneity makes nursing homes highly complex social and cultural systems, fraught with the potential for conflict. Is it reasonable to expect that racial and ethnic stereotypes nurtured over a lifetime will disappear upon entrance to a nursing home as a resident or employment as a staff member? Of course, this is unlikely, but the effects of these attitudes are not well understood. The case studies in this book were stripped of their class and cultural complexities in some instances, the better to focus on the ethical dilemmas they pose. But these markers of identity do not fade away when people get old and sick. So the issues remain, and they raise important ethical questions for managers.

Consider, for example, the implications of ethnicity in the case of Miss

Crochet's chair (Battin, this volume). In addition to issues of private property and public space, this incident would assume more menacing proportions were ethnic differences also present. If Miss Crochet was black and Miss Newly was white, might Miss Newly's unknowing assumption of Miss Crochet's chair be interpreted by Miss Crochet, and by some observers, as a racist act? And if the aide was Black too, could her support of Miss Crochet in the dispute further fuel racist attitudes? Other ethnic, class, and gender roles for the three participants in this dispute might be imagined and would have many different implications. The intrusion of these factors, which in real life are always present, could complicate many of the cases in this book. Further research is needed to identify the existence and effects of these factors on daily life in the nursing home setting, and to develop approaches to resolving the ethical dilemmas they pose.

Given the inevitable existence of differences in ethnicity, class, and gender among residents and staff, do nursing homes have an obligation to level these differences as much as possible in order to promote equality? Should, for instance, a white resident's objection to rooming with a Native American be ignored? Or is it better to accommodate such prejudices with the goal of preserving people's unique identities? Which strategy better promotes the autonomy of the residents? What obligation does the staff have to understand the diverse cultural and ethnic backgrounds of residents and to translate between people who fail to understand each other? Alternatively, is it appropriate, in the context of the increasingly multicultural society America is becoming, for some nursing homes to try to minimize these issues by restricting whom they admit and hire by religious or ethnic affiliation? Do restrictions of this sort amount to discrimination, particularly if such nursing homes are able to charge more for services and provide what may be better care? These are all basic issues of equality and justice. No simple answers exist to these kinds of questions in American society, so it is hardly surprising that answers are equally elusive for the nursing home.

The Nursing Home as Total Institution

What kind of a place is a nursing home to live in on a daily basis? From a sociological perspective the nursing home is a particular kind of institution, one that sociologist Erving Goffman (1961) labelled a "total institution." Goffman defined a total institution as "a place of residence and work where a large number of like-situated individuals, cut off from the wider society for an appreciable period of time, together lead an enclosed, formally administered round of life" (p. xiii). He identified five varieties of total institutions. An obvious type is the prison, which is organized to protect a community against what are perceived to be intentional dangers to it. In such institutions the welfare of the inmate is of secondary importance to the organization's function of community protection. Other types of total institutions are designed as voluntary retreats from the world, such as monasteries, or as organizations intended the better to pursue some worklike task, such as army barracks, ships, and boarding schools. There are also total institutions established to care for persons felt to be both incapable of caring for themselves and a threat to the community, albeit an unintended one. Mental hospitals are an example of this type of total institution.

Finally, there are institutions designed to care for persons thought to be both incapable and harmless. This type includes homes for the blind, the orphaned, the indigent, and the aged and disabled. Naturally, the ideology of this last type of total institution differs from that of prisons, monasteries, and army barracks. Mental hospitals and nursing homes are created with the goal of guarding or improving the welfare of their residents, and the staff in these establishments perceive their roles as helpers, facilitators, managers and aides, not as wardens or superiors. Moreover, the boundaries between the world outside and such institutions, especially nursing homes, are less rigid and more permeable. External groups and institutions—such as regulators, religious officials, physicians, and especially families—can influence the world inside the nursing home to some extent. It is not uncommon, for example, to find a nursing home resident's family members actively involved with his or her daily care. Some nursing homes encourage visits from family members and community groups as well as trips for residents. A family may seek to impose on the staff certain requirements for care to their relative. Nursing homes vary in the extent to which they are open to these external intrusions on their routines by families or other sources, and struggle and negotiation sometimes ensue. But one of Goffman's (1961) insights was to recognize, that despite variations in their permeability and their avowedly different purposes, there exist many underlying similarities among these different types of total institutions and that they all function as enforcers of social control.

It is a defining feature of modern, plural societies that individuals sleep, play, and work in different settings, with different co-participants, under different authorities, and without a comprehensive, rational plan. Individuals may typically escape the authority structure of one setting by moving to another one—from a rough day at work to a consoling evening with the family—where their relationships with other people may be separate and quite different. A central feature of total institutions, including nursing homes, is the breakdown of the barriers that usually separate these three spheres of life. In a total institution all aspects of life are conducted in the same place and under the same single authority. Each phase of the member's daily activity is carried on in the immediate company of a large group of others, all of whom are treated similarly and required to do mostly the same things together. All phases of the day's activities are scheduled, with one activity leading at a prearranged time into the next, the whole sequence of activities being imposed from above by a system of explicit formal rulings and a body of officials. And the various enforced activities are brought together into a single rational plan purportedly designed to fulfill the official aims of the institution.

Yet despite the cohesive and regimented character of these organizations, total institutions are not communities as that term is commonly used. The individuals within them are not linked by the kind of multifaceted relationships that characterize life on the outside. Field research on life in nursing homes reveals surprisingly few ties among residents and an absence of community-enhancing links such as kinship, reciprocity, politics, religion, and ritual (Shield, 1988). Even when a religious official, ombudsman, or family remains involved with a resident, the institution tries, and often succeeds, in subordinating this outside influence to its rules and authority. Rather, the total institution is a social hybrid, part residential setting and part formal organization. It is a bureaucratic entity. Unlike a community, which is typically united by one or more ideologies, the nursing home emerges from society's dominant ideology about how to manage the aged and the infirm. Goffman (1961) refers to life under these circumstances as "batch" living, to distinguish it from the social life of people in groups or communities.

This regimented handling by the bureaucratic organization of many human needs and of whole blocks of people—whether or not this is a necessary or effective means of social organization in the circumstances —is the key fact of total institutions. Regimentation of the large managed group, conveniently called residents, clients, or inmates, is accomplished by a small supervisory staff, whose job is as much surveillance of compliance with the institution's rules as it is guidance and care. The flow of information, especially about the staff's plans for the residents, is often restricted. As a result, a certain distance enters the relationship of residents and staff, and they tend to conceive of each other in terms of stereotypes.

Regimentation also mitigates against the extent to which a nursing home can assume the semblance of a resident's "home." In the nursing home, regimentation derives not only from the setting's characteristic as a total institution but also from its quasi-medical aspects. Many residents require some measure of medical care, and the senior staff member is typically a nurse, whose professional identity is linked to a medical model of relating to people. The application to the nursing home of the medical model increases the regimentation of human interaction and decreases the independence of residents, who are viewed as ill, incapable, and in need of externally imposed direction. Other staff members, most often the social workers, perceive the nursing home from a different set of assumptions. These assumptions de-emphasize the medical aspects of life in this setting, but the social workers may also regiment the lives of residents through activities and expectations for socialization.

Not surprisingly, individuals react in various ways to these circumstances. Admission itself may have many and varied meanings to individuals, depending often on the circumstances surrounding the decision to enter the nursing home, the way in which the new resident understands and interprets this decision, and the resident's anticipation of what life in the nursing home will be like. The admission is often perceived as a series of losses, leading to an unpredictable world in which the only certainty is further decline (Shield, 1988).

Once they are initially acclimated to the nursing home, new residents who are cognitively intact acquire information from which to devise strategies to negotiate the institutional bureaucracy. Different styles of adaptation may be identified. Some residents may withdraw into themselves, apparently losing interest in all events except those that impinge directly on their bodies. Psychologists describe this state as depression or regression. Others may take the opposite tack, becoming intransigent and uncooperative with the staff. These residents—an example in the case studies is Mrs. Finch—frequently resist identifying the nursing home as their home and fight all attempts to incorporate them into the routine round of activities (Macklin, this volume). Yet others may plunge into nursing home life, seemingly with considerable determination to make the best of it, sometimes to the point of claiming to prefer it to life on the outside. At an extreme this mode of adaptation resembles religious conversion, and such residents may be described as overly identified with the institution and its view of them.

Although the forms of individual adaptation vary, there is little doubt that the institution generates many changes in the resident's self-view and behavior. As Goffman (1961) writes of such establishments, "In our society, they are the forcing houses for changing persons; each is a natural experiment on what can be done to the self" (p. 12). Many of the case studies in this book demonstrate this aspect of the nursing home. A few examples may be illustrative.

Conformity, Efficiency, and Autonomy

Individuals build their lives on stable social roles and personal routines. When people age, they seem increasingly to need continuity between their past and present roles and routines. Unfortunately, admission to a nursing home leads to role dispossession and disruption of accustomed routines. The cases provide numerous instances of this process. Mrs. Hollinger is forced to eat breakfast for the first time at age 76 (Childress, this volume) and Mr. Brown can no longer read the newspaper before he has his (Mayo, this volume). Mr. Birkennen and Mr. Olsen, "regular fixtures" at a local tavern and coffee shop, must each stop their daily exodus (Priester, this volume). Mr. and Mrs. Stanley find it virtually impossible to work out time to simply sit together and hold hands (Tong, this volume). Instead, multiple and minute aspects of residents' behavior, from dress to deportment, are directed by a higher authority. Failure to cooperate is punishable in various ways, ranging from the fairly benign, such as the deliberate bureaucratic indifference visited on Mrs. Finch (Macklin, this volume), to the overt and intrusive, such as the application of restraints to Mr. Andrews, the otherwise cooperative "liberator" of his nursing home (Jameton, this volume). Any withdrawal or sullenness, frequent face-saving reactions to such affronts, leads only to interpretation as evidence of "poor adjustment" to nursing home life.

Everyone's sense of self, of personal integrity, rests on a certain level of privacy and personal space. These normally assumed rights are already in jeopardy for people whose age or disability generates dependence on others. But in the case studies, the nursing home appears only to exacerbate the violation of personal privacy and space already set in motion by residents' physical dependence. For instance, the nursing home breaches the customary informational preserve on one's social status and past behavior. Every resident has a "chart" with a "history" that is available to all staff. Mr. Birkennen's history of depression and violence, though never exhibited at his present home, is known to that home's staff and apparently becomes a factor in the decision to restrict his movements (Priester, this volume). Undesired interpersonal contacts may occur. Unpleasant roommates may be assigned, and one may even be asked to "watch over them," as with Mrs. Finch (Macklin, this volume). Mrs. Frank is threatened with being forced to eat with the "feeders" (Waithe, this volume). Even one's physical presence is subject to intrusion. Strange food must be eaten, sometimes in unaccustomed quantities. Most of one's personal possessions are shed upon entrance, and what little is left may be touched, mishandled, or removed. Mrs. Hollinger's shoe polish, aspirins, candle, and sherry are removed from her room (Childress, this volume). Even residents' rooms may be changed at the discretion of the institution. On the other hand, when Mrs. Smith seeks help to reach a commode quickly in order to retain the integrity of her bodily functions, she must wait anxiously, sometimes until it is too late (Fry, this volume).

The nursing home also disrupts the self-concept of individual adults by violating their self-determination, accustomed freedom of action, or sense of adult executive competency. Sometimes this occurs directly, as with the application of restraints or, as in the case of Mr. and Mrs. Stanley, the disruption of a lifelong personal relationship (Tong, this volume). Often, the violation is symbolic, with forced activities or abdication of accustomed patterns of behavior whose symbolic implications are incompatible with an individual's concept of self, leading to a feeling of being demoted in the age-grading system of American society. Clara Smith cares for her appearance despite (or perhaps because of) her amputations, but she must wear some of her dresses "ass-backwards," making her feel "foolish" (Benjamin, this volume). Mr. Birkennen's street clothes are removed and he is restricted to the grounds by being forced to wear his pajamas all day. Mrs. Finch feels infantilized by the activities at her nursing home and by being made to depend on the staff for medications that she has taken by herself for 15 years. Mr. Elwin is forced to "trail along miles of cord" for his oxygen in order to eat in the dining room. Birthday parties are all collapsed to once each month. Staff members enter residents' rooms with, at best, a warning knock.

The point of these examples is not to vilify individuals, whether aides or managers in the nursing home industry. Indeed, the case studies contain many examples of thoughtful, caring, and humane aides. Many aides and social workers attempt to provide individualized and decent assistance, within a framework of scarcity, to people who are not always easy to like or to take care of. Some social workers become diplomatic jugglers of individual needs and demands for rooms and dining arrangements. Kim Clark jeopardizes her job by "going over her boss's head" to reduce dosages for an overmedicated resident (Kjervik, this volume). And the example of Alice Bennett shows that aides are far from inured to the illness and death of residents (Wetle, this volume).

What the cases demonstrate repeatedly are two ubiquitous dilemmas of staff in nursing homes. One is a frequent need to weigh ends against each other. The necessity and desire to achieve certain ends may require a sacrifice of other ends. For example, Mrs. Harper's dislike of restraints and her aide's dislike of applying them must be weighed against the danger posed by her poor balance. Or the standard of treatment that one resident has a right to expect may conflict with the standard desired by another. Such is the dilemma of the staff regarding Mr. Birkennen's and Mr. Olsen's desire to leave the grounds. If the grounds are to be kept open out of respect for those who may leave the home safely, then other residents, who otherwise could have been trusted on the grounds, may have to be restrained to keep them from leaving. The staff is in a similar quandary in the case of Mrs. Frank, for they must juggle her right to eat in the company of cognitively intact residents against the right of these residents to eat apart from the unsavory Mrs. Frank.

A second staff dilemma is the constant conflict between institutional efficiency and humane standards or, put differently, between the ease with which residents may be managed and personalized, individualized care. The case of Mrs. Smith's toilet habits illustrates this dilemma. It would be humane to help Mrs. Smith to the commode whenever she feels she needs to use it, but this would be highly inefficient in view of other pressing needs. Changing her sheets or putting her in a diaper uses staff time more efficiently. Similarly, efficiency is the stated motivation of the aide who puts some of Clara Smith's dresses on backwards.

Instead of blaming human failure or the customary "few bad apples," the point is to recognize that there are patterns here that variations in individual nursing homes and the quality and caring of staff cannot explain. In fact, if one assumes that the staff in most nursing homes is caring and well motivated, it becomes even more difficult to explain why the kinds of cases found in this research arise. There is little doubt that substantial additional resources, in the form of better resident staff ratios, better-trained aides, and improved facilities and programming, would alleviate some of the conflicts and disappointments revealed in these cases. More and better-trained staff would, for example, ease the omnipresent dilemma between efficiency and individualized care. More staff and better facilities might help, in some instances, to reduce the conflict between contradictory ends.

But even vastly increased resources would not alter the character of the nursing home as a total institution. For no resource or technological "fix" can alter the function of the nursing home as an organization designed, in part, to manage the behavior of the invisible old and sick in American society. Conditions might be improved—not an insignificant achievement—but the nursing home would remain a place where the aged and the infirm, the socially and economically useless, are warehoused. And as Goffman (1961) helps us understand, the organization of this human warehouse subsumes the good intentions of individual actors within a bureaucratic social framework that functions to regiment the residents' daily lives in order to manage their behavior.

THE CONTEXT OF AUTONOMY

Given the characteristics of the nursing home as a total institution, it should be no surprise that the dominant theme raised by this project's directors is the search for "appropriate autonomy." But this is no simple task. As Lawrence Haworth (1986) points out in another context, the concept of autonomy embodies an entire theory of human nature. A comprehensive discussion of autonomy must focus on what is involved with being autonomous, why being autonomous is to be valued, and why it is proper to ascribe to people a right to autonomy and to those conditions without which autonomy cannot be achieved. Thus, any serious discussion of autonomy in a total institution is akin to reconsidering the human condition.

The philosophers who comment on the individual cases offer a variety of definitions of autonomy, that clarify certain aspects of the concept, such as the important distinction between "decisional autonomy" and "executional autonomy." Although each definition emphasizes different distinctions and subtleties, they share a common focus on the individual will. This focus may be expected from the intellectual history of the concept of autonomy as the characteristic of the moral being by virtue of which he or she is said to be a "law to himself." This does not mean the flagrant indulgence of personal desires or simply the expression of difference for its own sake but the law the individual recognizes as morally binding because it is the law laid down by that individual's own moral consciousness.

From that perspective, the cases raised by this study readily appear as instances of a conflict between a resident's individual autonomy, or will, and the institution's apparent indifference to this right. The commentators on the individual case studies offer useful suggestions on the specific issues in their cases but do not extend their analyses to what are often the originating institutional causes of the problem. This chapter argues, by contrast, that the frequent daily conflicts between the individual and the nursing home discussed in this book must be understood in the context of the nursing home as a total institution. Put differently, although autonomy may be a personal matter, people exist in a social context, and this context has much to do with both the individual's formation of autonomous will and his or her capacity to act on it.

The nursing home is not an isolated entity. It is a creation of the society in which it exists, which means that any serious attempt to enhance the autonomy of its residents must engage society at large in a discussion and clarification of the appropriate role of the nursing home. Because it is a total institution with the cultural sanction to manage behavior among its residents, promoting autonomy in the nursing home means reconceptualizing its role. This implies struggle, and in this struggle it may be useful to identify some strategies by which autonomy may be nurtured even in a such a setting.

What should be the expectations of the nursing home, as embodied in normative expectations and regulations, to act as an agent of social control? What kind and how much conformity is required of residents? Is the nursing home a residence or a medical facility or some hybrid of both, and what implications do these functions have for the authority structure of the institution? In what ways and to what extent is the staff, as employees of the institution, responsible to the residents? Who is the client of the nursing home and under what circumstances: the resident, the resident's family, the payer (if other than the resident), the physician? How should nursing homes deal with the increasingly multicultural and class-stratified characteristics of both resident and staff populations? Without greater clarity, if not consensus, on these difficult issues, nursing home managers have little guidance about the kind of institution society at large expects them to operate.

When confronted with the battle cry for fostering greater resident autonomy, nursing home managers and staff rightly protest that the reformers should back their demands for improvements with the resources to make change possible. More money—to buy better facilities, more and better staff, improved training and activities—is required to make improvement possible. Of at least equal importance, however, is the question of managerial intent. Additional staff may be used to increase surveillance and establish greater regimentation of daily life in the nursing home —in other words, to run a more efficient human warehouse. With the appropriate managerial intent, however, additional staff may serve to increase resident autonomy.

And it must be acknowledged that managers do not have a completely free hand. The nursing home industry is heavily regulated, often with the purpose of removing managers' freedom of action regarding various aspects of daily activities, out of a well-founded concern that residents have been and continue to be mistreated in some homes. Initial attempts to regulate nursing homes focused on physical safety and adequacy of treatment and services (Morford, 1988) but frequently reinforced nonperson people-work treatment of residents by staff at the expense of individualized and humane attention. Federal regulatory intent appears to be shifting toward emphasis on patient outcomes (Morford, 1988), but these and many current regulations need to be reexamined from the standpoint of their effect, albeit unintended, on the autonomy of nursing home residents. This need notwithstanding, the case studies demonstrate the routine manipulation of externally imposed rules and regulations to enforce conformity. When managerial intent is lacking to maximize autonomy, external regulations can be used to justify unwanted intrusions, as in the case of Mrs. Hollister's forced breakfasts.

Nursing home managers and staff who seek to increase the opportunity for autonomy of the residents in their homes must begin by focusing critical attention on the staff-resident relationship. Of concern are the methods by which authority and power are exercised on a daily basis.

This is an issue of process as well as substance; that is, how mundane exercises of power and authority are presented to residents is as important as the exercises themselves. For example, the social worker who sought the conformity of Mrs. Finch, the "bad resident," employed the metaphor of family as a coercive prod. No matter how well intentioned, this and similar kinds of interpersonal manipulation, common in nursing homes, have no more place there than in any other sphere of social life. As the cases of Mrs. Moorse and Mrs. Finch show, nursing homes, like many other institutions, have more or less clearly articulated models of "good" and "bad" behavior for their residents. It is an obligation of nursing home staff and management to avoid imposing their concept of appropriate behavior on residents and to avoid confusing their convenience with any model of "good" behavior.

This obligation must be a central focus of any training program for nursing home staff, together with efforts to focus the attention of staff on residents as real people with prior lives, achievements, and hopes—in other words, as more than human material to be kept clean, fed, and occupied. But as the dismal experience of training physicians to act more cost-consciously demonstrates, by themselves such training efforts have limited capacity to alter behavior, no matter how elaborate and well conducted the training program. People respond primarily to the incentives in the social contexts in which they operate, and unless the messages in the training programs are consistent with those incentives, any behavioral changes are inevitably ephemeral. This indicates the significance of orienting managerial intent in the direction of increasing resident autonomy and humane treatment.

The critical focus on the staff-resident relationship is the avenue by which managers and staff can begin to dismantle the most autonomy-restricting aspects of the nursing home. Where possible, attempts should be made to break down the barrier between the inside and outside worlds, to increase the permeability of the nursing home to the world outside. The importance of reducing the encompassing tendency of the nursing home is underscored by the editors' research findings about the choices residents prefer (Colatta, 1989). The residents' top two priorities, going out and phones and mail, which ranked above roommates, care, activities, and food, are ways to escape the nursing home. It is important to note that the staff survey revealed that the staff did not understand residents' priorities clearly. Obviously, additional resources and greater attention should be devoted to facilitating residents' access to the world outside the nursing home.

A consequence of increasing the permeability between the outside and inside worlds is the promotion of continuity between the previous and present lives of residents. Simply leaving one's home is change enough. It should not be necessary to learn a new and restrictive set of rules on entering a nursing home. This means reducing the authority of the nursing home over residents' possessions, deportment, schedules, and behavior. Both formal rules and tacit expectations should be reexamined with a view to eliminating all but those that are truly grounded in resident safety. Resources will never be sufficient to facilitate the execution of residents' every desire. People who are dependent on others must invariably wait for assistance, both inside and outside the nursing home, and reasonable people understand this. But most people also understand when an institution tries to facilitate or to hinder their will. The mission of the nursing home must be to assist residents in their attempts to exercise their autonomous will rather than to manage their behavior. Resident autonomy for all residents capable of asserting it must replace institutional efficiency as the central goal, and it must be more than an occasional, unintended by-product of an otherwise smoothly running total institution.

At base, the issue is one of governance. What justifies the assumption and exercise of authority in such a setting? The nursing home constitutes a highly heterogeneous, accidental community of largely poor, dependent people, and legal authority, as well as liability, resides with the management. The liberal political tradition of participative democracy, with its premise that free, rational individuals submit their will to the general will of the whole people, applies poorly to this setting. Yet rules must be negotiated that govern the common affairs of staff and residents, and the residents are at a clear disadvantage in these negotiations. In this unequal setting, one responsibility of the management must be to create opportunities among the residents and staff to explore and find common ground, to define and articulate their shared interests. When helped creatively to explore issues of public significance, people of all ages can usually identify their commonalities and act upon them. At the same time, management and staff have the responsibility to avoid homogenization and to acknowledge and deal with plurality and diversity. Diverse ethnic and class backgrounds, divergent life histories, and unique skills and personal preferences must be valued rather than suppressed. Even in this awkward setting, authority over the affairs of daily life must flow from the people who are the subjects.

ACKNOWLEDGEMENTS

The author gratefully acknowledges the assistance of Riv-Ellen Prell and the support of the Minnesota Department of Human Services.

REFERENCES

Colatta, G. (1989). Life's basic problems are still top concern in the nursing homes. *New York Times.* January 19, p. B14.

Goffman, E. (1961). *Asylums: Essays on the social situation of mental patients and other inmates.* Garden City, NY: Anchor Books.

Haworth, L. (1986). *Autonomy: An essay in philosophical psychology and ethics.* New Haven, CT: Yale University Press.

Morford, T.G. (1988). Nursing home regulation: History and expectations, In *Health Care Financing 1988 (Annual Suppl.):129–132.*

Shield, R.R. (1988). *Uneasy endings: Daily life in an American nursing home.* Ithaca, NY: Cornell University Press.

Chapter 3

THE MORALITY OF THE MUNDANE: Ethical Issues Arising in the Daily Lives of Nursing Home Residents

Arthur L. Caplan

The nursing home occupies a central position in contemporary discussions in health care ethics. Efforts to establish ethical boundaries for the use of medical technology often use demented or unconscious patients in nursing homes as paradigmatic examples.

The widely discussed Karen Ann Quinlan case, in which a young woman's parents sought court permission to remove her respirator once she had fallen into a permanent coma, took place in a New Jersey nursing home. More recent but equally widely discussed cases such as those of Clare Conroy, Paul Brophy, Nancy Cruzan, and Nancy Jobes, (Emanuel, 1988), all involving requests from family members that doctors discontinue the provision of food and fluids by artificial means, were based in nursing homes.

Cases involving questions of when to stop life-prolonging medical treatments for those who are unable to express their own wishes are among the most morally puzzling in health care. But, an exclusive focus on the highly dramatic issue of the ethics of stopping or withdrawing medical care draws attention away from the many other equally wrenching ethical dilemmas that those who live or work in nursing homes experience.

Many residents of nursing homes do not face the prospect of imminent death. Many are poorly served by images of frail, incompetent human beings who are bedbound and dependent on medical technology for their every breath. Many are quite capable of expressing their views and wishes about all manner of subjects, from what should have been done in the cases of Karen Ann Quinlan and Clare Conroy to what ought be done about the national debt, taxes, and environmental pollution.

On a day-to-day basis, the kinds of issues that the residents of nursing homes confront, as the cases described in this book show, are matters that at first glance appear mundane or banal: Can I eat what I want? Must I have a designated roommate? When can I go out for a walk? Why can't I wake up and go to sleep when I want to? Why can't I wash my clothes in the bathroom sink? What can I wear to dinner? Do I have to take a bath? When can I expect help in using the telephone? Must I sleep with a bed rail up? These are only a few among a thousand and one other seemingly minor moral matters.

It may seem odd at first even to describe such questions as moral or ethical. But ethics concerns not only questions of life and death but how one ought to live with and interact with others on a daily basis. The ethics of the ordinary is just as much a part of health care ethics as the ethics of the extraordinary. For the resident, the small decisions of daily life set the boundaries of his or her moral universe.

The range of ethical issues constitutive of this universe is both extensive and rich. The autonomy of competent residents to live their lives as they see fit must be constantly weighed against the value of maintaining and enhancing their health and well-being, especially when individual choices compromise an individual's health. The rights of individuals to live their lives as they wish must frequently be balanced against the need to maintain and enhance the interests of other, cognitively impaired residents who are not able to make choices about their own well-being. Individual choice often runs up against concerns for safety, efficiency, and even legal liability for injuries. Nursing home administrators, care providers, and those who regulate nursing homes are constantly faced with the challenge of weighing the interests of the individual resident against the interests and needs of the entire nursing home community. Nursing home policies must not only acknowledge the desires and wishes of individual residents, they must also attempt to deal fairly and equitably with the many situations in which the desires of residents come into conflict.

Similarly, the nursing home, by its very nature as a place where people live in close proximity to one another, imposes obligations, duties, and responsibilities on residents to behave in a considerate manner toward their fellow residents and the staff. Yet it is not at all clear where individual autonomy and dignity should end and duties to others ought to begin. The nursing home is also a setting in which the boundaries and limits of family responsibility and familial obligation are often put to their severest test. And the nursing home reflects society's willingness to treat its elderly and disabled citizens fairly and equitably. Social policies must be formulated that reflect ethical choices about who it is that should bear the responsibility for caring for the elderly and how much society should spend on their care relative to other pressing social needs.

The ethics of life in a nursing home for the competent, cognitively intact resident concerns decisions and policies governing matters that most of us spend little time worrying about—what we eat, when we bathe, using the telephone, seeing our friends. But we do not worry about these matters because we take our control over them for granted. Moreover, most of these choices can be made without seriously infringing on the rights and interests of others. We are more or less free to decide what the sequence and composition of events will be that make up our day-to-day life.

Those who live in nursing homes frequently feel that their control over the ordinary decisions of their lives, their autonomy, their dignity, even their sense of self, is lost in the routines, policies, and constraints of nursing home life. Ethical questions about the loss of autonomy over the ordinary or routine decisions of daily living or about obligations on the part of those who are competent toward those who are not may seem to pale when viewed from the perspective of ethical issues concerning the use or cessation of lifesaving or life-prolonging medical care. But it is simply wrong to think that they are less momentous or deserving of careful thought and deliberation. Ethical questions about the nature of autonomy, dignity, fairness, equity, obligation, duty, and responsibility, as they arise in the nursing home, are at the very heart of morality in health care and, indeed, of understanding basic ethical questions in the relationships that ought to prevail between human beings.

ETHICS AND THE QUALITY OF LIFE

It is the small decisions about the content and order of one's daily life that, when added together, determine something of fundamental ethical importance, whether one is in a nursing home or some other setting—the quality of life. If those who live in nursing homes have relatively little control over the content of their own lives, then a critical element of the quality of life—autonomy—will be absent.

Our society often gives low priority to questions in health care that bear on the quality of life. For every newspaper story written about the satisfaction of nursing home residents and their families with their environments,

10 are written about the moral dilemmas faced by patients and their families in intensive care units. For every article in the literature of bioethics that discusses the rights of nursing home residents to select their meals or the time they go to bed, 100 have been written about the right to receive a liver transplant or an artificial heart. Yet far more people will face the question of whether their wishes about meals and bedtimes will be respected than will have to worry about whether their views will be heard about accepting a liver transplant or artificial heart.

In one sense the disproportion of time and energy spent discussing transplants, artificial hearts, and other issues of high-technology, acute-care medicine is appropriate. Matters of when and whether life should be maintained are of fundamental ethical importance, but the seemingly small stakes involved in the nursing home context—setting mealtimes and bedtimes, use of the phone, the right to keep personal property in one's nightstand—should not lull anyone into thinking that daily life in a nursing home lacks either ethical content or importance.

Life-and-death decisions actually obscure a fundamental question that cannot be ignored for long in the setting of the nursing home or long-term-care facility: What is the goal of health care—merely to preserve life? Most providers and patients would argue for something more.

The point of providing medical care, even lifesaving medical care, is to preserve life in order to allow people the opportunity to enjoy their lives. This means restoring them to health or, at minimum, ameliorating the impact of disease and disability so that people may make choices about what to eat, whom to see, where to go, what to wear, when to rest—in short, to have the abilities, capacities, and opportunities to do those things that in their entirety make life meaningful. It is out of the thousands of small, ordinary, mundane components of our lives that the quality of life arises. It is only when we lose control over the content of our daily lives either as a result of illness or by living in conditions where little control is permitted—a prison, a monastery, or nursing home—that we notice their vital importance. And it is the perception of injustices regarding these small, ordinary, and mundane components of lives in nursing homes that is the source of many of the moral dilemmas that arise in such settings.

The concept of quality of life is not to be confused with the phrase "the quality of a life" (Arras, 1985). There is great danger in discussions of the comparative worth of the quality of various lives, as is evident from the crimes perpetrated by Nazi physicians and nurses who invoked the quality of life to justify euthanasia of the demented elderly and the severely disabled. Comparative value judgments about the relative worth of lives have no place in health care decisionmaking, management, or planning.

Although fears of comparatively judging the worth of people's lives, or sliding down a slippery slope once the concept of the quality of life is introduced, may be based on real abuses, they are not an adequate basis from a physician allowing them to stay up late enough to watch their favorite late-night television program!

Different legal principles also apply, depending upon whether a nursing home is seen as a residential environment or a medical environment. Staff members are concerned about their liability, or the institution's, for any harm befalling patients in medical settings. Staff in medical settings are expected to perform according to standards of practice recognized by their peers. And health care professionals are protected from certain forms of legal action when they follow requirements such as informed consent or maintaining confidentiality in interactions with patients.

None of these kinds of rules apply where residential environments are concerned. Residential environments are evaluated by their residents, not by their staffs. Unless there is a perceived threat to the neighbors, it is they who decide how much risk they are willing to bear while engaging in various behaviors. The residents also decide whether their needs are being met, and the standard that is used usually involves weighing the quality of life the environment permits against the amount of money one has to pay, rather than against improvements in health or the curing of illness or disease.

Nursing homes, of course, are special environments even if they are viewed primarily as residences. Few people choose to live in them, and those who do rarely can rarely afford to shop around and find the home they think best suits their needs. Moreover, residents are often dependent on others, family members or the government, to help pay their costs.

Once in a home, residents are dependent on the staff in ways that have few analogies in other residential settings. This dependency for the basic necessities of life has led some to classify nursing homes, along with prisons, monasteries and mental hospitals, as total institutions (see Foldes, this volume).

A total institution is a place where nearly every aspect of ordinary life is regulated by policies beyond the control of the individuals who live there. It is the involuntary dependency of residents on others within the institution of the nursing home that has led all states and the federal government to insist upon special regulations and oversight of nursing homes.

In many ways the nursing home environment seems more appropriately classified as residential rather than medical when viewed from the perspective of competent and healthy residents. Such persons are no more or less likely than anyone else to be concerned about their health status. Their goal is to have a safe and enjoyable place to live.

If this is so, then the standards against which nursing homes must be measured concern the ways in which they enhance or fail to enhance the quality of life enjoyed by those who live in them. This means that those concerned about the ethics of life in the nursing home must pay special

for ignoring the central role the quality of life plays in determining whether people can enjoy residence in long-term-care settings. Properly understood, not as a measure of the value of a life but of the opportunities and possibilities open to a resident, the quality of the life is a critical standard against which health care institutions must be assessed and evaluated. If the quality of life is dull, dangerous, or worse, then the institution and those who work there are failing the residents. If life in a nursing home does not give adequate provision for some individual choice and personal autonomy, then even a safe and clean environment may not score well in terms of the quality of life afforded those who live there. And if our society insists on judging the efficacy or worth of societal expenditures for various health and social services in terms of quality-of-life criteria such as the ability to work, to engage in activities of daily living, or to function independently without help from others, then these concepts must be carefully analyzed to establish their appropriateness to the setting in which nursing home residents live.

WHAT IS A NURSING HOME?

A relatively unexamined but vitally important question underlying our inquiry is, what kind of place is a nursing home? Is a nursing home a medical facility? Does the fact that doctors, nurses, nurse's aides, and other medically trained personnel supervise daily living and provide resident care create an ethical atmosphere in which residents should be treated like patients with the rights, responsibilities, and duties appropriate to that role?

Or is the nursing home more like a residential facility, say an apartment complex or hotel, where for a fee people can contract with others to provide various services to them, some of which can be medical but most of which are not? The responsibilities and rights of those who live together less by choice than cf necessity are far different from those that govern doctor-patient and nurse-patient relationships.

It seems odd to use the label "patient" to describe the cognitively intact resident of a nursing home whose health is stable. Many people do not enter nursing homes to receive acute medical care, nor do they see themselves as gravely ill or severely disabled. They enter because they cannot manage the functions of independent living or because their neighborhoods have become unsafe or because they hate living alone. Yet the daily life of the nursing home is permeated by a model of staff-resident relationships that is firmly rooted in an ethic drawn from acute-care medical settings. Residents must seek permission from a health care professional to undertake even the most mundane activities. The residents of nursing homes, even those who are manifestly competent, are too often treated solely as patients who are sick and who, as a result, must depend upon and trust their health care providers to make decisions for them about nearly every aspect of their daily lives. But is patienthood the only option for the roles assumed by those living in nursing homes? Should society expect the emphasis on nursing homes to be on the "nursing" or on the "home?"

Residents may feel reassured that competent medical help is readily available in the nursing home, but that assurance does not make it appropriate for those who staff such institutions to treat every resident literally as a patient. For at least some of the mentally competent residents, the nursing home is their home, not their hospital or hospice.

The goals of the staff of nursing homes will be very different depending upon whether the nursing home is conceived of as primarily a medical or primarily a residential environment. The goals of health care organizations such as hospitals, rehabilitation centers, and health maintenance organizations (HMOs) and of those who staff them is the maintenance and promotion of health and the relief, cure, or amelioration of disease and disability. These goals take priority over everything else that is done in such institutions.

On the other hand, the goals of those who staff residential facilities such as apartment buildings, hotels, and condominium complexes are to make the lives of residents as pleasant as possible in order to attract new residents while retaining the business of those who are already residents. It is also to assure that certain rules and policies (e.g., bag all of your trash, no loud music after midnight, no pets, no use of the pool without a lifeguard, no loitering) are in place to ensure the safety, well-being, and orderliness of the environment.

Perhaps the primary function of the staff of a hotel or apartment complex is to make sure rules are in force that will maximize the opportunity for privacy given to each resident. Some, perhaps many, residents will want interaction with their neighbors more than they want privacy, but it is the right to privacy that sets the boundaries against which all other activities are carried out.

It would be viewed as totally inappropriate for a doorman in an apartment building to decide who may leave the building and cross the street to visit a bar. It is well within the boundaries of medical relationships for doctors and nurses to tell their patients to stop drinking and to stay away from places that serve liquor. If the resident of a nursing home wants to go out and have an alcoholic beverage, which model is more appropriate —residential or medical?

In my home no one would view it as proper for anyone to tell me when or what I can watch on my television set. Yet in a nursing home setting it might be necessary for residents to obtain a written order

attention to the freedom, safety, and opportunities for choices afforded residents.

Ethicists sometimes refer to the liberty, choices, and opportunities a person possesses under the general rubric of autonomy. Autonomy is a critical component of the quality of life for Americans because they believe each person is his or her own best judge of what makes life valuable and enjoyable. If autonomy is necessary to assure the quality of life, then environments in which autonomy is vulnerable to the control or restriction of others merit special ethical scrutiny. The nursing home is one such environment.

THE MEANING OF AUTONOMY

Ethicists have struggled mightily to discover both a definition and a justification of autonomy that can command consensus in a pluralistic society such as the United States. The philosopher Larry McCullough (this volume) argues that autonomy ought be respected because it is the individual who best knows his or her own interests. Each of us knows our values and no one else can know them as well; so, he argues, the choices of the individual must be given priority over the choices of others even when the individual's choices seem outlandish, bizarre, unorthodox, or just plain wrong.

And the theologian Bart Collopy (1988), in a widely discussed article, "Autonomy in Long Term Care: Some Crucial Distinctions," advances six dimensions or what he terms polarities of autonomy: decisional versus executional, direct versus delegated, competent versus incapacitated, authentic versus inauthentic, immediate versus long-range, and negative versus positive. He is concerned to show that "autonomy is a philosophically complex and ethically problematic value, thick with distinctions, polarities, and interpretive variation" (p. 11).

Numerous other philosophers, lawyers, and ethicists (Beauchamp & Childress, 1983; Dworkin, 1976; Miller, 1981; Thomasma, 1984) have offered their own multidimensional definitions of autonomy. Whatever else the experts on autonomy have had to say, they all agree that the concept is not one that admits of a simple, clear-cut definition.

Behind each of these definitions is, nevertheless, a common presumption concerning autonomy—that individuals are the best judges of what is in their interest. The etymological origins of the concept of autonomy (Greek for self-rule) underscore the importance of personal, individual choice in understanding this much-discussed concept.

It is a powerful belief within most Western societies that the individual rather than the family, the local community, the church, or the state knows best what his or her interest is. Indeed, it can be a source of great confusion to health care providers to encounter families or patients who do not subscribe to this belief and, instead, put their trust in a spouse, religious leader, father-in-law, or even a health professional to make decisions as to what is or is not the best thing to do.

But for the most part, it is the presumption in our society that whatever autonomy is, the individual is in the best position to cash out its practical content. This leads to the conclusion that when the capacity for autonomy is present it must be respected and enhanced. It also means that the principle of respect for personal autonomy ought to be given the highest priority relative to other values or moral principles because if it is true that each individual knows what is best for himself or herself, then people ought to be able to control their lives and their environment in accordance with their personal values.

Most discussions of autonomy note that autonomy refers to actions of a very special sort—those that are the product or result of voluntary, uncoerced choice. For autonomy to exist, people must be capable of making informed, deliberative choices about what it is that they do or do not want to do. That is why the concept of competency is so closely linked to that of autonomy; if a person is incapable of informed deliberation, then it is hard to see how that person can act autonomously.

Competency is not in itself, however, sufficient for autonomy to exist. In order for people in any environment to act autonomously, they require not only the ability to think, deliberate, and choose but also the opportunity to make choices (Caplan, 1987).

Imagine a man parachuted into the midst of the Sahara Desert. Those who put him in this predicament give him nothing but the clothes on his back. Can we say such a person is autonomous? In one sense we can. A man alone in the desert is not being coerced, threatened, or pressured by anybody in any way. But it seems silly to speak of such a situation as one of full autonomy when in fact few options or choices are possible.

Philosophers sometimes distinguish between negative and positive senses of freedom. To be autonomous a person must be free from the threat of force or coercion—negative freedom. But to be autonomous a person also requires options, possibilities, and opportunities—positive freedom.

A nursing home can restrict the autonomy of its residents in two ways. It can restrict the ability of residents to make choices by coercive pressures of schedule or by force. It can also restrict autonomy by failing to provide a minimal range of choices, options, and opportunities—by failing to provide positive freedom.

Those who live in nursing homes and who possess the capacity to make rational, deliberative choices need to be given the opportunity to do so. This means that staff members, administrators, and society must ensure that those who have the ability to act autonomously have the chance to do so. It also means that those conditions required to act voluntarily—the absence of coercion, threats, manipulation—must be ensured. Those who can act autonomously must also have the privacy, information, and time to enable them to make choices about their lives.

There is a final element of autonomy that has captured the attention of many writers in the field of bioethics. Some would argue that it is not sufficient to assure autonomy that choices be available and that those who act on them have the ability to think, deliberate, and choose what they wish to do or not do. If I wake up one day and, after thinking long and hard, decide to join the circus, my family and friends would be right in challenging my decision even though it may indeed be the result of a rational, uncoerced decision on my part.

Similarly, if the resident of a nursing home suddenly decides one day to move out of a home where he or she has lived happily and without complaint for 10 years or decides not to accept phone calls from family members with whom the resident has talked on a regular basis for many, many months, questions can legitimately be raised about the autonomous nature of those choices. Such questions have nothing to do with doubts about the competency of those who make them; rather, they seem inconsistent with the behavior, attitudes, and choices that have preceded them.

Autonomy seems somehow to be linked to actions that are not only the result of voluntary, deliberative action but that are also a result of someone's deeply held values. A philosopher who has a nice job who suddenly announces that he is joining the circus or a contented resident of a nursing home who one day decides to move out rightly gives others pause as to the authenticity of what it is the person proposes to do.

Actions that are inconsistent with the deeply held beliefs and values of a person may not be autonomous in that they may represent a passing fancy or a moment of depression or despair. To know if an act is truly autonomous it may be necessary to determine whether the act is the result of an authentic choice. The assessment of authenticity is not simple because it requires an intimate knowledge of an individual's values and conduct over a sustained period of time. Nursing homes desirous of enhancing the autonomy of their residents must be in a position to know the values and desires of each resident so that some assessment can be made of the authenticity of their choices and decisions.

WHY IS AUTONOMY VALUED?

These preconditions and elements of autonomy point toward a set of important distinctions that must be made in thinking about autonomy in the nursing home setting. The most common reason given for valuing autonomy is that it is a prerequisite for viewing people as moral agents. Only those who freely, voluntarily, and deliberately choose to act can be said to be subject to praise or blame for the actions.

The resident who is given no choice about what she will eat cannot be praised for her prudent selection of a healthful diet. The resident who refuses to take a shower because of an irrational fear of falling is not acting autonomously and thus may not be held accountable for such actions. The resident who works in the gift shop for fear that the staff will punish her with fewer privileges if she refuses is not deserving of praise for her altruism. Only those who rationally choose to act and who have options to choose among can be the subjects of ethical approbation or condemnation.

Autonomy, seen from this perspective, has value because it allows us to hold others responsible for their actions. It is of instrumental value in that its value derives from the value we assign to the importance of being able to hold people responsible for what they do to themselves and others. If we want nursing home residents to be moral agents, then we must ensure that those who are competent are given the opportunity to act autonomously.

Autonomy in this instrumental sense is present only to the degree to which staff members, families, and administrators strive to create conditions in which autonomy is possible. If no autonomy at all is possible, if residents are kept restrained all day or placed on rigid, inflexible schedules that permit no deviations at all, then it will be difficult to maintain that residents can be praiseworthy or blameworthy for what they do. They have no choice, not because they lack the capacity to act in a responsible and accountable manner but because they live in situations where they lack the opportunity to act autonomously.

Autonomy is also valued in its own right. Some people would argue that the ability to act autonomously is good not because of the good feelings that it brings or because it allows others to hold people to account for what they do but because it is inherently good to act from one's own values under one's own volition. In this view autonomy is an intrinsic, not an instrumental, good. It is good in and of itself not because it promotes some other value that people think is good.

In the interpretation that sees autonomy as an intrinsic good, it is better to wear a dress everyday because you choose to do so as against having someone make you wear one, not because you pick out a dress that others like but because it is you who does the picking.

Conversely, it is wrong to force someone to wear a dress she does not want to wear simply because it makes life easier on the staff, other residents, or the resident's family. One might decide to override autonomy in the interest of a person's safety, or health or for aesthetic reasons, but although the overriding of personal autonomy may be justifiable, it would still be wrong simply because the autonomy is overridden and that in itself would be wrong.

Finally, some commentators argue that autonomy is good because it enhances the health and well-being of those who are allowed to act autonomously; that is, autonomy is not an intrinsic good but an instrumental good, valued not because it allows people to be treated as responsible agents but because it benefits them by enhancing their health.

There are numerous reports in the literature of gerontology noting that nursing home residents who are given more choice in their environment live longer, are healthier, and seem happier than other residents (Lawton, 1980). There seems to be an association between the range of action throughout which autonomy is possible and overall health and well-being. If this is true, then autonomy has value as a means of enhancing other values such as health or well-being.

On both rationales instrumental and intrinsic—autonomy scores quite high relative to other values that command our respect. It is hard to imagine any characteristic that a cognitively intact nursing home resident would want more and deserve more than to be treated as a responsible moral agent. When residents complain that they are being treated like children or that they do not like being told what to do every waking moment, they may be complaining that their ability to be moral agents is being threatened. In a pluralistic society such as ours it is important to realize that not every nursing home resident may come from a cultural or social background that stresses the value of autonomous action as intrinsically good. But many do, and for them autonomy is a good thing in and of itself.

WHAT PRIORITY SHOULD BE GIVEN TO AUTONOMY IN THE NURSING HOME SETTING?

The toughest moral dilemmas of daily life in the nursing home do not arise because the staff is indifferent or uncaring. Such conduct is clearly wrong and creates no ethical puzzles or dilemmas. Moral problems arise when moral principles or values come into conflict. They conflict in nursing homes when the staff is committed to values that are not the same as those that guide the lives of residents.

Conflicts are particularly likely when the staff attempts to advance the values of health and safety, and some residents give lower priority to these values. The staff may be concerned to protect the interests and welfare of the most vulnerable residents, whereas individual residents who have high levels of physical and mental function may feel constrained by regulations aimed at others more in need of protection.

Legal and financial constraints may create value conflicts between staff and residents that are motivated by legitimate concerns on both sides. Fear of lawsuits resulting from injuries to residents may lead staff and administration to restrict mobility for certain patients or to tightly regulate trips outside the facility. Residents may feel their freedom unjustly infringed by regulations and policies that do not allow them to make their own choices about facing risks or dangers.

The centrality of autonomy, on both instrumental and intrinsic grounds, to the quality of life enjoyed by residents points strongly in the direction of according great weight to this principle. Ordinary citizens are allowed to place safety, health, and well-being at a lower priority than they give to other values or interests. There is no reason to think that a competent person in a nursing home should have any less presumption of scope or degree of autonomy. The burden of infringing autonomy must be borne by those who wish to override autonomy, not by those who desire to exercise it.

Autonomy is and ought to remain a central value in the daily lives of nursing homes. The greater the extent of personal choice accorded residents in matters of daily living, the easier it will be both to hold them accountable for their actions and to encourage them to play an active role in cooperating with staff rather than battling them.

But even if it is granted that autonomy is a central value of both intrinsic and instrumental value for every person and that nursing homes and those who regulate them must make every effort to ensure that this value is accorded respect, the moral problems raised by autonomy will not be solved, for the fact remains that the exercise of autonomy can create conflicts, not just with staff or administrators but between residents.

Daily living among the autonomous residents of a nursing home may be no less free of moral problems than is daily life in an environment that is coercive, paternalistic, or offers few options. Problems of justice, fairness, and dignity will move to the forefront of ethical concern in direct proportion to the degree to which the autonomy of nursing home residents is enhanced by the staff and residents of such facilities.

The staff will have to decide how to resolve conflicting demands made by residents who want to sit in the same chair or watch different television programs at the same time. They will still have to decide how to weigh the desires of those residents capable of autonomous action against the interests of those residents who are so impaired as to be clearly incapable of such behavior.

But this is as it should be. The problems of justice, equity, and dignity, the weighing of conflicting claims, decisions about the rights and interests of the incompetent and the extremely vulnerable confront all of us in our daily lives. The moral situation ought be no different for those who live or work in nursing homes.

REFERENCES

Arras, J. (1985). Ethical principles for the care of imperiled newborns: toward an ethic of ambiguity. In T. Murray & A. L. Caplan (eds.), *Which babies shall live?* (pp. 83–136). Clifton, NJ: Humana.

Beauchamp, T. & Childress, J. (1983). *Principles of biomedical ethics.* New York: Oxford University Press.

Caplan, A. L. (1987). The termination of medical interventions for the elderly: Who should decide? In G. Maddux & E. Busse (eds.), *Aging: The Universal Human Experience,* (pp.636–648). New York: Springer Publishing Co.

Collopy, B. J. (1988). Autonomy in long term care: Some crucial distinctions. *The Gerontologist*, 28, (Suppl.), 10–17.

Dworkin, G. (1976). Autonomy and behavior control. *Hastings Center Report, 6,* 23–28.

Emanuel, E. (1988). A review of the ethical and legal aspects of terminating medical care. *The American Journal of Medicine, 84,* 291–301.

Lawton, M. P. (1980). *Environment of Aging.* Belmont, CA: Brooks/Cole.

Miller, B. L. (1981). Autonomy and the refusal of lifesaving medical treatment. *Hastings Center Report, 11,* (4), 22–28.

Thomasma, D. C. (1984). Freedom, dependency and the care of the very old. *Journal of the American Geriatrics Society, 32,* 906–914.

PART II

CASES AND COMMENTARIES

Chapter **4**

ABOUT THE CASES

Rosalie A. Kane and Arthur L. Caplan

These 18 cases were crafted from real-life material. They are made from the experiences, predicaments, and reactions of the residents, nurse's aides, and social workers whom we interviewed. They also reflect the views of residents, family members, staff members, and other interested parties, who spoke to us through the records of metropolitan nursing home ombudsman offices.

The cases themselves represent both some of the most frequently arising ethical issues and a broad range of ethical issues that emerged from the data we collected. They tend to be complicated cases. They often present the perspective of more than one resident and occasionally more than one staff member as well. The cases are almost always played out against a backdrop of scarce resources.

The commentators have diverse backgrounds. They are physicians, nurses, lawyers, theologians, gerontologists, and philosophers. Many of them are dually qualified in several fields—for example, philosophy and medicine, philosophy and nursing, law and nursing. The philosophers themselves reflect diversity in viewpoint—for example, libertarian, communitarian, utilitarian, and even feminist. As a result, the everyday problems in nursing homes are approached from a variety of moral perspectives. Multiple definitions of autonomy are scattered throughout the case commentaries, as each author sets the stage for his or her analysis. We also find different authors giving different weight to particular values—for example, maintaining family ties, personal identity, loving relationships, dignity, or fairness.

In the opening case, "Good Citizen, Bad Citizen," Macklin considers basic issues about the nursing home setting that are applicable to all of the cases in the set. She raises questions about the nature of the nursing home community—is it a medical setting, a housing complex, a neighborhood, a family?—and, therefore the types of obligations that residents owe to each other and to the management.

"The Chair and Other Public Space" speaks to the conflicts over property, possessions, and space that nursing home residents and staff mentioned to us so frequently. With both private and public space wrenchingly scarce, residents struggle for places to be alone and places to entertain. Bereft of personal possessions or a safe place to put them, or even room to keep a meaningful selection of clothing, some residents struggle to stake out territory in the facility. Under these circumstances patience wears thin and tempers flair. Nurse's aides report they are continually breaking up quarrels over chairs or choice of television channel. Battin applies an ethicist's lens to these ordinary but emotion-laden issues that too often literally give rise to fights that must be settled in a hurry. She suggests that each resident needs, and is perhaps owed, a publicly visible vehicle for self-expression. It is not the chair per se, Battin argues, but the meaning of the chair that should be offered to each resident.

More often, problems in nursing homes are expressed not in fights but in quiet resignation to restricted lives. Many examples in this category have a genesis, or at least a rationale, in the regulations that govern nursing homes. The regulations, we are told, require that the environment be safe for those who are the most impaired. Regulations breed the sterile environments, the routines, and the restrictions that go along with a "life by care plan." In Chapter 7, Childress explores this contention in a case involving a resident who seems beset and bested by regulations—regulations that require her to rid her room of potentially dangerous substances and regulations that force her to rise early each morning for a breakfast she prefers not to eat. The case commentary squarely faces the tension between respect for autonomy and beneficent wishes to protect the residents. The impulse to protect underlies much of the problematic behavior of nursing home staff and many of the regulations as well.

The next three cases involve matters of room and table assignments—two items that nursing home social workers told us account for many of the vivid dilemmas of their jobs. Residents, too, are hardly indifferent to these issues. They expressed strong resentment about being paired with incompatible or difficult roommates and tablemates. Some residents preferred to eat alone in their rooms but were discouraged from doing so in the name of rehabilitation and social activity. In Chapter 8, Miles and Sachs propose a hierarchy of criteria for allocating the scarce supply of single rooms and a process for settling the competing claims both to single rooms and to preferred roommates. In Chapter 9, Tong considers a similar case of room allocation with the added complication that the claims of a newly admitted married couple to live together must be juggled with other claims of long-standing residents. Tong's analysis gives great weight to the importance of upholding people's rights to sustain loving relationships.

In Chapter 10, Waithe examines the dilemmas surrounding meals for two residents: one who values the social circumstances of eating in the dining room but whose eating habits are repugnant to tablemates, and another who would prefer—if only the staff would allow it, to avoid the dining room entirely and eat in the greater peace of his own room. Waithe's case commentary is also instructive as an example of a step-by-step application of the "polarities" of autonomy recently introduced by Collopy. In addition, another section of the chapter illustrates how a "consequentialist" argument might play out if autonomy in dining routines were examined, not in terms of absolute values to achieve but of the positive and negative results for all concerned.

Our respondents, particularly nursing home social workers, identified many instances in which the wishes of family members were at odds with those of the resident, and sometimes family members were at odds with each other. Complaints to the ombudsman also reflected family disagreements. Chapter 11, "Phone Privileges," is an example of how nursing home staff can be caught in the middle between family and resident. Commenting on the case, McCullough takes the reader through a formal analysis of the ethical principles of autonomy, beneficence, and family responsibility as a prelude to his specific arguments that staff should engage both resident and family members in a process of clarifying their values as they relate to the conflict. McCullough's case comment, perhaps more than any other, introduces *procedural* aspects of ethical decision-making and distinguishes between substantive and procedural ethical principles.

The next three cases revisit the issue of autonomy versus beneficence, and each has legal ramifications. Schwartz, an attorney, discusses the legal and moral implications of three situations involving either a petition for guardianship or the actions of a guardian or conservator. Priester, also an attorney, discusses two situations of residents who wish to leave a facility unattended and, in each case, are at some risk.

Jameton's case deals with physical restraints in nursing homes, a sadly ignored subject, given the prevalence of various restraining devices, the disagreements among family about their use, the difficulties some staff have in applying restraints, and, most of all, the way many nursing home residents dread and abhor the prospect of physical restraints. In both the Priester and Jameton chapters, the issue arises: How can the nursing home protect itself against legal liabilities if something goes amiss as a result of an effort to respect a resident's autonomy?

Next comes a cluster of six cases that, all bring to the fore questions about the rights and responsibilities of nurses' aides as well as the need to further delineate the obligations of staff to residents. In "Bathing: On The Boundaries of Health Treatment," Aroskar explores whether daily care routines, such as a shower, are, in fact, treatments that may be refused. In a related case, Fry examines the question of how far nurses' aides must go to permit an immobile woman the dignity of remaining continent. Kjervick's case, "Beyond the Call of Duty: A Nurses' Aide's Judgement," raises questions about the limits of the rights and responsibilities of a paraprofessional nurses' aide (who nevertheless is the person on the spot) to counteract the care plan or to intrude her own viewpoint about what is best for the resident.

In "Death of a Resident," Wetle discusses the obligations of staff to those worried about impending death, to those actually dying, and to "newly dead" bodies. Somewhat to our surprise, these issues loomed large in the thoughts of the nurses' aides whom we interviewed. This cluster concludes with "Dressing For Success," a case in which Benjamin addresses the dignity of a resident versus the convenience of a staff member. In his discussion, Benjamin introduces his view of compromise, an approach that has relevance to many of the other cases.

The last three cases move toward matters of money and use of resources. Mayo explores the correctness of private contractual arrangements between residents and staff, and the custom of tipping. Moody analyzes criteria that nursing homes might justifiably use to decide who should have the scarce resource of the next available nursing home bed. Here business interests, compatibility of the resident group, and justice to potential residents who are poor, members of ethnic minority groups, and or difficult to tend all figure in the analysis. Finally, Lomasky examines the ethical justification for evicting residents from nursing homes, responding to a case that involves a home that is converting to "private-pay" only. Lomasky's commentary gives consideration to the concerns of both the nursing home operators, as well as the nursing home residents. He also offers a trenchant critique of the Medicaid program from his particular ethical perspective; unabashed libertarianism. Both the

Moody and Lomasky papers force consideration of systemic issues in the way nursing home care is allocated.

Taken together, these cases and case commentaries represent a faithful representation of the range of ethical problems in everyday life in nursing homes and, we hope, a rich resource for ethical reflection. At the end of each chapter, we have included further questions that are raised by the cases and the commentaries. They illustrate the diversity and interrelationship of ethical issues that this material provokes. We are hopeful that philosophers and practitioners alike will begin a process of refining the questions as well as attempting answers.

Chapter 5

GOOD CITIZEN, BAD CITIZEN

A "GOOD RESIDENT"

Mrs. Moorse has spent the last 5 years at Xavier Nursing Home. She is an 83-year-old widow who has had a number of strokes. She uses a wheelchair, and her left arm is very weak. She refers to herself as a quiet lady and says, "I don't like to make trouble."

Even though she has been at Xavier for 5 years, she still does not have the single room she requested when she entered. She is philosophical about it and says, "Other poor souls are much worse off than I am." She's become sort of used to having a roommate.

Mrs. Moorse takes part in many activities. She believes that as long as she is living in a place, she should pitch in and try to help make the program succeed. Though she has trouble getting about, she tries never to bother "the girls" about taking her to activities. The director of nursing describes Mrs. Moorse as a "model resident."

Mrs. Moorse helps out in the gift shop twice a week. She really doesn't like it there because she doesn't like to deal with money. But someone has to keep the gift shop open, and not everyone is capable. The home's administrator never fails to praise her for helping out.

Carolyn, Mrs. Moorse's present roommate, is 92 years old. She cannot talk intelligibly or write, and the aides must help her with almost everything. She is ambulatory, but since she is also confused, she needs to be gently guided around. Mrs. Moorse helps Carolyn as much as possible and keeps an eye on her when they are in the room together. The staff are grateful because they can use the help.

Mrs. Moorse doesn't like the responsibility for Carolyn but has not said anything to anyone about it. For that matter, she feels responsible just by having a roommate who is so helpless. "I don't think it is quite fair," she says mildly, "for us to be in the position of being there all the time with someone who needs so much help. It is a big responsibility when your roommate is so helpless; most of the time there is nobody around but me, and I don't quite know what to do. Sometimes it scares me." But Mrs. Moorse knows she'd like someone to help her if she was like poor Carolyn.

A "BAD RESIDENT"

Mrs. Finch has been at Xavier for only 6 months. She moved in after her husband died and she could no longer manage their home alone. She is 81, and her diabetes is managed with oral medication. Although somewhat frail, she is capable of independent activity. She believes in speaking her mind.

Mrs. Finch can't understand why she was given a double room when she specifically requested a single in the application. Her roommate is a docile but slightly demented lady who is always singing and who pesters her with repetitive questions. An aide once asked Mrs. Finch if she could help out by reminding her roommate about meals and going to the toilet and watching to keep her from wandering off. Mrs. Finch was indignant at the request. She pointed out that the aides are paid to do this kind of thing, and with the "high rent" charged here, residents should not have to do the work. She believes you should get what you pay for. She wants a single room and a chance to spend her time as she pleases, and she is willing to pay for that.

Mrs. Finch refuses to work a shift in the gift shop. She says, "I've done my share of volunteering." Besides, she likes to pick the conditions of her philanthropy. For example, for years she has been active in an annual phone drive for the American Cancer Society and hopes she can work at this from her private telephone at the home.

Mrs. Finch cannot understand why she is not allowed to keep her diabetes medicine in her room. She has taken it for 15 years and never missed a pill. Now she must depend on the staff to bring her the pill in the morning, or she must go to the nursing station to get it. She thinks this is ridiculous. Mrs. Finch also complains loudly about the food, and she claims that there should be choices even on her restricted diabetic diet. She also thinks most of the activities are for babies and is very selective about what she will do.

The social worker has talked to Mrs. Finch about her adaptation, suggesting that she think of the residents and staff group as a large family where "we all make allowances for each other" and "we all pull our weight." Mrs. Finch responds that she is in the nursing home because she needs health care. She already has a family and does not want another one. She hopes she *never* adapts if it means "losing your common sense or settling for the kind of life so many here have." She thinks that many residents would appreciate being treated like adults but are afraid to say so. Though most of the activities seem foolish to her, Mrs. Finch is considering getting active in the resident council to do something about the problems she sees.

The direct care staff largely ignores Mrs. Finch's complaints, saying "Give her another few weeks and she'll get used to the place and quiet down."

CASE COMMENTARY

Ruth Macklin

In the acute-care hospital a "good patient" is one who is compliant and makes no trouble for the staff, and a "bad patient" is one who is defiant and makes demands on medical and nursing personnel. A suspicion lurks that the same rating system applies in nursing homes. "Good residents," as judged by the staff, are ones who assume responsibility for other residents, participate in activities in the facility, and are uncomplaining and understanding when their wishes are not granted. "Bad residents" are uncooperative, defiant, unwilling to assist others, and complain about everything.

Should these traits be viewed, respectively, as virtues and vices? Does becoming a resident of a nursing home invest a person with a set of responsibilities toward the staff and other residents? Is it appropriate to expect nursing home residents to adopt new attitudes and behaviors or abandon old traits that have been part of their lifelong personality? And how do these questions relate to the autonomy of nursing home residents?

MRS. MOORSE AND MRS. FINCH

Mrs. Moorse assumes more responsibility than she is happy with. She watches over her frail, confused roommate but feels burdened by that responsibility. She works in the gift shop despite her distaste for dealing with money. She does not impose on the staff to assist her in moving about, although she has physical difficulty in managing on her own.

There is an inclination to feel sorry for Mrs. Moorse. Because she doesn't like to make trouble, as she herself puts it, she seems too easily exploited. In helping her 92-year-old roommate, Mrs. Moorse is relieving the paid staff of additional burdens yet taking on those burdens herself. In her own judgment the burden on her is "unfair." If she were more assertive, perhaps she would already have been given the single room she requested 5 years earlier. Out of a sense of obligation she is doing things she doesn't like to do. Do her attitudes and behavior deserve commendation? Should she be pitied because she is continually placed in situations she does not like? Or are these situations partly of her own making, ones that Mrs. Moorse could remedy if she showed more strength of will?

Before attempting to answer these questions, let's conduct a thought experiment: What would life be like for Mrs. Moorse in Xavier Nursing Home if she acted otherwise? What if she withdrew from the many activities she takes part in, began to demand assistance in getting about, refused to help out in the gift shop, and failed to keep an eye on Carolyn, her roommate, or help her when needed? In all likelihood Mrs. Moorse would feel guilty about not making a contribution to the facility's programs and remorseful about not living up to what she feels is her obligation to work in the gift shop. She would feel like a nuisance if she began making demands on the staff when she could remain more independent. She would see herself as abandoning her helpless roommate, with the prospect of harm befalling her. Would Mrs. Moorse truly be better off with these feelings and attitudes than with the ones she currently experiences?

Of course, these suppositions are merely hypothetical. Even if we concluded that Mrs. Moorse should be more assertive on her own behalf, there is the question of whether she could be. An old philosophical adage states that "ought implies can." Before it can be said that a person ought to do something, it must be established that the person has the capacity to do that thing. Mrs. Moorse's actions and attitudes toward the staff and other residents in Xavier Nursing Home are most probably not newly acquired pieces of behavior, isolated from her past self. Instead, they are manifestations of a personality developed many years ago and exhibited in a lifelong pattern in a variety of settings.

In contrast, consider Mrs. Finch's attitudes and behavior. Outspoken and demanding, Mrs. Finch not only takes no responsibility for her slightly demented roommate, but she feels put upon when asked to assist the roommate in small ways. She refuses to work in the gift shop, wants more independence in taking medicines than the rules allow, and complains about the lack of choice on her restricted diabetic diet.

Everyone knows someone like Mrs. Finch. A chronic complainer, she would probably be unhappy no matter what the nursing home provided. If she were given the single room she wants, she might very well find some feature of it unsatisfactory. We hadn't met Mrs. Finch before she entered Xavier Nursing Home, but those who have known her for a long time could no doubt confirm the supposition that the traits she now exhibits are long-standing features of her personality.

It is true that the nursing home restricts Mrs. Finch's freedom and independence in a number of ways, transforming her situation from what it was in the recent past. As a capable adult living alone, or with her husband, she was accustomed to managing her own diabetes medication. Now, however, she must comply with a rule of the nursing home intended not for people like her but for impaired or demented residents. No wonder she feels somewhat demeaned, even infantilized.

Apparently, Mrs. Moorse and Mrs. Finch have quite different conceptions of what it means to be a nursing home resident. Mrs. Moorse sees herself as part of a community and, as a result, believes that she has obligations to the community as a whole as well as to individual members, such as her roommate, Carolyn. Her participation in numerous activities is one expression of her feeling part of a community, as is her work in the gift shop.

Mrs. Finch, on the other hand, sees the nursing home as a place where she resides out of necessity. She's there because she needs health care, not because she volunteered to join a community. She rejects the social worker's analogy between the nursing home and "a large family." According to this conception, she owes nothing to the institution as a whole or to individuals in it, staff or fellow residents.

ROLE RESPONSIBILITIES AND MORAL RULES

To conceive of the nursing home as a community raises the question of whether a set of obligations flows from membership in the community, as is true of better-defined social groups. It also requires an assessment of just which model of community best applies to the nursing home. The usual, prevailing model is that of a medical facility. Other possibilities include a neighborhood, an apartment complex, a hotel or resort, or even a family.

Family members owe each other more than is owed to a stranger, for example, and employees of a company are expected to show more loyalty to the firm and to fellow workers than they would to a rival organization. In some social contexts, rather strong obligations flow from specific roles: health professionals owe duties to their patients, parents have responsibilities to their own children that they lack toward a neighbor's children, and elected officials are obligated to uphold the public trust. It is characteristic of these situations that people who take on certain roles are expected to assume responsibilities attached to those roles.

It might be thought that moral responsibilities of these sorts arise because the roles are assumed voluntarily. People choose to study to enter a health profession, decide to run for elective office, and plan to found a family. In choosing these roles, they choose the obligations and responsibilities attached to them. But it is a mistake to assume that responsibilities and obligations attach only to voluntarily chosen roles. The unwed mother who had an unplanned, unwanted pregnancy has parental obligations toward her baby just as the mother of a much-desired child does, and a draftee in wartime has obligations connected with being in military service as much as does the peacetime volunteer.

Does becoming a resident of a nursing home carry with it any such role responsibilities? Are there obligations attached to residency, whether or not an individual acknowledges or accepts them? A comparison with other social roles may be instructive.

A decision to become a nurse obligates the person to comply with the Code for Nurses, and the decision to participate in organized sports commits an individual to being a team player. The nurse who routinely discloses confidential information about her patients fails in her obligation both to the profession and to the particular patient. And the athlete who plays in a self-interested manner, undercutting the larger interest of the team, violates the sporting code. Even if the nurse or the athlete do not see themselves as having certain role obligations, those obligations exist nonetheless.

In addition to imposing role responsibilities, professions and social organizations have rules that govern the conduct of members. One kind of rule stipulates what is good practice in that particular activity. The nurse who tends to her patients' needs efficiently and in a caring manner, who enters full and clear nursing notes, and who provides details about patients' condition to the next nursing shift and to the physicians follows the rules of good nursing practice.

Having greater moral weight than rules of good practice are the ethical rules peculiar to a profession or activity. The Code for Nurses is a formal set of the moral rules that bind nurses, as is the Code of Professional Responsibility for lawyers. In athletics, informal codes of sporting conduct have ethical content. The moral rules governing a specific activity exist side by side with the ordinary ethical precepts that guide conduct between people in everyday life.

Are these rules of good practice and codes of ethical behavior applicable to the situation of being a resident in a nursing home? I claim they are not. There is no set of rules stipulating what counts as good "nursing home resident practice," analogous to good nursing practice. And unless the Residents' Council of a nursing home decides to establish a set of ethical rules that residents should abide by, there are no implicit moral rules peculiar to residents of a nursing home other than those that apply generally to human beings in their interactions.

WHAT KIND OF COMMUNITY IS A NURSING HOME?

Despite the absence of moral rules that are peculiar to nursing homes and the lack of role responsibilities on the part of residents, a nursing home is still a community of sorts. What kind of community is it? Even if the traditional conception of a medical facility is rejected, the alternative models of a neighborhood, a hotel or resort, and a family remain. Each of these models implies a different set of virtues for the residents.

Mrs. Finch is not violating an implicit moral rule by declining to work a shift in the gift shop. Nor is she failing in her obligations if she refuses to engage in other activities for residents, choosing to remain picky about what she will do. She could properly challenge the social worker's admonition by denying that she has any particular "weight to pull" in the nursing home. Nonetheless, Mrs. Finch lacks the virtue of being a willing contributor to the overall good of the community in which she resides.

As for Mrs. Finch's having an obligation to her slightly demented roommate, the situation is roughly equivalent to what would be morally required of a next-door neighbor in an apartment building or on a city block, if the neighbor (or the roommate) were in danger of harm but the harm were not imminent. Mrs. Finch would have an obligation to assist the person or notify someone who could take charge. These are general moral obligations people have toward one another. Such obligations flow from being in physical proximity with others, rather than from the voluntariness of entry into the community. Being a roommate in a nursing home places one in a situation where potential harm to another is more likely to be noticed than it would be in the privacy of individual homes or apartments. But Mrs. Finch would be morally culpable only if she failed to notify the staff that her demented roommate was in need of more assistance than she was getting.

Mrs. Finch is quite right to reject the social worker's suggestion that the nursing home be viewed as "a large family." A family is a well-defined social and cultural institution. People may choose to "adopt" unrelated persons into their own family, and biologically related family members may choose to "disown" one of their members (which doesn't sever the kinship ties, though it may sever relations). But an organization or institution does not become a "family" because members or residents are exhorted to treat each other in the way family members should. The social worker's well-intended chat with Mrs. Finch is an exhortation to virtue rather than a proper reminder about the resident's obligations to her new "family."

Mrs. Moorse is a "good citizen" of Xavier Nursing Home, and Mrs. Finch is a "poor citizen." Mrs. Moorse exhibits virtues, ordinary human virtues: compassion, altruism, civic responsibility, self-help. These are not virtues peculiar to being a resident in a nursing home but rather virtues of citizenship in any community.

Mrs. Finch, on the other hand, shows a distinct lack of virtue in these same respects. Yet to lack virtuousness is not equivalent to manifesting vices. Perhaps her conduct is even lacking in propriety. As the eighteenth-century philosopher Adam Smith (1759) noted, "There is a considerable difference between virtue and mere propriety; between those qualities and actions which deserve to be admired and celebrated, and those which simply deserve to be approved of." Mrs. Finch is complaining, unhelpful, demanding, and uncooperative, qualities that are typically disapproved. At the very least, she fails to comply with certain social rules of etiquette. But etiquette should not be confused with morality. Mrs. Finch is not actually harming others, and her offense to others is mild, albeit unpleasant.

A relevant moral distinction in these models of citizenship is between duties or obligations, on the one hand, and virtues, on the other. I contend that being a resident of a nursing home does *not* carry with it a set of moral obligations peculiar to that role. Whatever duties are binding on residents stem from their being members of a human community living in close proximity. That is no different from residents of a neighborhood or transient occupants of a hotel or resort.

Nevertheless, as members of an ongoing community, one like a neighborhood or apartment complex, residents of a nursing home can exhibit virtues of citizenship that go beyond what is expected of people thrown into proximity in a temporary arrangement, such as guests in a hotel or resort. There is no expectation that hotel guests exhibit the virtue of contributing to the general welfare of the institution. There is a financial obligation to pay the bill at the end of the stay and duties of courtesy (etiquette rather than full-blown ethics) to others encountered during the stay. Residents of a nursing home may choose to become more or less involved as contributors. If they choose to remain uninvolved, they are not morally blameworthy. If they choose to contribute, they are praiseworthy on account of their virtue in helping to promote the general welfare of the community.

It is a mistake to fasten on a single, pure model of a community for determining the obligations, virtues, and appropriate behavior of nursing home residents. Three overlapping models, existing simultaneously, afford a better picture of this complex reality: a home, inhabited by people who may come to view each other as members of an extended family; a medical facility, particularly for those residents who need medical treatment, nursing care, or supervision; and a small neighborhood or apartment complex in which communal goods can be identified and promoted.

AUTONOMY IN THE NURSING HOME

Now we come to the question of the autonomy of these two nursing home residents. Is the autonomy of either Mrs. Moorse or Mrs. Finch being restricted? If so, in what ways? Before replying, a brief foray into theory is necessary.

Bruce Miller (1981) has observed that both ordinary language and moral philosophy embrace several different notions of autonomy. Miller identifies four different senses of the concept, three of which are relevant to our case. The simplest notion of autonomy is Miller's first sense: autonomy as free action. "Autonomy as free action means an action that is voluntary and intentional" (p. 24). This is a thin notion of autonomy, one that does not do justice to the concept. It confuses autonomy with freedom or liberty.

Autonomy must mean something more than mere freedom to act. The etymology of the word literally implies "self-rule," what the philosopher Immanuel Kant referred to as a "self-legislating will." What is required for self-rule? There are two basic ingredients: first, an authentic self that can be identified; and second, the capacity to rule the self. These ingredients begin to shape a full-bodied concept of autonomy, richer than the thin notion of freedom to act.

Miller's second meaning is autonomy as authenticity: "Autonomy as authenticity means that an action is consistent with the person's attitudes, values, dispositions, and life plans. Roughly, the person is acting in character" (p. 24). The autonomous person is one who is self-directed rather than one who obeys the commands of others. To be autonomous is to be the author of one's own beliefs, desires, and actions, however weird or deviant those beliefs and actions may be. There must, however, be a consistent pattern of beliefs and actions over time. The beliefs and actions must flow from a self that can be identified. Examples of people who lack these characteristics are those who suffer a sudden onset of mental illness or who have been subjected to what is commonly called "brainwashing" or "thought reform."

But there are other ways a person can lack autonomy. To fail in the most elemental capacity to reason results in lack of autonomy. Miller's third meaning of autonomy—autonomy as effective deliberation—captures this concept. In his words: "Autonomy as effective deliberation means action taken where a person believed that he or she was in a situation calling for a decision, was aware of the alternatives and the consequences of the alternatives, evaluated both, and chose an action based on that evaluation" (p. 24). This is a standard description of reasoning capacity. Having autonomy presupposes an ability to marshall relevant reasons for action.

We now have some conceptual apparatus for analyzing how autonomy fits into the cases of Mrs. Moorse and Mrs. Finch. If autonomy is taken to be synonymous with free action, it is clear that all residents of a nursing home are subjected to restrictions of their autonomy. Although both women are in double rooms despite their wish for a single room, this may have little to do with restricting autonomy. Not every instance in which people's wishes cannot be fulfilled counts as a limitation of their autonomy.

Curiously, although Mrs. Finch is more outspoken and defiant than Mrs. Moorse, the restriction on her ability to self-administer her diabetes medicine limits Mrs. Finch's freedom more than any of the nursing home's regulations appear to limit Mrs. Moorse. But I have already suggested that the "thin" interpretation of autonomy, making it equivalent to the concept of freedom, ought to be abandoned.

To apply Miller's second interpretation, autonomy as authenticity, we would have to know more about both women's values and behavior before they entered Xavier Nursing Home in order to assess the authenticity of their current attitudes and conduct. But it is safe to assume that both residents are exhibiting traits that have long existed in their adult personalities. Mrs. Moorse was, no doubt, a "quiet lady" who didn't like to "make trouble" for much of her life. As for Mrs. Finch, it is likely that she always believed in "speaking her mind," choosing her activities, and selecting her companions. Both residents appear to be acting "authentically," consistent with their attitudes, values, and dispositions over a lifetime.

The social worker's talk with Mrs. Finch about her adaptation could be seen as an attempt to interfere with her autonomy. In trying to inculcate traits and behavior deemed more suitable to nursing home residents, the social worker was actually trying to alter Mrs. Finch's authentic self. Having family of her own, Mrs. Finch could never view the nursing home community as "another family." And it would mark a radical departure for her to "settle for the kind of life so many here have," as she put it.

Mrs. Moorse's authentic self leads her to do some things she doesn't really like to do because of her felt obligations and sense of responsibility. Her feeling of duty to help out in the gift shop, as one of the residents capable of the task, outweighs her dislike of handling money. The responsibility she takes for her frail roommate, despite feeling burdened, has a moral underpinning: she'd like someone to help her if she were in that situation. If the nursing home staff coerced Mrs. Moorse into doing these things, that would constitute an interference with her autonomy. But people who choose to do things they dislike because they believe it is their duty are those who best fulfill Immanuel Kant's conception of the autonomous moral agent with a self-legislating will.

Both Mrs. Moorse and Mrs. Finch manifest Miller's third meaning of autonomy, autonomy as effective deliberation. Each woman is in an overall situation calling for decisions and actions. Each appears to be quite aware of the alternatives open to her and the consequences of these alternatives, evaluates the situation, and chooses accordingly.

A crucial feature of this sense of autonomy is the ability to give reasons in support of actions chosen. Mrs. Moorse believes that residents of a place should pitch in and make a contribution, and she acts according to that belief. She accurately assesses her roommate's helpless condition and need for her watchful assistance. Her reason for bearing this responsibility is a version of the golden rule: She'd like someone to help her if she was "like poor Carolyn."

Mrs. Finch also gives reasons in support of her behavior, reasons that evince an accurate assessment of her situation. She is in the nursing home because she needs health care, not because she wants a new family, a place to spend her time as a volunteer, or a new community of friends. Her disdain for her fellow residents is based on not wanting to become like them. We may dislike Mrs. Finch's attitude, but we cannot doubt that she retains her autonomy. If Mrs. Finch were to become more of an "ideal resident" of Xavier Nursing Home, displaying some of Mrs. Moorse's traits, we might begin to wonder whether she was losing her autonomy.

RESOLVING THE ISSUES

It is unrealistic and perhaps also inappropriate to expect any change in the attitudes and behavior of Mrs. Moorse and Mrs. Finch. However, in the case of each resident, a possibility exists for changing matters for the better.

In Mrs. Moorse's case, she deserves the long-awaited single room. The nursing home has single rooms, and Mrs. Moorse has waited 5 years, longer than some residents who arrived after her. Because she is not a loud complainer, her quiet requests for the single room may well have been ignored. And it is in the staff's own interest to keep her in the double room with Carolyn, who receives the help and monitoring she needs as long as Mrs. Moorse is there. It would be doubly fair to Mrs. Moorse to offer her the next available single room. First, she has waited long enough for that room; and second, the "unfair" burden she assumes in carrying the "big responsibility" for her roommate will be lifted. This change would dispel any lingering suspicion that Mrs. Moorse is being taken advantage of in the nursing home.

In Mrs. Finch's case, given the present administrative structure of the nursing home, there is nothing the staff can do directly that would improve her situation or change her attitude. Trying to get her to adapt would be more for the staff's convenience and comfort than the resident's. But encouraging her intention to become active in the Resident Council might prove to be the best solution. Mrs. Finch might channel some of her discontent into useful action and spend less time complaining about matters she can't change. For her to "quiet down" might be a sign of declining autonomy. But for her to remain vocal by becoming an active leader in the Resident's Council would be to express her autonomy in a constructive way.

The nursing home could respond to Mrs. Finch in other ways that would enhance her autonomy. This would involve some changes in administrative structure. As a first step, it is worth considering whether the rules are more rigid than they need to be. Could Mrs. Finch be given some control over her own medications? Rules designed for demented patients need not be applied to mentally alert, capable residents like Mrs. Finch. And why are residents not encouraged to continue to participate in outside activities? There may be no good reason why Mrs. Finch cannot continue to serve as a telephone volunteer for the American Cancer Society, despite her residency in Xavier Nursing Home.

An individualized approach to medical and nutritional consultation might reveal that some of the dietary restrictions for Mrs. Finch are unnecessary. Allowing more variety and more choice in her diet would not only improve her well-being, but also show respect for her autonomy. In addition to deviating in these ways from its standard practice, the nursing home could also seek to introduce recreational activities that are more meaningful to adults. Mrs. Finch's complaint that most of the activities in the home "are for babies" is probably justified. It need not involve great ingenuity or expense to bring more challenging programs for residents into the home.

It is always tempting to resolve an ethical problem by proposing a "technological fix": changing the circumstances so that the ethical problem is lessened or eliminated. Of course, it is often not possible to make such changes. But greater efforts to introduce flexibility might yield surprising results. An improvement in some of the features of the community could better enable the residents of this and other nursing homes to exhibit the virtues of citizenship.

REFERENCES

Miller, B.L. (1981). Autonomy and the refusal of lifesaving treatment. *Hastings Center Report*, 11(4), 22–28.

Smith, A. (1759) *The theory of moral sentiments*. Reprinted in D.D. Raphael (Ed.), *British Moralists*. Oxford: Clarendon Press, 1969.

FOR FURTHER DISCUSSION: EDITORS' QUESTIONS

1. What virtues should a nursing home resident display? What is the ideal resident?
2. What obligations do nursing home residents have to each other? What are the limits of such obligations?
3. Should the home expect residents to help out with other residents? Or is there always a tinge of exploitation in a facility seeking help from residents?
4. Is the home obliged to find ways that residents can be helpful and altruistic?
5. Which attitudes are more commendable, Mrs. Finch's or Mrs. Moorse's? Why?
6. Which resident—Mrs. Finch or Mrs. Moorse—is likely to do most good for the nursing home community?
7. What model of community is relevant to the nursing home? Should the facility be viewed as a family, a hotel, or a hospital, or is some other analogy helpful for understanding this kind of community? Does the notion of community make any sense at all in this kind of setting?

Chapter 6

THE CHAIR AND OTHER PUBLIC SPACE

MISS CROCHET'S CHAIR

Miss Crochet is a heavyset woman who is acknowledged to be a leader. She is viewed as kindhearted but quick-tempered. Miss Crochet always sits in the armchair in the dayroom next to her friend Emily. Other residents leave the armchair for her, and they also let Miss Crochet decide what television channel to watch.

One day the nurse's aide heard screaming and shouting emanating from the dayroom. She rushed in to see what the trouble was and saw that Miss Newly, a resident just admitted a few days before was sitting in "Miss Crochet's chair." Miss Crochet was protesting loudly and making menacing gestures at Miss Newly. Emily was adding to the confusion, trying to explain, despite a speech impediment, that Miss Newly was in "someone else's chair." The latter looked puzzled and was weakly stating that "I thought the chairs belonged to all of us."

The aide made peace as best she could, explaining to Miss Newly that Miss Crochet usually sat in the big armchair and pleading with Miss Crochet to make allowances for the fact that Miss Newly had just arrived and didn't know that she was in someone else's chair. When asked later why she sided with Miss Crochet, the aide gave a mixed reply. First, she had to act to resolve the fight quickly, and she calculated the best course for restoring peace. Second, "Some people are more powerful than others, even in nursing homes." It would be best if Miss Newly did not alienate Miss Crochet. Third, the aide thought that in some ways the chair did belong to Miss Crochet: "It was almost part of her."

WHO OWNS THE DAY ROOM?

At a Residents' Council meeting later in the week, the discussion turned to all the bickering that had been going on lately about the day areas. Emily questioned some of the informal rules that had grown up. Her friends and relatives had come to the home with a cake and the makings of a party to celebrate Emily's 75th birthday. In this facility the men who smoke tend to congregate in the dining room. Emily's birthday party was held in the much smaller dayroom, and some residents who were not invited were hovering around. Emily had felt at the time that it would have been wrong to ask the four men who were smoking to leave the dining room, but now she wonders. Her birthday party was somewhat spoiled by being held in such a congested space. The activities director, who represents the staff at the meetings and helps convene the Residents' Council, reminded the group that there had already been a birthday party on May 15 for all of those born in May and that family members had been invited to that party, as is facility policy. For that regularly scheduled event, the dining room was used, and, of course, the smokers were invited to the party. The activities director wondered if exclusive parties were fair to other residents. In any event, she thought that "if everyone wanted to do it, it would be disruptive."

MUSIC ON THE PUBLIC ADDRESS SYSTEM

A few months later Emily was bothered by yet another space issue—this time air space. The administrator had initiated a new policy of hooking the radio into the public address system and leaving the station at "gentle listening" for large parts of the day. The music was audible in the corridors and in the bedrooms. Emily complained and was told that music is relaxing. The administrator had recently read that frequent, hummable music can reduce agitation among confused residents. He said that Emily was the only person who had complained so far.

As for Emily, she said she likes music as much as the next person, though she probably would not choose that station. But she finds it "nerve-wracking" to have the music floating through the air as a perpetual background. She did not bring this up at the Residents' Council but is thinking of circulating a petition and asking residents who do not appreciate the music to sign it. Miss Crochet does not plan to sign the petition because she likes the music, though Emily asks, "What about the principle here?" Emily argues that those who want music can have their own radios on.

CASE COMMENTARY

Margaret P. Battin

THE MUSIC

Let's start with the easy part: the music. Though Emily doesn't express it quite this way, we suspect she recognizes the strategy: piping the "easy listening" station into the nursing home is a thinly veiled strategy for behavior control. Like Musak in elevators and shopping centers, it is intended to produce a certain behavioral result. In this case, its purpose is to "reduce agitation" among confused residents; and insofar as this purpose is a legitimate goal, it may be a better way to do so than by using tranquilizing drugs or other means.

But not all of the residents are confused; certainly Emily is not. Insofar as the residents who are not confused cannot escape the music (especially since it penetrates into the corridors and bedrooms as well as the dayroom), it must be viewed as an extension of illegitimate control over persons for whom this is not required. It would be morally intolerable to impose tranquilizing drugs on all of the residents, not just those who needed them; it is equally intolerable to impose tranquilizing music on those who do not need it either.

THE BIRTHDAY PARTY

Emily's birthday party also doesn't present much of a moral problem, at least not at first. First, it involves only a temporary disruption for the men who smoke, not a serious, sustained one. Second, the hypothetical "What if everyone did it?" is a red herring because (unfortunately) not every resident has a large, boisterous family eager to visit. Third, there is no real reason why all of the residents need be invited to Emily's party; despite the usual rhetoric, nursing homes are not communes or families, which have some understanding about mutual participation; they are involuntary assemblages of persons who live in a single space for reasons other than the intention to share their lives. No one enters a nursing home in order to share his or her life with the other residents. Rather, a person enters a nursing home because he or she can no longer live anywhere else. Although residents may develop relationships with other residents once they enter a nursing home, it cannot be assumed that residents' primary relationships are with each other or that all residents' relationships are equally close. This is a message the official once-a-month birthday party, to which all are invited, seems to convey.

On the contrary, some residents will continue to have primary relationships with family or friends outside the home. Such ties are of positive intrinsic value, not just of extrinsic value, in contributing to these residents' mental health or manageability, and these ties should be offered as much protection and furtherance as possible. Consequently, functions within the home should be arranged to be the least disruptive of these ties as possible because they are often the only intimate, personal, significant relationships older persons have left. Under the hypothesis of the story, the principle that primary relationships of intrinsic value should be given as much protection as possible would have meant using the dining room for Emily's birthday party even if it meant moving the smokers elsewhere. The smokers should have been provided with an alternative place to smoke while the party was going on. No primary relationship of intrinsic value is being disrupted by asking the smokers to move for an evening. On the other hand, crowding Emily's party into the dayroom or, worse still, combining it with the official monthly affair would certainly do so.

There is no serious, immediate moral dilemma here; all this case really shows—besides the appalling fact that there is so little common space in the home—is that Emily was a little too meek in not taking over the dining room to begin with. Since the staff failed to support her in exercising a basic right, perhaps she should have employed her friend, the powerful Miss Crochet, to do the dirty work.

THE CHAIR

The hard case is Miss Crochet's chair. (Notice how the case seems to change is you think of her as Miss "Crochet" as in "knit a doily," or as Miss

"Crotchet" as in "crotchety," said of a person who gripes or complains.) Our initial egalitarian impulse may be to say that Miss Newly was right: in the common area of nursing home life every resident must have equal rights. As Miss Newly said, "I thought the chairs belonged to all of us."

In this egalitarian view, for the aide to side with Miss Crochet was wrong. She was adopting a morally unjustified way to maintain peace because it simply served to perpetuate Miss Crochet's little tyranny. Not perpetuating crotchety residents' tyrannies, it might further be argued, is particularly important in a nursing home, where resources are usually so limited that the tyranny of one resident means substantial deprivation for the others. Thus, the institutional suppression of Miss Newly's attempt to maintain equality, as in the aide's siding with Miss Crochet, simply adds to the other deprivations, constrictions, and indignities of nursing home life and, morally speaking, cannot be tolerated. It is particularly important to protect the rights of residents like Miss Newly, who have just been admitted to a nursing home and are therefore at a disadvantage in power interactions with other residents and cannot protect their equal rights alone.

But although I think this argument is right, the conclusion it draws, that Miss Crochet must let Miss Newly sit in the chair, is wrong. The inference has been drawn in an erroneous way. Although the *principle* of equality is right—and, indeed, especially important in the limited contexts of nursing homes—drawing the conclusion that Miss Newly may sit in the chair results from applying the principle in a mistaken way. What must be done prior to the application of the principle is to identify the good at stake because it is a good, not a thing, that all residents have equal rights to enjoy. It is this step that has been omitted and that results in the erroneous conclusion to which the egalitarian view seems to lead.

The good at stake is not the chair. It is, rather, what the chair represents: a zone of privacy, control, "ownness." The chair is merely a physical thing that serves as the tangible expression (the "objective correlative," as old-fashioned literary critics used to say) of an individual's personality in an otherwise leveling environment. The aide seems to recognize that the chair serves this function for Miss Crochet. "It's almost a part of her," says the aide. Although this might seem an inflated claim in other contexts, it cannot be taken lightly in the context of nursing homes precisely because this environment is not only limiting but also has most likely been entered involuntarily. Sitting in the chair provides Miss Crochet with virtually her only opportunity for self-expression and assertion of her own unique personality. There is nothing else she can do in the nursing home that can achieve this for her.

Thus, what the chair represents is a substantial good. Like maintaining primary relationships with family and friends, it is a good that is of positive, intrinsic value. No person ought lightly to be deprived of a good of this sort unless that person's enjoyment of the good seriously harms someone else. To deprive Miss Crochet of the chair would be to accelerate that process of dehumanization for which nursing homes are often notorious, and it must be weighed against the comparatively trivial good of allowing Miss Newly to sit in the chair. The chair has no antecedent significance for Miss Newly. For Miss Crochet, it is all.

But if the chair represents a positive, intrinsic, significant good, then in an egalitarian view it is something to which *all* residents, including Miss Newly, have equal rights. It would seem, then, that not letting Miss Newly sit in the chair does harm her after all because it is depriving her of whatever benefit the chair may come to offer. But here we see that the distinction between the chair and the good that the chair represents is crucial. It is what the chair represents, not the chair itself, to which all residents have equal rights. Thus, the principle of equality can be preserved, as well as the equally important principle, derivative from the more general principle of beneficence, that what is a positive, intrinsic value in the lives of persons should be given greatest protection. The conclusion to be drawn is not that all residents may share Miss Crochet's chair equally but that each resident has an equal right to the furtherance and protection of some object or circumstance that serves the same function as does the chair for Miss Crochet. This is just to say that each resident has the right to the kind of good the chair provides for Miss Crochet but not to Miss Crochet's chair itself.

When we try to think of examples of other items that might provide the same sort of good for other residents, only a few come to mind: a windowbox to tend, perhaps a piano to play, but not much else. Nursing homes are remarkably devoid of the kinds of items in public spaces that can serve roles such as these—a particularly unfortunate circumstance because there is no automatic limit to them except the flexibility and inventiveness of the administration and staff. It is not enough that residents can keep knickknacks or special mementos in their rooms. In talking about Miss Crochet's chair, we are talking about an object that serves as a vehicle of self-expression, and self-expression involves an audience. Self-expression is a matter of conveying one's own personality to other persons, of characterizing oneself vis-à-vis other persons, of establishing oneself as a person among others. The same chair installed in Miss Crochet's room could not possibly serve the same function.

Thus, in showing that what is crucial about Miss Crochet's chair is the role it plays in her life, this case also serves as an indictment of the restricted, depersonalizing environment many nursing homes present: they do not make possible and do not protect the kind of individual self-expression Miss Crochet has been able to achieve. In the environment she has been placed in, she can do it only because she is powerful, and she can do it only at the expense of other residents. But the proper conclusion is not to limit her opportunities as well but to expand such opportunities for everyone else. It might be suggested that the nursing home should dispose of the troublesome armchair and refurnish the dayroom with chairs that are all alike; then, it is true, disputes like these would not break out. But that solution would compound what is really wrong with this nursing home (and nearly all others) and leave the egalitarian problem unsolved.

The chair is a little like Dad's Chair in the Traditional American Family. We all know the stereotype: Dad sits in the chair (of course, a Barca-lounger) when he comes home from work, while Mom brings him a drink, the kids show him their schoolwork, and the dog fetches the newspaper. In this stereotype Dad's chair is the visible symbol, the "objective correlative," of his position as head of the family. Here too the good is not the chair itself, as material object, but what the chair represents.

We also know what is wrong with this picture. But if it consigns an inferior, subservient role to Mom, getting rid of Dad's chair is not the appropriate egalitarian answer; instead, Mom should be entitled to a similarly substantial chair—or more correctly, to the sort of position within the family that a similarly substantial chair or other "objective correlative" might represent. In just the same way, the nursing home makes a mistake in principle if it evicts Miss Crochet from her chair; instead, rather than imposing a misguided uniformity by policing everyone's opportunities to sit in the chair, the nursing home ought to protect whatever equally idiosyncratic items might also serve as vehicles for the intrinsic good of self-expression for each of its other residents.

INTRINSIC GOODS FOR ALL

Seeing what to do about Miss Crochet's chair also allows us to see that there is a very real moral issue associated with Emily's birthday party after all, though not the one that seemed to present itself at first. Just as it is unwarranted to get rid of Miss Crochet's special chair by insisting that all seating in the home be uniform or that every resident have an equal chance at every place, it would be equally unwarranted to discourage birthday parties like Emily's big, boisterous one on the grounds that other residents had no outside friends or family they could invite to similar parties for themselves. Restricting parties like Emily's to the uniform, official, once-a-month affair is precisely the same moral maneuver as getting rid of Miss Crochet's chair; it disposes of the good the chair and the birthday party represent because they cannot be equally shared by all.

But this is just the wrong move. Rather, an attempt should be made to make the same kind of good available to other residents. If some unfortunate people in the home no longer have family or friends to celebrate their birthdays with them, are there outside volunteers who might like to do so instead? Could the staff plan something special—an outing or a favorite meal—for those who have no one else? Or is there some other way to make special the day that at some deep emotional level often still remains one's own even if one has had literally scores of birthdays already? If the home cannot find some small way of giving *personal* recognition to something that may have such significance, some way of substituting for the basic, intrinsically important relationships that are traditionally active on these occasions, then it is morally callous. If it compounds this failing by restricting those who still do have such relationships to official once-a-month birthdays, even to serve a conception of equality that is right in theory but wrongly put into practice, then its moral errors are more substantial still. Let Miss Crochet sit in the chair and let Emily have the birthday party. The home has a basic moral obligation not to restrict basic, intrinsic goods for them but to find some way to make the same sort of goods available to all.

FOR FURTHER DISCUSSION: EDITORS' QUESTIONS

1. These incidents—Miss Crochet's chair, Emily's party, the piped-in music—all involve various uses of the common space and property. What is common space in a nursing home setting? What is public and what is private?

2. What, if any, zone of privacy is each resident entitled to? What notions of property make sense in the nursing home context?

3. Is entitlement to privacy or to property somehow based on the length of time the resident has lived in the facility?

4. Given all of these considerations, is it right for Miss Crochet to stake claim to a chair and for staff to back her on it?

5. How far should staff go to facilitate Emily's birthday party? Should they ask the men to leave their accustomed spot to accommodate a private event? Is a private birthday party in any way inappropriate?

6. Does the practice of the monthly, collective birthday party (which is widespread in nursing homes) promote the sense of importance of each resident, or does it somehow dehumanize the residents?

7. Who should make decisions that affect living space, such as the music or use of the dayroom, and how much agreement is necessary before an action is taken or a change implemented?

Chapter 7

IF YOU LET THEM, THEY'D STAY IN BED ALL MORNING: The Tyranny of Regulation in Nursing Home Life

At Mansion Manor the nurse's aides pretty well all agree that residents need to get up for breakfast, which is served at 7:30. Some of the aides feel bad waking the residents up, especially knowing that many residents have little in particular to do all day. Mildred, one of the senior aides, says she sometimes makes an exception and lets a resident sleep through breakfast, especially if the resident was feeling poorly the night before. But "If we left the residents alone, some would just stay in bed all morning." Not only is it bad for residents to get "lazy," but also the facility must get everyone up so that the baths and morning routines can be done after breakfast.

BATTLE OF THE BREAKFAST

Mrs. Hollinger, aged 76, is one resident who really is not a breakfast fan. She has lived in the home for 2 years, ever since her first stroke, when she also started using a walker. Lately, she had a second stroke and now uses a wheelchair for mobility. She finds that making the effort for breakfast is almost intolerable—she has been feeling so tired lately. All of her life she has skipped breakfast, preferring just a cup of coffee. The aides insist on having her up, washed, and dressed for breakfast by 7:20.

Partly because of her disregard for breakfast, and partly because she is slow in navigating the wheelchair, Mrs. Hollinger has been late for breakfast every morning for the last 2 weeks. The aides say that her late arrival disrupts the feeding of other residents. Also, Mrs. Hollinger is a slow eater and doesn't finish if she comes late. The floor nurse warned Mrs. Hollinger that if she continues to be late for breakfast, they will have to put her with the "feeders" (those unable to feed themselves) in a separate dining room. Mrs. Hollinger now has trouble sleeping at night because she worries about being late for breakfast. This stress tires her even more and makes the morning more difficult.

OTHER BATTLES

This is not the first time Mrs. Hollinger has run afoul of nursing home policy. When she first came to the facility, she thought she could keep a bottle of sherry in her room to use in the evening and to entertain guests. The nurse put a stop to that. She said the sherry could be kept in the medications area, and if the doctor agreed, an evening drink could be prescribed.

Mrs. Hollinger has also objected to the way staff "poke around" in her room. Just before the inspectors came 6 months ago, a staff member actually looked in the drawers to see if anything was unsafe. Mrs. Hollinger's shoe polish and her bottle of aspirins were taken from her night table drawer, and the decorative candle she was given for Christmas was also removed. When she protested, staff explained that although Mrs. Hollinger could handle these things safely, someone who was confused might wander in and harm themselves with these poisonous substances. Regulations stipulated what could be kept in a resident's room.

All of these matters were upsetting, but the breakfast situation was the worst thing that had happened to Mrs. Hollinger since her admission.

THE REGULATIONS DID IT!

This week when Mrs. Hollinger's son James came to visit, he found his mother nervous and teary. When he learned about the breakfast problem and the threat to put his mother with the feeders, he furiously confronted the floor nurse and director of nursing (DON). He said that his mother was not one of their "seniles." Moreover, Mr. Hollinger questioned the reasoning behind the breakfast policies. His mother lived very well for years without having breakfast, and he himself never ate in the morning.

Mr. Hollinger exerted so much pressure that the DON took him to her office to show him the regulations about feeding. She explained that federal requirements state that no more than 14 hours can elapse between a "substantial evening meal" and the first meal of the next day. Dinner gets served at 4:30 for some residents and at 5:15 for a second group. Therefore, to be in compliance with the regulations, the residents must have an early breakfast.

CASE COMMENTARY

James F. Childress

TIME IN ETHICAL ANALYSES OF LONG-TERM CARE

Several features of long-term care in nursing homes generate ethical problems and dilemmas that often differ from those encountered in critical care, the primary focus and locus of biomedical ethics. These problems and dilemmas frequently involve routine care in which no course of action is life-threatening, at least in the short run. The situations often evolve over time and do not require immediate, definitive answers. Both of these features point to the significance of time in long-term care and to the lack of urgency of most decisions in that setting.

In long-term care there is often time for trial and error and for rational resolutions, negotiated settlements, or compromises (on negotiated consent, see Moody, 1988; on compromise, see Benjamin, in press). In addition to the significance of the present and the future, the past is also important in various decisions in long-term care. For example, what has happened in the recent past in the care of Mrs. Hollinger is important for interpreting and assessing the actions of the different parties. Because of a series of conflicts, or "battles" as the case report calls them—over the bottle of sherry and over the staff "poking around" in her room, looking in the drawers, and removing shoe polish, a bottle of aspirins, and a gift decorative candle—the staff appears to view Mrs. Hollinger as a difficult and uncooperative resident. The very language—"battles"—indicates the perceived intensity of the conflict. In turn, it is not unreasonable that Mrs. Hollinger would view the staff as hostile intruders and meddlers, bent on breaking her independence and establishing control over every aspect of her life.

Agents make their moral judgments not only in light of various moral principles but also in relation to their interpretations of situations in which they have to act (Niebuhr, 1963). In this case it is probable that neither party's interpretation of the current situation is fully adequate; but their interpretations are surely shaped by their memories and images of past actions and conflicts, and their interpretations include assessments of the motives, intentions, attitudes, and traits of character of the other party.

The staff's view that Mrs. Hollinger is a difficult and uncooperative resident may stem from their sense that she is asserting rights without accepting her obligations and responsibilities within the institution. Her responsibilities (see Jameton, 1988) include respecting the rights of other residents as well as the legitimate demands of institutional order.

One major source of uncertainty in analyzing this case is whether Mrs. Hollinger's actions really infringe on the rights of others and disrupt institutional order. Even if Mrs. Hollinger's actions cannot be characterized in these terms, the staff may nonetheless attempt to persuade her to act in ways they deem appropriate. However, for forcible actions (such as removing her valuables) and coercive threats (such as threatening to put her in a separate dining room with the "feeders," who are unable to feed themselves"), it is essential that the staff meet a heavy burden of proof in overriding her autonomous choices, privacy, and liberty.

The aides could respond that they are not overriding Mrs. Hollinger's autonomy but respecting it because, after all, she accepted the rules and regulations that restrict privacy and liberty when she voluntarily entered the nursing home. Thus, she has a duty of compliance, not only because of the need for institutional order but because of her consent.

Before such a claim can be sustained, we need to know exactly what Mrs. Hollinger (and her son) were told at the outset about the rules and regulations. If they were not adequately informed, they would have additional grounds to complain about some of the interventions. However, even if they were adequately informed and accepted admission on those terms, they may still legitimately complain about those terms and seek to have them changed. In this case, their complaints could be directed at the nursing home's excessively legalistic and narrow interpretation of governmental and institutional rules and regulations.

State and federal regulations also set the context for what the long-term care facility may require of admittees. It is important to determine whether some of the institution's demands themselves violate federal and state regulations, which serve as the background and justification for several of the nursing home's restrictions of Mrs. Hollinger's liberty and privacy. As Ambrogi and Leonard (1988) note, federal regulations and some state regulations contain a "patients' Bill of Rights" designed to protect nursing home residents by "preserving the dignity and individual liberties that are central to residents' autonomy." Even though the law usually does not require that potential residents or their proxies receive notice of those rights when executing the admission agreement, the acceptance of the proffered terms of admission cannot be construed as *ethically* valid without clear notification of those rights. In short, then, appealing to Mrs. Hollinger's acceptance of the rules in the past, upon entry, will not necessarily dispose of her current complaints.

THE NATURE, VALUE, AND LIMITS OF RESIDENT AUTONOMY

The principle of respect for autonomy (hereafter referred to as the principle of autonomy) implies *individualized care* in the nursing home setting; it suggests that the provision of care, within limits, should follow the tracks set by the resident's autonomous choices, and it establishes both negative rights (e.g., liberty and privacy) and positive rights (e.g., to information and assistance).

Neither this principle of autonomy nor the rights (and correlative duties) that express it can be construed as absolute, that is, as outweighing or overriding all other ethical principles and values. At most the principle and the rights that specify it—particularly, for our purposes, liberty and privacy—are only prima facie binding. Insofar as respect for autonomy, liberty, or privacy is a feature of an action, that action is right or obligatory, all things being equal. However, in any situation it may be outweighed or overridden by competing prima facie principles, such as beneficence, nonmaleficence, and justice. A judgment that a prima facie principle can be overridden or outweighed in particular circumstances requires justification. In accord with the logic of prima facie principles, the process of justification—here stated in terms of overriding the principle of respect for autonomy—requires satisfying the following conditions:

1. The competing principle(s) is considered stronger or weightier in the situation than the principle of autonomy.
2. Infringement of the principle of autonomy protects or respects the competing principle(s).

3. Infringement of the principle of autonomy is necessary to protect or respect the competing principle.
4. The principle of autonomy is infringed as little as possible consistent with the protection of the competing principle(s).
5. Efforts are be made to minimize the negative effects of the infringement of autonomy.
6. Where possible, the infringement is explained and justified to the person whose autonomy has been infringed.

Even when the principle of respect for autonomy (or liberty or privacy) is justifiably overridden, it still exerts pressure. It is not canceled, as the above conditions make clear. Consider, for example, the autonomy-based rights of liberty and privacy. When a agent justifiably overrides another's liberty, he or she should choose the least restrictive alternative; and when an agent justifiably overrides another's privacy, he or she should choose the least intrusive alternative. Furthermore, respect for autonomy requires an explanation and justification to the person whose autonomy, liberty, and privacy are justifiably overridden.

The above conditions are not rigid, but they identify relevant considerations in the justification of the infringement of a principle such as autonomy in situations of conflict. Two sorts of limits are involved, one internal and the other external.

Determining when the principle of autonomy actually applies raises a question of internal limits. If residents lack autonomy—for example, the capacity for effective deliberation—then it is inappropriate to talk about respecting their autonomous choices even though they are due other forms of respect. If an intervention is designed to protect the nonautonomous agent, it is a form of weak or limited paternalism and is more easily justified than strong or extended paternalism that overrides an autonomous patient's choices in order to protect him or her. In this case, there is no evidence to suggest that Mrs. Hollinger is not autonomous in the sense of having the capacity to deliberate rationally and to choose freely.

Some philosophers have proposed authenticity as another criterion of autonomy (Dworkin, 1976; Miller, 1981). The intuitive idea is "acting in character." Even though I do not accept authenticity as a criterion of autonomy (Childress, 1982), I think it important to consider whether a person's actions are in accord with that person's character. Actions apparently out of character alert us to press for justifications and explanations in order to determine whether they are actually autonomous—for example, whether the agent has undergone a change in settled preferences, basic values, and life plans. In this case, Mrs. Hollinger's actions regarding breakfast are in character; she has skipped breakfast all of her life, preferring instead a cup of coffee each morning. Thus, there is no reason on grounds of inauthenticity to suspect that her choices are not autonomous.

External limits may justify overriding the principle of autonomy. In this case, as in real life, different reasons are mixed together. First, in the breakfast battle, one senior aide notes that she sometimes makes an exception to the rule about awakening residents in time for breakfast but that residents, if permitted to do so, would stay in bed and get lazy (a paternalistic justification), and the staff needs to take care of baths and morning routines after breakfast (institutional and staff needs). Furthermore, Mrs. Hollinger's late arrival allegedly disturbs other residents at breakfast. Finally, there is the institution's stated concern for compliance with the federal regulations (which will be discussed later). Other external limits include costs to the institution and to the society of respecting autonomy, as well as the society's interest in preventing exploitation of vulnerable people in settings that cannot be adequately monitored. These reasons are all *relevant,* but whether they are *adequate* will depend on whether the procedure of justification can be met.

The paternalistic justification seems insufficient in this case for requiring Mrs. Hollinger to have breakfast. Paternalism may be defined as nonacquiescence in a person's wishes, choices, and actions for that person's own benefit (Childress, 1982). The alleged benefits in this case may include (a) Mrs. Hollinger's health and (b) her future autonomy of action. It is not clear that breakfast is essential to protect Mrs. Hollinger's health, particularly in view of her eating habits over many years, and requiring her to eat under the circumstances may actually harm her physical and psychological health.

Another benefit that may be invoked in a paternalistic rationale is autonomy itself. One argument is that respecting Mrs. Hollinger's autonomy of choice or decision—to refuse breakfast—would fail to promote her future autonomy of action. A version of this argument appears in the claim that residents would just stay in bed all morning and get lazy if permitted to do so. However, there is no evidence that allowing Mrs. Hollinger to skip breakfast and get ready for the day with less stress would lead her to want to stay in bed all morning or to become lazy. Here again much depends on the interpretation of Mrs. Hollinger's actions. If we interpret her actions narrowly (i.e., as having to do with problems surrounding breakfast), there does not seem to be a sufficient paternalistic justification based on future autonomy of action to override her current autonomous choices by requiring her to be ready for breakfast at the set time.

The staff's stated justification for examining Mrs. Hollinger's personal property and removing some items—shoe polish, a bottle of aspirins, and a decorative candle—was to protect others in the nursing home, not to protect her. (The removal of sherry may have had both justifications.) Personal property falls within the zone of privacy, which can be defended on the basis of the principle of autonomy, but neither autonomy nor privacy is absolute. However, as prima facie binding they establish presumptions against interventions that infringe them. Thus, both the examination and the removal of personal property, without Mrs. Hollinger's consent, require justification, along the lines indicated by the process sketched above. In particular, it is important to determine whether there are alternative ways to protect other vulnerable residents without infringing Mrs. Hollinger's autonomy, privacy, and liberty by examining and removing her personal property without her consent. (The case report is not clear about whether the regulations that govern what may be kept in a resident's room are only institutionally developed or also governmentally imposed, but the demands of justification apply to both sources of regulations.)

Among the various infringements of autonomy, there is the staff's threat to put Mrs. Hollinger with the "feeders" in a separate dining room if she continued to be late for breakfast. This coercive threat engendered great stress on her part. Even though she could still make some choices in this context, her range of choices was so limited and the alternatives were so dismal that she was under great stress and had trouble sleeping. Attempts at persuasion and even positive inducement to eat breakfast with the other residents would not have been illegitimate in this case, but it is far from clear that the staff had adequate reasons, despite the appeal to governmental regulations, to justify a coercive threat in this case.

ETHICS, POLITICS, AND GOVERNMENTAL REGULATION

As Aristotle and others have noted, ethics and politics are inseparably connected. Politics may be internal to the institution of the nursing homes or external to it (for example, through the larger community's interest in what happens in long-term care). It is now necessary to consider the adequacy of the final justification offered by the nursing home staff for the refusal to acquiesce to Mrs. Hollinger's and her son's request that she be exempted from the requirement to take breakfast in view of her dislike for breakfast and the distress the situation is causing her. This justification identifies federal regulations as the culprit in restricting the discretion of nursing homes to provide individualized care that could meet Mrs. Hollinger's needs and wishes.

Although these federal regulations determine much of the context of health care, it is difficult to view them in this case as any more than a rationalization—even a form of "bad faith"—for the nursing home's conduct. As this case is presented, the nursing home personnel appear to have other reasons for their refusal to accede to Mrs. Hollinger's requests. Despite the various proffered reasons—concern for Mrs. Hollinger, concern for other residents, institutional needs, and governmental regulations—it is tempting to view the real reason as an effort to control the independence and individuality of Mrs. Hollinger, who is viewed as a somewhat difficult resident because of several previous "battles."

What about the regulations themselves? First of all, federal and state regulations are needed to ensure the protection of residents of nursing homes, who are often weak and vulnerable and unable to assert their rights. What Robert Dahl (1970) notes about government also applies to rules and procedures in nursing homes: "It seems wiser to design a government on the assumption that people will not always be virtuous and at times surely will be tempted to do evil, yet where they will not lack for the incentive and the opportunities to act according to their highest potential" (p. 137).

It is also appropriate that nursing home regulations encompass matters that become the source of concern and distress for Mrs. Hollinger: (1) what residents may keep in their rooms and (2) the frequency of meals for residents. Such regulations may strike an uneasy balance between generality (e.g., safety and adequate nutrition) and specificity (e.g., a detailed list of what may not be permitted in residents' rooms and the number of hours between served meals). Insofar as they tend in the latter direction, as they often do for reasons of clarity and enforceability, they may not permit as much latitude or discretion as would be appropriate to provide individualized care, in accord with residents' needs and preferences.

However, in at least one instance, and perhaps others, the nursing home chose a stringent rather than a lenient interpretation of the regulations. The regulation that no more than 14 hours elapse between a "substantial evening meal" and the first meal the next day could be interpreted to establish an option right or a mandatory right on the part of nursing home residents. This distinction, as drawn by Joel Feinberg (1978), affects what the rights-holder can do with his or her rights. An example of a mandatory right is the right to education, which also imposes a duty to obtain an education at least up to a certain level.

At a minimum the federal regulation regarding the time between meals establishes the institution's obligation to *provide* meals at those intervals, but it would be surprising if the regulation also required that residents accept or receive all meals. And yet that is how the nursing home interpreted the regulation. The logic of this interpretation would even require force-feeding of resistant autonomous residents, not only to protect their life and health. The implausibility of such an interpretation is another reason to suspect that the institution is displaying bad faith in its conflict with Mrs. Hollinger.

If the regulation is as strict as the nursing home suggests, then political efforts should be undertaken to create a more satisfactory balance among the principles of autonomy, beneficence, nonmaleficence, and justice (Beauchamp & Childress, 1983). One way to achieve such a balance is to include autonomy-based exceptions in the formulation of rules intended to express the last three principles (e.g., the requirement of the provision of food at certain intervals). If the regulation is strictly construed and cannot be altered, however, then selective noncompliance would be justified in order to respect residents' wishes and needs.

If the nursing home follows the plausible interpretation of the regulation as imposing an obligation to provide food at set intervals but not the obligation to force residents to eat, then it will probably need to establish procedures to let residents exercise their option right to refuse to eat at times. For example, the nursing home might require Mrs. Hollinger and her son to sign a statement of their wishes in this matter, rather than awakening her each morning to determine her wishes for that day. Another possibility is to test her regularly (e.g., by weighing her) to make sure that her weight is remaining adequate. At any rate, the moral pressure to find alternatives to protect Mrs. Hollinger, short of infringing her autonomy, stems from the logic of the prima facie principle of respect for autonomy.

REFERENCES

Ambrogi, D.M. & Leonard, F. (1988). The impact of nursing home admission agreements on resident autonomy. *The Gerontologist, 28* Suppl., 82–89.

Beauchamp, T.L. & Childress, J.F. (1983). *Principles of biomedical ethics* (2nd ed.). New York: Oxford University Press.

Benjamin, M. (in press). *Splitting the difference: Integrity - preserving compromise in ethics and politics.* University Press of Kansas.

Childress, J.F. (1984). Ensuring care, respect, and fairness for the elderly. *Hastings Center Report, 14,* 27–31.

Childress, J.F. (1982). *Who should decide? Paternalism in health care.* New York: Oxford University Press.

Dahl, R. (1970). *After the revolution? Authority in a good society.* New Haven, CT: Yale University Press.

Dworkin, G. (1976). Autonomy and behavior control. *Hastings Center Report, 6,* 23–25.

Feinberg, J. (1978). Voluntary euthanasia and the inalienable right to life. *Philosophy and public affairs*, 93–123.

Jameton, A. (1988). In the borderlands of autonomy: Responsibility in long term care facilities. *The Gerontologist, 28* (Suppl.), 18–23.

Miller, B. (1981). Autonomy and the refusal of life-saving treatment. *Hastings Center Report, 11*, 22–28.

Moody, H.R. (1988). From informed consent to negotiated consent. *The Gerontologist, 28,* (Suppl.), 64–70.

Niebuhr, H.R. (1963). *The responsible self.* New York: Harper and Row.

FOR FURTHER DISCUSSION: EDITORS' QUESTIONS

1. What values and whose interests should be advanced by regulations?
2. At whom should the regulations be aimed—the most vulnerable and needy residents and the most unscrupulous nursing homes, or the average resident and nursing home?
3. What rights do residents have regarding regulations that affect their lives? If, perhaps, a regulation is needed—say, to ensure that food will be served at reasonable intervals—is the resident required to appear to eat it?
4. Can a resident refuse a regulation? Which sort might be refused?
5. Is the regulation about the sherry and shoe polish of a different sort than the one about breakfast?
6. In Mrs. Hollinger's case, should she have been required to get up for breakfast regardless of her preference? Is it a reasonable expectation that residents make themselves available for the morning routines?
7. Is the government justified in regulating the lapsed time between meals?
8. Does the facility comply with the regulation by having a meal available, or are residents also required to eat it?
9. Is the intent of the regulation distorted by facilities that have the last meal so early?
10. If the facility's obligation stops at having a meal available and offering it to the residents, how much effort is needed to complete the offer? For example, must Mrs. Hollinger be awakened to receive the offer?

Chapter 8

INTIMATE STRANGERS:
Roommates in Nursing Homes

THE MANY ROOMMATES
OF MRS. ANDERSON

During the 3 months since Mrs. Anderson, age 91, was admitted from her home to the nursing home building of Happy Manor, a multilevel facility for the elderly, she has had four roommates. She wanted a private room from the outset so that she could do as she pleased, but none was available. Although eventually she will spend down to Medicaid, she can now afford the private room and is on a waiting list.

Since "they are going to give me roommates," Mrs. Anderson would prefer "a quiet one." Her first roommate sang all night. She continually poked into Mrs. Anderson's things and once opened up and sampled a box of chocolates that had been left as a surprise on Mrs. Anderson's bed. She went into the hospital one night, and "I think she died." The next woman seemed pretty nice. She was in for only 3 weeks and then went home. Her last roommate, Mrs. Watson, was the worst. She had "lost her mind, poor soul. She left the bathroom door open when she was using it, and she never flushed. She threw my clothes all over the floor."

Mrs. Anderson complained to the staff, and after a month Mrs. Watson was moved to a single room that became available. Mrs. Anderson's current roommate is better. She seems a little confused, but mostly she sits and looks out the window.

THE CHALLENGE OF ALLOCATION

Happy Manor has 110 beds and only 15 single rooms. The social worker is responsible for allocating rooms and roommates, taking into account such factors as disability levels (people must be located in the areas with staffing levels that meet their needs) and payment source (only 10 beds are certified for Medicare recipients, and neither Medicare or Medicaid will reimburse for a single room unless a medical need is established). A single room can be justified on medical grounds for someone who is dying or perhaps for someone very difficult to live with, such as Mrs. Watson. Nevertheless, the social worker tries her best to match people well and to handle problems creatively. Once, for example, she put a noisy person in with a deaf person.

MOVING A RESIDENT IN A VEGETATIVE CONDITION

But the social worker does not like to move people around like dominoes. She recalls Bessie, a regressed, almost vegetative resident who the nurses thought should be moved down the hall to where they could watch her better. This also gave Bessie's roommate a chance for normal companionship. After the room change, Bessie assumed a fetal position and stopped responding at all. The social worker felt guilty every time she saw Bessie. "Just because she couldn't tell us her feelings, it doesn't mean her room wasn't important to her, does it? It was her room longest, and she lived here too. It probably wasn't fair to move her."

A SINGLE FOR MR. PETERSON TO DIE IN

On the other hand, the social worker was proud of a recent room decision: Mr. Peterson, "a very independent gentleman of 72," had been living in the independent apartments and, in fact, had a woman friend who lived on the floor below. He suddenly became ill, was diagnosed with a virulent form of cancer, and was told he had only months to live. It was apparent to the social worker, to Mr. Peterson's daughter, and even to Mr. Peterson himself that he rapidly would need the additional care available in the nursing home. Mr. Peterson refused to be admitted except to a single room where he could enjoy his privacy and continue his relationship with his woman friend. Considering his limited prognosis and his special circumstances, the social worker arranged for him to move into the next available private room, where he lived until his death 6 weeks later. The social worker felt pleased that she could "individualize" Mr. Peterson's care and that she had recognized the sexual needs of an elderly dying man. "It feels good to be able to do the right thing sometimes." The social worker acknowledged the existence of a waiting list for transfers to single rooms (in fact, Mrs. Anderson was on that list) but said that nobody had been complaining particularly. Assessing the whole waiting list would have been impractical, and Mr. Peterson had a very good case for a single room.

CASE COMMENTARY

Accommodating Room and Roommate Preferences

Steven H. Miles and Greg A. Sachs

Although conflicts about assignment of rooms and roommates arise in colleges and hospitals, those in nursing homes present especially poignant difficulties. The vignettes given above are familiar to those who know daily life in nursing homes. Underlying the difficult accommodation of room and roommate preferences in nursing homes is the essential fact that, amid the communal and regimented life in nursing homes, private personal space is both vitally important and hard to come by. The supply of private rooms is inadequate to the preference for them; bedrooms must often be shared.

The heterogeneity of the nursing home residents complicates the allocation of private rooms and assignment of roommates. Residents differ in their illnesses, disabilities, cognitive function, financial resources, marital status, expected length of stay, ability to express preferences, and needs for caretaking, special architectural modifications, or behavioral control. Some differences merit a "communitarian" allocation of rooms, in which rooms are assigned to serve communal purposes that override the importance of individual preferences. For example, residents who are infectious may need to be isolated in a highly desired private room to protect other residents. Allocating rooms for communitarian purposes diminishes opportunities for resident autonomy in room and roommate selection. Policies for allocating rooms and accommodating roommate preferences must take account of both the heterogeneity of residents and communitarian needs even as they maximize opportunities for resident autonomy.

PERSONAL SPACE

The concept of personal space has been a difficult subject in psychological research for 20 years (Hayduk, 1983; Mishra, 1983). Despite the absence of studies done directly in nursing homes, this research sheds some light on the importance of room and roommate allocation. Hall's (1966) pioneering work described four interpersonal distance zones: an intimate zone (0-1.5 feet), a personal zone (1.5-4.0 feet), a social zone (4-12 feet), and a public zone (12-25 feet). These zones are important for communication and to prevent a feeling of being violated or threatened. If desired, having someone within one's intimate space can be pleasurable, as in making love. If undesired, the same proximity results in anger, bewilderment, or the urge to flee (Hall, 1966). Others have found that prisoners who desire a large interpersonal distance are more often involved in fights with other inmates (Walkley & Gilmour, 1984). Long (1984) found that college students prefer a larger interpersonal distance in stressful situations. Perhaps more directly applicable to nursing homes was Cooper's (1984) finding that chronically institutionalized nonverbal patients with a heightened sense of vulnerability tried to control a larger space around their bodies. She concluded that such clients need to be allowed "individual control and enjoyment of personal possessions and private living space" (p. 5).

The possibility for controlling personal space in a nursing home is limited. Nursing homes are largely communal spaces. Dining rooms, dayrooms, activity rooms, and often bathrooms are spaces that are shared by many residents. These communal spaces are crowded; residents often must tolerate other residents entering their personal and even intimate spaces. Even trips outside the facility are group activities. The regimented timing and conduct of many of the activities in communal spaces, including eating and recreation, heightens the loss of autonomy as creative self-expression.

In this setting, residents' rooms are the last frontier of privacy. The room is the one place that residents can "own" and personalize with their belongings. The room is where residents can attempt to define a personal space and establish interpersonal boundaries to be respected by others. Such privacy or space is not equivalent to autonomy. Rather, room and roommate selection is an important area where self-expression (the end result of autonomy) can be realized. Thus, nursing home staff should respect, as much as possible, the personal space and boundaries that residents establish in their rooms. As a corollary, room allocation and roommate assignments should accommodate residents' preferences to as great a degree as possible.

SCARCITY

Opportunities for choosing a nursing home room or a roommate, let alone being able to define and defend a personal space, are severely limited. Happy Manor, with 110 residents and only 15 single bed rooms, is typical. Assuming that more than a handful of residents desire or require private rooms, it is clear that there is a shortage of single rooms. Even in a facility where all but 30 of the 188 residents live in private rooms, there are still numerous complaints and requests for single rooms (Carol Peck, personal communication to GS, June 11, 1988). Though single rooms are the focus of the allocation problem, the accommodation of roommate preferences is an important similar concern.

Winslow's (1982) analysis of the ethics of allocation and scarcity is helpful in addressing this issue. Regarding the allocation of life-sustaining treatment, "scarcity" includes the following: (1) a shortage of a resource that is desired by many people, (2) a shortage that is obvious and expected to continue, and (3) a resource that cannot be divided and still retain its value. "Dire scarcity" is present if a misallocation of a scarce resource harms people; otherwise, scarcity is said to be relative to the preference. Single rooms are scarce in that they are desired, in short supply, and indivisible. In some instances, the scarcity of single rooms is dire because failing to allocate a single room to an infectious or assaultive person can result in harm to other persons. Thus, an ethic of scarcity for room and roommate policies in nursing homes allows weighing of communitarian needs and resident preferences.

HETEROGENEITY

Understanding which differences between nursing home residents bear on the allocation of rooms is important. First, certain medical conditions justify a priority for a private room. Having an infectious illness, like newly diagnosed tuberculosis, or being assaultive or disruptive, like Mrs. Watson in the case, are justified reasons for giving priority. (As discussed above, those are examples of assigning rooms to meet communitarian needs.) Residents who are near death, like Mr. Peterson, may also be preferentially allocated a private room according to the social deference to the privacy claim of dying residents and their families or to shelter roommates from having another person (usually a stranger) die within their social interpersonal distance zone.

Second, our society highly honors the institution of marriage and endeavors to support it in many ways. It would be an urgent priority to unite married couples. Other close relationships should also be given preference in allocation according to the priority given to any autonomous wishes.

Third, permanent nursing home residents have a greater priority of preference for rooms or roommates than do short-term residents. In most facilities it is possible to distinguish two groups: short-stayers (admitted for rehabilitation, convalescence, terminal care, or caregiver respite) and chronically disabled long-stayers, who stay longer than 6 months. The nursing home is *home* for long-stayers, not an intermediate institution, as it is for the short-stayers (Kane & Kane, 1987). Thus, long-stayers' claims for single rooms and particular roommates as a part of "homemaking" carry greater weight than the claims of short-stayers. The short-stayers' prospect of return to the freedom and personal space of their own homes means that infringement of their autonomy is less grave than infringement of the privacy and personal space of permanent nursing home residents.

Finally, the financial resources of nursing home residents may play a role in the allocation of rooms. Although many permanent residents eventually depend on public aid for their care, diversity of wealth is seen in nursing home residents. This is particularly true early in a resident's stay, before personal assets are "spent down." Though an egalitarian view might hold that wealth should not play a role in room allocation, equal access to equal-quality housing is not a right that our society recognizes. People who have more money can and do purchase more spacious or better appointed houses. In the absence of dire scarcity, wealthier long-term residents may be allowed to have priority for the costlier single rooms. Nevertheless, given that nursing home residents are in some way a captive population, the relative surcharge for private rooms should not be determined by demand but by a fair estimate of the modest incremental cost to the nursing home of servicing a private room.

PRINCIPLES FOR ALLOCATING ROOMS AND ROOMMATES

Two principles for room and roommate allocation emerge from the foregoing discussion: autonomy and communitarian priorities. Respect for autonomy as creative self-agency means that residents should be given an opportunity to express their values and preferences about rooms or room-mates. As residents become more dependent on caregivers and even lose some of their mental abilities, respect for autonomy can be difficult. The concept that decision-making capacity is *task-specific* reminds us that persons who are unable to reflect on or manage health care decisions or personal finances may still retain strong preferences about rooms, room-mates, or personal space. These preferences should be honored. Because of the intimate immediacy of room and roommate preferences, preferences that are not directly and contemporaneously expressed by a resident (those derived from advance directives or the substituted judgment by proxies, for example) do not have the same weight as contemporaneously expressed wishes. Thus, claims made by a family on behalf of a severely demented relative who cannot express or hold a current preference should give way to the contemporaneously expressed preferences of other residents contending for the same room or roommate.

The communitarian use of rooms refers to the assignment of rooms and roommates for purposes that originate outside the resident's preferences. Respect for patient autonomy means that communitarian allocation applies *only* in situations of dire scarcity, where a compelling interest in avoiding harm is present. Communitarian allocation accords priority for single rooms to infectious, assaultive, or dying residents and to double rooms for married couples.

In the absence of dire scarcity, resident preferences must be accommodated. Thus, the decision by the Happy Manor social worker to pair a noisy, confused resident with a deaf individual is inappropriate if the deaf resident was not given an opportunity to ratify this arrangement. The social worker treated the hearing-impaired resident as if she were incapable of preferences. Another inappropriate communitarian use of rooms or roommates is allocation as a reward for good behavior, as punishment for bad behavior, or to promote nursing convenience in a manner that does not serve essential communal ends. If resident preferences are not solicited and serious harms are not at issue, then communitarian allocation of roommates or rooms is simply manipulation, which arbitrarily subordinates resident autonomy.

Waiting lists and lotteries are two ways to decide allocation issues when residents with claims to the same resource cannot reach agreement on their own. Queuing, with entry to the waiting list on expression of a preference rather than by duration of residency, seems a reasonable basis for nursing home room allocation. It is orderly and avoids the periodic commotion of a lottery. Queuing allows residents to develop reasonable expectations as to when a room or roommate request might be granted.

IMPLEMENTING A ROOM AND ROOMMATE POLICY

Explicit room and roommate policies offer several advantages over ad hoc allocation. They should help convince residents of the fairness of decisions and lessen complaints. By promoting autonomy and a sense of personal empowerment, they may ameliorate the disabling phenomenon of learned dependence. Table 8-1 outlines a room and roommate policy that balances autonomy and communitarian needs.

Residents and family members should be informed of the room and roommate allocation policy at the time of admission to the facility. The staff member who implements the policy should be identified and accessible to residents. Appeals of unfavorable room assignments might be considered by a residents' committee empowered to make nonbinding recommendations to an ombudsman. Publicizing the allocation principles need not entail publicizing individual residents' characteristics. Room changes that involve dislocating residents like Bessie, who are aware of their surroundings but incapable of articulating a preference, should be minimized in light of recent data suggesting that transfer shock can cause increased morbidity and mortality to this subset of nursing home residents (Pruchno & Resch, 1988).

It would be easier to appreciate the importance of individual preferences in the roommate situation if all administrators and staff tried to put themselves in the place of a nursing home resident. Imagine how

TABLE 8-1

Room and Roommate Policy in Long-Term Care

	Single-bed rooms	Roommate
Dire scarcity (communitarian priorities)	Preventing injury, infection control, assaultive residents, dying residents	Married persons
Relative scarcity (autonomy)	Resident preference waiting list Long stay, able to pay Long stay, unable to pay Short stay, able to pay Short stay, unable to pay	Resident preference waiting list[a] Long stay, able to pay Long stay, unable to pay Short stay, able to pay Short stay, unable to pay

[a] Greatest priority for allocation goes in order of highest to lowest from top to bottom within each column. The place on the waiting list is established by the time at which a specific room or roommate request is made, not simply by duration of residence in the nursing home.

much more difficult it would be if one could not even choose or define one's bedroom, perhaps being placed with someone whose particular idiosyncrasies were offensive. Room and roommate assignment is one area where residents' preferences can and should be respected.

REFERENCES

Cooper, K. H. (1984). Territorial behavior among the institutionalized: A nursing perspective. *Journal of Psychosocial Nursing and Mental Health Services, 22*, 6–11.

Hall, E. T. (1966). *The hidden dimension.* New York: Doubleday.

Hayduk, L. A. (1983). Personal space: Where we now stand. *Psychological Bulletin, 94*, 293–335.

Kane, R. A. & Kane, R. L. (1987). *Long term care: Principles, programs, and policies.* New York: Springer Publishing Co.

Long, G. T. (1984). Psychological tension and closeness to others: Stress and interpersonal distance preference. *Journal of Psychology, 117*, 143–146.

Mishra, P. K. (1983). Proxemics: Theory and research. *Perspectives in Psychological Researches, 6*, 10–15.

Pruchno, R. A. & Resch, N. L. (1988). Intrainstitutional relocation: Mortality effects. *The Gerontologist, 28*, 311–317.

Walkley, F. H. & Gilmour, D. R. (1984). The relationship between interpersonal distance and violence in imprisoned offenders. *Criminal Justice and Behavior, 11*, 331–340.

Winslow, G. R. (1982). *Triage and justice: The ethics of rationing life-saving medical resources.* Berkeley and Los Angeles: University of California Press.

FOR FURTHER DISCUSSION: EDITORS' QUESTIONS

1. What values should guide the allocation of single rooms in Happy Manor? What values should guide assignment of roommates and response to complaints?
2. In assigning rooms, what priorities from the viewpoint of staff, administration, residents, and family should be given to safety, benefit to residents, merit, seniority, medical needs, psychological needs, ability to pay, age, marital status, handicapping condition,

quality of life, compliance with the rules of the facility, lobbying power of the family, virtuousness of the resident?

3. What arguments could be launched for and against length of occupancy as a relevant factor in deciding who should move if roommates request a change.

4. What ethical considerations are raised by the specific cases: Mrs. Anderson's experience with her roommates as she waits for a single room? Mrs. Watson's transfer to a single room because she was disturbing to live with? Bessie's relocation for the sake of her roommate and more convenient nursing? Mr. Peterson's assignment to a single room despite others ahead on the waiting list? How can the claims and interests of all of these people be appropriately reconciled? Does Mr. Peterson's wish for privacy for a sexual relationship exert a higher claim than Mrs. Anderson's general wish for privacy and relief from undesirable roommates?

5. What *procedures* should be followed in making such allocation decisions? Who should be involved? What are residents rights to refuse? What procedures for appeal should exist?

6. Does an obligation exist to "mainstream" mentally intact with cognitively or emotionally impaired residents? Or does an obligation exist to protect cognitively intact residents from the burdens of intimate and frequent association with the demented? What is the foundation of any duties to mainstream or protect from mainstreaming? Are the duties in a nursing home setting different from other settings—for example, hospitals, schools, or ordinary community settings?

7. How legitimate is speculative consideration about the meaning of Bessie's room to her, given that Bessie is so cognitively and physically limited?

8. Is privacy necessary for autonomy? Can a moral argument be constructed for or against having double rooms predominate in nursing homes?

9. Explore the claim that a private room to die in is justified on communitarian grounds. Would this claim be justified if it meant that *all* private rooms were reserved for dying in, leaving none left to live in? How close to death must a resident be to claim this privilege of privacy?

Chapter 9

TILL DEATH US DO PART:
Married Life in Nursing Homes

THE COUPLE

Mr. and Mrs. Stanley have been married for 60 years. Mr. Stanley was admitted to the Faraway Center with symptoms of congestive heart failure. Mrs. Stanley is herself not very well. Given her multiple ailments, the difficulty she has in keeping up the household, and her desire to be near her husband, she began considering entering the Faraway Center as a minimal-care patient. Mrs. Stanley's plans were accelerated when she broke her hip a few months later. After 2 days in the hospital, she entered Faraway Center.

Mrs. Stanley's room was on the first floor and Mr. Stanley's in a male-only section on the second floor. No rooms suitable for couples were immediately available. Mr. Stanley developed a pattern of visiting Mrs. Stanley in her room for most of the day while she was still in a cast. They spent the time talking together. Sometimes they held hands, and in the evenings they would sit together on Mrs. Stanley's bed watching television.

After a few days of this, Mrs. Stanley's roommate, Alice, complained to the nurse about men visiting in the room. In fact, Alice preferred that

Mr. Stanley not visit at all and absolutely objected to his presence in the evenings. An arrangement was ultimately negotiated that allowed Mr. Stanley to visit Mrs. Stanley between 3 and 5 P.M. each day, a time when Alice often had her own visitors. Nobody was satisfied with the arrangement, but Mrs. Stanley thought she could put up with it until a room was available for her to share with her husband.

THE ROOM

The best room in Faraway Manor was a large corner double room that had its own bath. (All of the other rooms shared a bath with the adjoining room.) Phyllis Partridge, a retired schoolteacher, had lived in that room for 3 years with her sister, Alma Partridge. About 4 months after Mrs. Stanley was admitted, Alma Partridge died after a brief illness.

The staff thought that the room would be ideal for the Stanleys because of its location and its bathroom. But Phyllis Partridge had a different opinion. This room was her home, the home she had shared with her sister for 3 years. Moreover, during the last weeks of Alma's life, the Partridge sisters, and Mrs. Mayne, a bridge-playing friend, discussed Mrs. Mayne's moving into the room. The idea that her sister would be with a friend gave Alma comfort in her last weeks. Phyllis Partridge was outraged that the staff could be so insensitive as to discuss this with her only two days after she returned from Alma's funeral. The social worker apologized and tried to explain the severity of the Stanleys' predicament. Furthermore, a lot of room juggling would be necessary to allow Mrs. Mayne to move in with Phyllis and still find a double room for the Stanleys. The easiest thing would be to move Phyllis to Mrs. Stanley's place. This outraged Phyllis even more. She thought that Alice was "prissy" and "a pain" and didn't want to live with her in *any* room.

When it seemed as though the staff might make Phyllis move in spite of her objections, Phyllis called the ombudsman office. She said that she sympathized with the Stanleys—Mrs. Stanley was a nice lady and deserved to be with her husband and away from that wretched Alice— but Phyllis didn't think it was fair for *her* to be moved out of her own room after so many years. She also didn't see why the married couple automatically deserved the best room in Faraway. There were double rooms that shared a bath and where the view was less spectacular. When Phyllis and Alma first moved to Faraway, they had to wait a year before they got the corner room. She asked the ombudsman to intervene on her behalf.

CASE COMMENTARY

Rosemarie Tong

When a person enters a nursing home, he or she generally does so reluctantly. Leaving behind many worldly possessions, the incoming resident may feel like a displaced person. One's space is limited to a room, perhaps half a room; one's time is regulated by the group's needs and/or by the staff's convenience; and one's identity is tied to a few memorabilia and to the visitors who drop by more or less frequently.

Given these constrictions, it is not surprising that nursing home residents are often preoccupied with the size, location, and ambience of their rooms and with the personality, habits, and guests of their roommates. Because many nursing homes were built before health care professionals identified and acknowledged the environmental needs of long-term nursing home residents, and because private or semiprivate rooms are high-cost items in the current pricing structure, fully adequate rooms are a scarce commodity. Whereas the ideal nursing home would probably cluster four or five single rooms, each with a private bathroom, around some sort of common room, the reality is a row of doubles, triples, and/or quadruples, with shared bathrooms, strung down a long corridor. Similarly, whereas the ideal nursing home would group people together according to compatibility and/or levels of personal intimacy, the reality is a system that tends to sort people out according to ailment, making for more than a few "odd couples."

Of course, people do not always enter a nursing home alone. Husbands and wives, siblings, and close friends sometimes enter a home together or at intervals, as in the case of the Stanleys. The expectation of such couples is that they will be able to maintain their relationship. Although some nursing homes are able to meet immediately the expectations of couples who wish to live in the same room, many are not. Depending on the level of care they require, even husbands and wives may be required to live apart from one another for several months or more.

The case of the Stanleys, Phyllis Partridge, Alice and Mrs. Mayne is complex. Our intuitions conflict. Obviously, it is a real hardship for Mr. and Mrs. Stanley to be separated from each other. After 60 years of marriage their identities are so intertwined that any separation, however short, is experienced as a cruel cleavage. Their time together should not be reduced to a daily 2-hour visit with no privacy. The fact that the Stanleys agreed to this arrangement, as temporarily necessary, does not justify its prolongation.

But even if it is unfair to restrict the Stanleys' time together, it seems no more fair to impose the Stanleys on Alice all day long. Despite Alice's unappealing personality—no one seems to want her as a roommate, a problem in and of itself—she does deserve some space and time that is not filled with the Stanleys. Likewise, despite the fact that Phyllis's desire to have both the best room at Faraway Center[1] *and* a congenial roommate may strike some of us as asking for too much, it seems callous to deprive Phyllis of both her room and the possibility of living with a friend. Although Phyllis and her deceased sister Alma lacked the authority to promise Alma's bed to Mrs. Mayne, we can sympathize with their desire to make their living arrangements as homelike as possible. Alma died with the thought that Phyllis would not be entirely alone, and Phyllis more easily accepted Alma's death because of the same consoling thought.

Clearly, someone is going to have to move somewhere if the Stanleys are ever to share the same room. On first inspection, the staff's solution to the plight of the Stanleys seems self-interested because it is articulated in terms of its ease and convenience. Simply move Phyllis out of her room and the Stanleys into it; any other solution requires too much effort. On closer inspection, however, the staff's solution may be motivated by something other than their own convenience. Alternative resolutions to the Stanleys' plight may require the staff to dislodge many persons rather than one person—in this case Phyllis—from their rooms.

But, we may ask, why should anyone be forced out of his or her own room so that the Stanleys can be together? William May (1982) reminds us that rooms in nursing homes are not like ordinary bedrooms: Ordinarily, people live in a number of different environments—home, workplace, streets, parks, gardens, and sidewalks. The bedroom is only part of a total world, often a sanctuary from it. But for the immobile or the impaired the world shrinks to a single room (p. 34). To be sure, some nursing home residents will be less possessive about their rooms than others, but they all have a right to some personal space.

Nursing home rooms, especially those of long-term residents, should not be regarded as hospital rooms. The common good of hospital patients is served, for example, by moving them as quickly as possible in and out of a limited number of intensive care rooms, but the common good of nursing home residents is not served by moving them in and out of the rooms they

---

[1] William May (1982 has observed that the medievals "identified avarice as the chief besetting sin of the aged." May comments:

> The closer one gets to the final disposition of death, the more fiercely one may be inclined to clutch at possessions, holding, grasping, managing, manipulating. Avarice has always been the sin of the hands. It strikes those are most insecure and least mobile except for the reach of the hands. (p. 36)

regard as their own. Moving is always a disruptive experience; it is virtually intolerable when the person making the move has not made the decision to change locations. If a nursing home room is comparable to any other kind of room, it is to a residential hotel room. To be sure, this comparison is not exact. Whereas a hotel manager is not at liberty to move hotel residents out of the rooms they have chosen as their own, a nursing home director may move residents out of their chosen rooms and into others *if* this is the least disruptive way to serve the common good.

The claim that Phyllis and everyone else at Faraway Center has a right to some private space and time is rooted in the right each person has "to withhold information or experience of oneself from others" (Richards, 1977). Ordinarily, this right is invoked when a person is subjected to illegal searches and seizures, when a person's life story is entered into a data bank, or when a person's private life is made excessively public by the media. This right is also operative in the case at hand. Nursing home residents are not in the prime of their lives. They suffer from a variety of physical ailments and mental impairments. Understandably, they do not always wish to expose their bodies to just anyone, nor do they always wish to see, smell, hear, taste, and touch other people's bodies. Likewise, they do not always wish to share their thoughts with any and all comers; nor do they always wish to hear the confessions, complaints, and criticism of people for whom they feel little affinity. The fact that Phyllis does not like Alice is not insignificant. Ordinarily, adults who do not like each other are not forced to share bedrooms and bathrooms for extended periods of time. To be sure, there are exceptions. Prisoners and soldiers have no choice about their roommates, but this is a matter of punishment or discipline. Since the aged—and for that matter, the diseased and/or impoverished—have neither committed a crime nor signed up for a tour of duty, they have a right to exercise some control over their physical and psychological environment.

Of course, Phyllis is not the only person who has rights in this case. The Stanleys not only have the same rights as Phyllis has, they also have additional rights because they are married. It is not the state of matrimony per se that ought to be privileged, however; rather, it is the love relationship it implies. In order to be full human beings, people have the right to establish and maintain love relationships. But such relationships are not the exclusive prerogatives of married heterosexual couples. Unmarried heterosexual couples, homosexual couples, and lesbian couples are not strangers to love relationships. In addition, parents and children, siblings, and close friends can also form love relationships. In general what distinguishes these familial and friendly love relationships from those that couples have is the lack of a strong sexual component, which is not to say that they lack a physical dimension.

In the course of doing research for this analysis, I read a report on social policy and everyday life in nursing homes. The report narrated the story of Claudia, aged 66, and her mother, Maria, aged 88, who were both residents of the same nursing home though on different floors. This mother and daughter duo were forbidden to visit each other at night because Claudia and her mother frequently cuddled each other in bed. Dismayed by this "lesbian" activity, the staff refused to permit it (Diamond, 1988). Not only is the staff's reaction to Claudia and Maria homophobic, it is also symptomatic of an apparent inability to appreciate the human need for physical as well as psychological intimacy. Physical expressions of intimacy range from cheek pecking to hand squeezing to shoulder rubbing to foreplay to sexual intercourse. For people who have relatively few opportunities for sensual satisfaction and who have a great deal of affection for each other, cuddling is a good way to derive solace, comfort, and pleasure.

Although the U.S. Supreme Court had been moving to expand the right of sexual privacy for purposes of procreation to include all sorts of physical intimacy—indeed, any significant relationship that love makes possible—movement in this direction has apparently ceased. As the court moved from *Griswold v. Connecticut* (1965) to *Roe v. Wade* (1973), it came to the position that whether adults are married or single and whether they wish to procreate or to remain childless, they have the right to engage in sexual relations and, presumably, other physical intimacies. More recently, however, the court has taken back what its former logic implied—namely, that the right to sexual privacy belongs to homosexual as well as to heterosexual couples. In June 1986, the court ruled that Georgia's anti-sodomy statutes were constitutional. In response to the argument that according to the Fourteenth Amendment due-process requirements it is unconstitutional to deprive homosexual lovers of the right of sexual freedom that heterosexual lovers have, Justice Byron White responded that there are "rational" state purposes behind this asymmetry—namely, this nation's traditional rejection of homosexuality as taboo and the court's greater historical respect for privacy around reproductive decisions as opposed to privacy around sexual decisions unrelated to begetting and bearing children (Greenhouse, 1986).

My conviction is that the court erred by once again connecting procreation, or at least its *possibility*, with legitimate sexual intercourse and by perpetuating arbitrary moral judgments of the past regarding the acceptability of different types of love and human relationships. Love is a fundamental good. Without love, life loses its sense of direction and purpose, and although loving people can forsake sexual relations (think here of religious celibates) or engage in them strictly for procreative purposes, most people want these relations simply because of the pleasure and intimacy they provide.

According to reigning legal norms as well as the line of reasoning I have adopted, had the Stanleys requested the opportunity for privacy for sexual intercourse, the staff would have been bound to find some way to facilitate this. Either Alice would have had to leave the room or an empty room would have had to be found for the Stanleys. But this is where my concurrence with the court stops. Had a homosexual or lesbian couple, instead of the Stanleys, requested privacy for sexual intercourse, I would have honored their request. Indeed, I would try to honor any request motivated by a love commitment; at minimum, I would take it very seriously in any decision-making deliberation.

Had Phyllis asked to room with Mrs. Mayne on account of deep emotional bonds to her, I would have taken her request as seriously as that of any heterosexual, homosexual, or lesbian couple. As it stands, however, the love issue is clouded in Phyllis's case. We are not certain whether it is Mrs. Mayne or the best room at Faraway Center that is the dominant object of Phyllis's attention. We may even wonder whether Mrs. Mayne is merely a congenial bridge partner for Phyllis. In contrast, for the Stanleys, it is their relationship that is paramount. We sense that they would settle for a room of their own even if it did not have a private bath. Togetherness, more than privacy, seems to be the object of the Stanleys' desire.

Certainly this is a matter for the ombudsman and the Residents' Council (if Faraway Center has one) as well as the staff to resolve. In thinking about the different ways to solve the problem, it is helpful to examine Carol Gilligan's (1982) theory that there are two very distinct methods used to deal with moral problems in human relationships. One approach can be thought of as an ethics of justice and involves evaluating the problem in terms of a hierarchy of rights. The rights of each individual are weighed and tallied, and whoever is seen as having the most rights or the most important rights is deemed the one whose demands are to be fulfilled over those of the others, who have less of a right. In this case, the Stanleys' right to maintain a very long-standing love/sex relationship probably trumps Phyllis's right to keep the best room at Faraway Center and to move in a congenial neighbor, Mrs. Mayne.

The problem with this hierarchy-of-rights approach is that it may inflict unnecessary hardship on Phyllis, and worse, that it may create tension or even enmity between the Stanleys' supporters and Phyllis's supporters. If instead the problem is evaluated through what Gilligan refers to as an ethics of care, extreme conflicts and hard feelings may be avoided. An ethics of care bypasses the hierarchy-of-rights approach in favor of a network-of-relationships approach. It is no longer a matter of looking at each participant in the conflict individually and evaluating his or her rights, separated from the rights of the rest of the people involved.

Instead, the situation as a whole is evaluated, taking not just individual rights but other factors into account. What is sought is a solution, usually much more complex and multifaceted than that which an ethics of justice provides, one that takes each individual's needs into account and tries to satisfy each one as best it can. In this case a solution might involve Alice changing places with Mrs. Mayne. That way Mr. Stanley could move in with Mrs. Stanley, and Mrs. Mayne could move in with Phyllis. Phyllis would have both the room she calls home and a friend to share it; the Stanleys would have a less than fully adequate room, but enough time and space to share their thoughts, feelings, and bodies.

Admittedly, Alice may refuse to move. Indeed, everyone else in the nursing home may refuse to budge on the Stanleys' behalf. Although I like to think better of Faraway Center's residents, should such a deadlock occur after all other alternatives have been exhausted, the staff is morally justified in moving either Alice or Phyllis in order to accommodate the Stanleys. But even if morality permits the staff to handle the immediate crisis situation by asserting their authority of oversight, it does not permit the staff to go on handling such disputes in this fashion. Indeed, the staff, together with the ombudsman and the Residents' Council (if Faraway Center does not have one, it should establish one), are obligated to devise mutually agreeable policies to resolve future conflicts of this type.

Nursing homes are not intentional communities. Residents come with a common need—to be cared for—but they do not come with common ends, aims, or goals. They can transform themselves into something like an intentional community if they are given the opportunity to legislate policies for themselves. Only then will nursing home residents discover their common end, aim, or goal: to make their limited time together and their limited space together as livable as possible for each and every individual. This is a noble purpose and one whose value any age group, but especially the elderly, can appreciate.

REFERENCES

Diamond, T. (1988). Social policy and everyday life in nursing homes: A critical ethnography. *Social Science and Medicine, 23*, 1287–1295.

Gilligan, C. (1982). *In a different voice.* Cambridge, MA: Harvard University Press.

Greenhouse, L. (1986, July 1). High court, 5-4, says states have the right to outlaw private homosexual acts. *The New York Times,* p. 14.

Griswold v. Connecticut, 381 U.S. 479 (1965).

May, W.F. (1982). Who cares for the elderly? *Hastings Center Report, 12,* 36.

Richards, D.A.J. (1977). *The moral criticism of law*. Encino, CA: Dickenson
    Publishing Company.
Roe v. Wade, 410 U.S. 113 (1973).

FOR FURTHER DISCUSSION:
EDITORS' QUESTIONS

1. Was the home correct in its initial arrangements with the Stanleys
    and Mrs. Stanley's roommate, Alice?
2. What rights do married couples have, and should they supersede
    rights to privacy of other residents?
3. If the Stanleys had requested the opportunity for privacy for sex-
    ual relationships, what would the facility's obligation be?
4. Would the obligation differ if this were an unmarried couple? A
    same-sex couple?
5. Could Alice have been fairly asked to leave her own room to allow
    conjugal privacy to her roommate?
6. What rights did Phyllis Partridge have to remain in the room that
    she was enjoying after her sister's death?
7. Were the Partridge sisters overstepping their bounds by making an
    arrangement with Mrs. Mayne to move into the room after Alma's
    death?
8. Should the Partridge sisters have been considered like tenants
    who often have the right of first refusal with their property, or
    should their room have been considered more like a hospital room
    and thus at the staff's disposal?
9. Compare the criteria for room allocation developed in this chap-
    ter to the hierarchy developed by Miles and Sachs in Chapter 8.
    Would the recommendations be the same using both schemes?

Chapter 10

THOUGHT FOR FOOD:
Nursing Home Meals

MRS. FRANK'S PREDICAMENT

Mrs. Frank's physical condition makes her an unsavory table companion. She eats with effort, frequently drooling, spitting, and making unpleasant sounds. She is also a well-educated, mentally intact woman who states that she enjoys the conversation that accompanies food and looks forward to each mealtime as a diversion from a dull routine. (She does not contribute much to mealtime conversation, however, partly because of a speech impairment.) And though she tries to be careful, she sometimes inadvertently splatters food on her table companions. Other residents have complained to the social worker. One said, "It turns my stomach to eat with her." Others were politer but made the same point, suggesting that Mrs. Frank should be assigned to first shift in the dining room, with people who need considerable supervision during meals because of their cognitive or physical limitations.

Mrs. Frank objected to this idea. She did not want to be relegated to spending her time with people who have "lost their marbles," and she said that the total lack of sense and decorum at the other sitting is disgusting. One day she looked in and saw that someone was actually throwing food.

She had heard that many residents in that group have regressed to infantile eating habits, smearing their food with their hands. Besides, the more supervised meal is much too early for Mrs. Frank. Always a late diner, she considers 5:30 too early for dinner and certainly objects to starting dinner at 4:30.

STAFF VIEWS

The social worker, who in this facility is responsible for table arrangements, is troubled by this situation. She can see no good solution. Table assignments are one of her least favorite jobs. "After complaints about roommates," she said, "complaints about table places are my next biggest headache." The recent increase in requests for table transfers were mostly attributable to discomfort with being seated near Mrs. Frank. Finally, after much discussion with nursing staff, the care team decided to assign Mrs. Frank to take her meals at the early sitting. Mrs. Frank was told that the change was necessary because of the possibility that she might choke and aspirate her food. The social worker knew this was a fiction but couldn't bring herself to hurt Mrs. Frank even more by telling her that her presence was repugnant to so many other residents.

In discussing the situation, the staff considered that Mrs. Frank might take her meals on a tray in her room. Although Mrs. Frank was not, strictly speaking, a "feeder"—that is, someone needing to be spoon-fed—a minimal amount of supervision was needed for safety. The director of nurses said she could not spare a nurse's aide to watch Mrs. Frank eat.

Besides, as a general policy, the facility tried to discourage residents from taking meals in their rooms unless they were acutely ill. A running debate was already going on between the staff and Mr. Elwin, a gentleman with chronic obstructive pulmonary disease, who said it hurt to walk and that he disliked "trailing along miles of cord" for his oxygen. As Residents' Council chairman and an active member of a regular poker group on his floor, Mr. Elwin stated flatly (using staff jargon), "I get plenty of socialization without having to drag myself to the dining room. Besides I like to eat alone. It's more conducive to my digestion." The staff were reluctant to create a precedent with Mrs. Frank that might interfere with their struggle with Mr. Elwin. The social worker did perceive some irony in the situation: Mrs. Frank liked to socialize at meals and was being discouraged, whereas Mr. Elwin was being discouraged from eating in solitude as he preferred.

CASE COMMENTARY

Something To Chew On

Mary Ellen Waithe

The general perspectives taken with respect to cases like this tend to fall into two camps: concern about people's rights and concern about the financial and other consequences of changing the status quo. Sometimes, if we are willing to question some of our own and others' underlying assumptions about what nursing home residents really want, what's good for them, and how much trouble it would be to make radical changes in the customary ways of doing things in nursing homes, we can find solutions to problems such as those depicted in the case. If we are careful (and also somewhat lucky), the solutions we propose will protect everyone's rights and will also have consequences that are financially and otherwise acceptable to all concerned.

In the latter half of this century moral philosophers, or ethicists, have developed consensus about the nature of individual rights. Nevertheless, this much can be said about the current state of moral theory. There is general agreement that a just society is one that respects individual moral autonomy. A society that is basically just (although it may not be perfect) will permit restrictions on individual liberties only to the extent necessary to permit equal liberty to all and to maintain institutions of justice that protect the liberties of all. That means that you can do whatever you want to do as long as I can do likewise and as long as whatever you do doesn't have the effect of destroying the very system of justice we've set up to govern our interactions. Violating contracts and disobeying institutional rules that we've agreed to abide by would be viewed as ultimately threatening our basic system of justice.

Do the dining preferences of Mrs. Frank and Mr. Elwin represent their autonomous decisions? If so, is the nursing home acting unjustly toward Mrs. Frank and Mr. Elwin if it interferes with their implementation of those decisions? Is the nursing home acting unjustly toward its staff or toward its other clients if it does not so interfere? Or are Mrs. Frank and Mr. Elwin required to abide by the institutional rules concerning meal assignments? I turn first to the issue of autonomy and limit this portion of the discussion to an examination of the autonomy of Mrs. Frank and Mr. Elwin, assuming that questions of autonomy of staff and other clients of the facility arise primarily as questions of justice toward them.

AUTONOMY CONSIDERATIONS

Different people understand autonomy differently. The analysis of autonomy offered by Collopy (1988) is particularly useful because it runs the gamut of prevalent views. Collopy distinguishes six contrasting polarities of autonomy: decisional versus executional, direct versus delegated; competent versus incapacitated, authentic versus inauthentic, immediate versus long-range, and negative versus positive. This array of interpretations represents the array of views about autonomy held by health care providers, courts, moral philosophers, and others who have enunciated them. Because such an array of views exists, it is likely that no one view is wholly adequate to defining the autonomy of Mrs. Frank or Mr. Elwin. In some respect, each of these polarities is relevant to the situation depicted in the preceding case.

Decisional versus Executional

Mrs. Frank and Mr. Elwin may be executionally constrained by their respective physical limitations, yet both appear to be fully autonomous in the decisional sense. The extent to which the executional autonomy of either Mrs. Frank or Mr. Elwin is constrained requires some further analysis. Would Mrs. Frank be better able, with appropriate therapy, to avoid splattering others during meals or to keep the number of incidents to a tolerable few? Does her messiness stem from limited ability or from either a lack of understanding or lack of concern about the way she eats? In this case it appears that the social worker was either unwilling or unable to find a way to direct Mrs. Frank's attention to the real reason she is being requested to change her dining arrangements. If Mrs. Frank is aware of her messiness and its negative effect on her companions' ability to enjoy their meals, is she lacking in appropriate concern for their sensitivities and making no attempt to make mealtimes less unpleasant? If she has the capacity to recognize her behavior, then her messiness ought to be pointed out to her and a determination made as to whether or not she is physically capable of controlling herself. If she cannot control herself and is in some sense handicapped (rather than mentally incompetent), further analysis is required. If Mrs. Frank's executional autonomy is impaired, then an important moral concern would be to protect her from paternalistic intervention or from coercion.

Mr. Elwin's executional autonomy is definitely not impaired. He manages his mobility requirements for events, like poker and Residents' Council, that interest him. His wish to dine alone is a personal preference, not a product of any physical or intellectual impairment or constraint. Requiring him to take his meals in community with other residents cannot be justified solely on grounds that he is either unable to make a decision or unable to execute his decision. In the sense of executional autonomy, he is clearly autonomously doing both.

Direct versus Delegated

A second polarity in the concept of autonomy identified by Collopy is that between direct and delegated autonomy, between the individual who has strong authorial control over choices and actions and the individual who has delegated certain decisions and actions to others who function as surrogates or agents.

The polarity between direct and delegated autonomy is relevant to most competent adults who consider themselves to be the authors of their own actions while clearly recognizing the prudence of delegating authority to a plethora of others who function in a surrogacy or agency capacity. We authorize stockbrokers to make investment decisions; we authorize accountants to consider those transactions and report the profits therefrom to the Internal Revenue Service; and, when necessary, we authorize counsel to devise the best defense when choices our agents made were unfortunate. We assert our autonomy by exercising choice in the selection of our agents. We maintain our autonomy by terminating agency agreements when our surrogates' decisions do not reflect our directives or our intentions or when they appear to have acted incompetently on our behalf. Thus, we effectively retain authorship of our own decisions. Except in cases of surrogate incompetence, fraud, deception, or coercion, we maintain authorship of our surrogates' decisions.

Capacitated versus Incapacitated

In the past two decades much of the discussion concerning autonomy has focused on discussions of competence and incompetence in the context of determining whether paternalistic treatment of others is morally justified. Definitions of competence abound; they have been articulated by the courts, by philosophers, and by psychiatrists. For a bibliography of the legal definitions, see Brooks (1980); for philosophical bibliography, see Waithe (1982a, 1988) and Faden and Beauchamp (1986). Psychiatric definitions are found in DSM-III (American Psychiatric Association, 1980) and Brooks (1974, 1980).

The question of whether Mrs. Frank and Mr. Elwin are competent or incapacitated is not addressed in the vignette. The assumption, there-fore, is that they are competent. Yet the prospect that such questions will be raised in the near future, particularly regarding Mrs. Frank, cannot be ruled out. Consider two possible answers to the question raised earlier regarding whether Mrs. Frank is aware of her messiness. On the one hand, she may be aware of her messiness and may care about the dis-turbing effects of her behavior on her tablemates. However, it may not be within her ability to control herself. If that is the case, we would say that she lacks executional autonomy but is competent.

On the other hand, if Mrs. Frank is unaware of her messiness, then we must ask whether she has or lacks the ability to acknowledge how she behaves. If she lacks the ability to recognize what she is doing, then legitimate questions may be raised regarding her competence, at least regarding this specific, unintentional, perhaps compulsive behavior. A determination of incompetence does not in and of itself provide answers about how we might treat her, however. It merely alerts us to the possi-bility that issues of paternalism might also merit consideration (Waithe 1982a, Sartorius, 1988).

Authentic versus Inauthentic

Based on Dworkin (1976), Collopy describes authentic autonomy as that which ". . . results in choices and behavior that are deeply in character, that flow from past moral career and ethical style, as well as from present values and immediate self-shaping" (p. 14). Nothing in the behavior of Mrs. Frank suggests that her preference for her present dining arrange-ment over dining at an earlier hour with companions who are consider-ably more impaired than she, is inconsistent with her past preferences or with her present values. Indeed, her present self-possession and self-understanding indicate that she has very clearly and correctly identified conditions present in the alternative dining situation that are unaccept-able to her and are inconsistent with her view of who she is and how her life is to be lived in the circumstances in which she now finds herself.

The authenticity of Mr. Elwin's decision is not as immediately apparent but no less certain. Although his decision to dine alone is a relatively recent one and represents a departure from his habitual arrangement and from the institutional norm, his reasons for his decision are clearly con-sistent with what we know of his values and personality. He finds the activity of getting to the dining room to be an unpleasant one, and once there, he finds that community dining experiences provide him with no compelling reason for enduring the arduous, albeit healthy, commute. He simply prefers to pursue some activities of daily living in privacy. Small talk and chatter are for the poker table; serious business gets conducted at Residents' Council. He has his "socializing" nicely compartmentalized and has found his way of achieving a balance of interests and activities.

Immediate versus Long-Range

Collopy's fifth polarity regarding autonomy is between immediate and long-range autonomy. He notes that the tension between immediate and long-range autonomy must be sustained and that immediate freedom should not automatically be restricted for the sake of achieving long-range goals. Tension between the two is most serious if caregivers automatically thwart immediate decisions for the sake of a future good that the resident does not agree is a good worth forgoing immediate freedoms for. Long-range autonomy may be meaningful, therefore, if and only if it is a good that is chosen as a good by an individual or, in the case of a person who is no longer competent to choose, if that long-range good is consistent with the person's moral history as he or she has tended to revise it (Waithe, 1982a). In this latter case, the short-term good can be imposed as an autonomy-preserving good on a nonautonomous person *only* if there is some degree of certainty that forgoing immediate choices is very certain to achieve the long-range good. This imposition on an incompetent person of a long-term, autonomy-preserving good that restricts immediate freedom to pursue short-term or immediate goods is justified paternalism (provided other conditions are also met) (Waithe, 1982a).

Mrs. Frank is not being reassigned in order to facilitate her long-term rehabilitation, although that is the reason she has been given. She is being reassigned out of concern for the sensibilities of others and, presumably, to contribute to *their* well-being. When the social worker deceived Mrs. Frank about the real reason she is being reassigned, Mrs. Frank was denied authorship of the decision and was denied the opportunity to cooperate autonomously in her own daily living activities.

With Mr. Elwin, deception is not practiced. Despite the existence of a "rule" to the contrary, despite possibly legitimate concerns about his long-term interests in physical rehabilitation, and despite staff concerns that widespread requests by residents for room service will impede the safe and efficient function of the facility, the staff is willing to engage Mr. Elwin in debate over his decision to dine in his room. Mr. Elwin is treated like an autonomous adult who maintains direct authority over self-regarding decisions. This is the case even though his decision is inconsistent with a treatment plan for his long-term stabilization or even recovery. He is treated like a competent, autonomous adult even when the staff is adversely affected because his decision stretches staff resources. There was no attempt to persuade him to delegate that authority to the institution. There also is no attempt to seek his cooperation through fraudulent appeals to his concern for his rehabilitation.

Positive versus Negative

I turn now to the final tension regarding autonomy identified by Collopy, that between positive and negative autonomy. Negative claims regarding autonomy assert rights *against* interference, coercion, and paternalism. Positive claims regarding autonomy assert rights *to* liberty, empowerment, opportunity, assistance. Negative claims regarding autonomy usually arise in discussions of autonomy of the elderly and the physically and mentally handicapped. Positive claims regarding autonomy usually arise in discussions of autonomy of children and of so-called underdeveloped cultures. Although it is important to clarify the rights of the elderly against coercion and against being interfered with, it is equally important to address the rights of the elderly to basic entitlements and to opportunities, assistance, and resources.

A Fair Share of Resources

Claimants to autonomy, such as Mrs. Frank and Mr. Elwin, may claim a fair share of those resources that are conducive to the preservation and enhancement of their autonomy. They are the best and proper identifiers of what their autonomy consists in and how their moral personality is to be expressed autonomously in their daily lives. The fair share of resources they may claim will be determined in part by their need and in part by the availability. Their fair share must not unfairly disadvantage other claimants of the resources. Thus, whether the community one lives in is global or the third floor of a nursing home, claimants must mutually share disadvantages of limited resources. And when the resources are extremely limited, triage would appear to be a fair and familiar rule of apportionment.

CONSEQUENCES OF AUTONOMY

Moral theories permit individual rights to be limited when they conflict with like rights of others. Should Mr. Elwin's right to make a dining decision be restrained because, if other clients exercised a similar right, the rights of all to safety and the rights of staff to fair conditions of employment would be violated? Should Mrs. Frank's autonomy be limited by the rights of other clients to choose more congenial dining arrangements? Can some solution be reached that will not require limitations on anyone's rights? Is it possible that concern for fairness to other residents (whether for their sensibilities or for their dining assignments) would motivate both Mrs. Frank and Mr. Elwin to act differently? What consequences to clients (including Mrs. Frank and Mr. Elwin), to staff, and to the institution ought to limit Mrs. Frank's and Mr. Elwin's rights to autonomously choose their dining arrangements?

When we look at the consequences of actions, we want to consider consequences to the well-being of the parties to the situation, as well as the financial and other costs. For the purposes of discussion, we can assume that achieving good morale is, morally speaking, a good "consequence" for nursing home residents, including Mrs. Frank and Mr. Elwin. Here a brief synopsis of findings from literature on morale of nursing home residents is relevant.

Making their own decisions about activities of daily living long has been identified as one of the strongest influences on the morale of elderly nursing home residents (Chang 1978a; Hulicka, Morganti, & Cataldo, 1975; Langer & Rodin 1976; Ryden, 1984). Scores on Chang's Situational Control of Daily Activities (SCDA) Scale (Chang, 1978b) showed that of the eight areas of daily activity, grooming and eating were seen by most residents as the areas of their daily lives where they had the least control (Ryden, 1984). If these findings are reliable, then freedom to make autonomous decisions about dining may strongly influence morale of elderly nursing home residents.

More important, perhaps, Ryden (1984) found that perceived situational control was the only variable that had a significant direct effect on the morale of residents on skilled care. According to Ryden, the greater the functional dependency, the less sense of control and the lower morale score. These results suggest to Ryden that the morale of competent residents could improve through interventions designed to increase their perception of situational control. Given that grooming and eating are areas over which large numbers of residents perceive that they lack control, increased autonomy in making grooming and eating decisions would be an important contribution to increasing resident morale. Protecting residents' rights to autonomous decision making—specifically, to decision making regarding dining—has good and therefore morally desirable consequences. However, the consequences to the principal parties, Mrs. Frank and Mr. Elwin, are not the only consequences we must consider.

Note that this line of argument does not examine what autonomy might consist of for either Mrs. Frank or Mr. Elwin, nor does it ask which conception of autonomy might be, morally speaking, the most defensible. It is a consequentialist argument: Given that high morale is a good thing for most people and given that we are satisfied that it has been empirically demonstrated that control over dining decisions contributes directly to morale and indirectly through a perceived sense of control over one's daily activities, then sustaining Mr. Elwin's and Mrs. Frank's control over their own dining decisions will have good consequences for them. And if they and other residents are able to control their daily living activities, good consequences will ensue for everyone unless such control brings with it unintended harmful consequences to others, such as the staff.

This is not an unfamiliar argument and is one that consequentialists, including John Stuart Mill (1961), make. According to Mill, the consequences we must consider include long-range goods and "trickle-down" goods. If we consider our actions in terms of long-range and trickle-down goods, we find good consequences ensue from generally unpleasant activities like going to the dentist and paying taxes. Mill's view was that better consequences almost always ensue when you respect individual autonomy (Waithe, 1982b). In order to determine whether, on balance, better consequences will result from respecting Mrs. Frank's and Mr. Elwin's autonomous dining choices or from not respecting those choices, we must identify the bad consequences of allowing residents to make their own dining choices. Then we will need to see if there is some way of avoiding those consequences while protecting residents' autonomy.

The most obvious negative consequences of prohibiting Mrs. Frank and Mr. Elwin from choosing their own dining arrangements concern the negative effect on their morale because of loss of control over an important activity of their lives. The most obvious positive consequence respecting Mr. Elwin is that disruption of staff activities will be minimized and that likely similar requests from other clients will be forestalled by making a clear example of him. In addition, we may assume that the walk to the dining room is beneficial to his health, and perhaps even the additional socializing would be good for him. These reasons appear not to be compelling; however, neither his physical condition nor his emotional state is so precarious as to warrant paternalistic coercion (Waithe, 1982b).

The most obvious positive consequences of prohibiting residents from making their own choices are, respecting Mrs. Frank, a pleasant and comfortable dining experience for her companions. However, the vignette does not explore the possibility that different companions might not find her messiness so objectionable. Further, it does not explore the possibility that merely bringing the matter to her attention and, if needed, providing her with some skills for minimizing the messiness will resolve the problem as far as her companions are concerned. Nor does the vignette explore the possibility that Mrs. Frank is simply being ostracized by a clique for reasons unrelated to dining. Likewise, we do not know whether the social worker is giving less consideration to or being less flexible regarding a client who is disliked than she would be for a client who is liked.

WHAT SHOULD THE NURSING HOME DO?

How might the institution accommodate Mrs. Frank and Mr. Elwin in their dining preferences without causing too many or too severe bad effects on others? Who are the other parties to the drama, and what are the consequences to them when residents make autonomous dining decisions? Certainly, other residents and nursing home staff are directly affected by any policy or practice allowing residents rather than staff to make dining decisions. The efficient and cost-effective functioning of the institution can be disrupted if clients eat when and where they choose. Confused clients who need the regularity of unvaried routine may become more confused and disoriented. Staff may be spread too thin to provide adequate assistance to confused residents and to those who require physical assistance. Accommodating client choices may create a staff scheduling nightmare as well as unfair and unsafe conditions of employment for staff. What the consequences are and whom there will be consequences to depend on the actual choice made by residents.

Choices can be severely circumscribed by the institution in order to maximize good consequences and minimize undesirable consequences to residents and staff. The ways in which those choices are circumscribed will depend in large part on how we view a nursing home. If we view it as a medical facility, sweeping infringements of individual autonomy are likely to be imposed in the name of therapy or routine. For those residents whose psychological or medical condition is very delicate, who require either a fixed routine or constant medical supervision, such infringements might be necessary for their exercise of autonomy. This is particularly true when function, safety, and health are viewed by the resident to be of paramount importance. However, other residents, whose needs and expression of autonomy are different, may view the nursing home as a neighborhood or as a retirement community that makes a variety of services available at limited hours and in limited ways. An institution conceived along these lines will impose fewer infringements on its residents. At the other end of the spectrum is the view of nursing home as a commercial hotel that must provide a wider variety of choices and cater to the whims of residents who will otherwise go elsewhere. This latter concept of a nursing home is clearly unfamiliar because of both the financial status of many residents and the lack of alternative choices of residences available. Nevertheless, some lessons may be learned from the commercial hotel model.

In a successful commercial restaurant, staffing schedules, staff and patron safety, and patron seating convenience are managed effectively and cost-efficiently by limiting hours of operation, by use of a reservation system, and by the physical parameters of the dining room itself. In better restaurants, hours are limited, staff-patron ratios are high, and patrons can assure satisfactory accommodations by making advance reservations for parties of a fixed size. In cafeterias and fast-food restaurants this is often not the case. Instead, dining decisions are limited by a "first come, first served" system and by a choice of takeout meals or on-site dining in limited-capacity booths or at tables with a fixed number of chairs, which are often bolted to the floor. In both types of commercial establishment patrons' exercise of autonomy is limited by institutional design and by policy. Restrictions on autonomous dining decisions at a commercial facility are not made on the basis of institutional assessment of individual patrons' needs and interests; patrons are assumed to be the best judge of these.

In a nursing home, many of the negative consequences to the institution and to the staff of client dining decisions can be minimized through institutional control of the hours of operation, the physical parameters of the dining room, and the type of reservation system the institution adopts. Arranging the physical plant so that choices of different sizes of tables are available would allow Mrs. Frank, as well as her present table companions, options to seek more agreeable tablemates. A system of reservations may not only be a dignifying morale booster by itself but would enhance opportunities for those patrons to whom it was important to dine at a particular hour or to whom it was important to have a particular companion for dinner. Clients who are confused and whose expression of autonomy requires a fixed routine can be offered "fixed reservations": the traditional system of meal assignments.

Recall that the social worker had complained that table assignments were one of her biggest headaches. This common complaint among nursing home social workers merits serious attention. Perhaps radical changes, such as the suggested system, could have beneficial consequences to residents and staff alike. On the other hand, setting up a system whereby clients effectively made their own assignments may have some costs attached to it. An efficient system would need to be established, and opportunities to make reservations would themselves need to be allocated in some way, either by taking reservations in rotating alphabetical order, room order, or some other system that would provide all residents with equal opportunities to effect choice. On the other hand, the time expended by social work staff in implementing such a system would likely be less unpleasant, and less than that expended in addressing client complaints about dining assignments. Furthermore, such arrangements would probably be highly cost-effective as well as efficient, provided they are well developed and properly administered, with the varying needs of residents and staff kept in mind. I assume the cost-effectiveness and efficiency of both the reservations and "as available" systems because they are the models for commercial dining facilities everywhere.

If the staff time spent and stress endured by dealing with client dissatisfaction with the present system decreases efficiency and therefore cost-effectiveness, the model I am proposing for nursing homes should be efficient and therefore cost-effective for two reasons. First, those residential institutions, such as nursing homes and prisons, that rely exclusively on assigned dining arrangements are widely reputed to be those that are perceived by their clientele to least serve their interests. Valuable staff time is consumed and client cooperation and goodwill lost as a result of resident dissatisfaction. Second, those residential institutions, such as hotels, that combine the three systems I am suggesting (reservations, availability, and in-room private dining) are widely reputed to be perceived by their clientele to best serve their interests. Although there will certainly be snafus in any system, which will result in some client complaints, the incidence of client dissatisfaction with dining arrangements in commercial institutions is directly related to the commercial success of the institution. One therefore concludes that some of the success of those commercial ventures is due to the industrywide implementation of one or more of the three systems mentioned above.

By combining a reservation system with seating on a space-available basis, clients who preferred less formal arrangements or who were indifferent to the time at which they ate, or who neglected to make a reservation, would not be constrained by the institution but by options that they themselves had limited. And although this might sound like a cruel consequence to impose on a confused resident, the reader will keep in mind that the reservation system I have in mind would include "fixed" as well as "daily" reservations. Some elements of the traditional fixed-assignment system would therefore be retained so that confused residents who require a fixed routine would have one.

In addition to the positive consequences for client morale, many positive socializing activities could result from residents making dining choices. The mere process of making arrangements with others to lunch together and of seeking out and coming to agreements with companions and neighbors requires some degree of friendliness and some amount of thought about whom one likes and why. Even wandering into a dining room and seeking out (or being sought out by) someone who would like company requires a commitment to breaking down barriers of unfamiliarity and to sharing of oneself. This system is compatible with the various concepts of a nursing home, whether that of medical facility, retirement community, or commercial hotel.

Of course, dining arrangements can be made only within the limits of institutional resources. There is no suggestion that the institution ought to make 24-hour dining available or even extend its dining room hours. By limiting the hours at which private dining is available to those who do not require special assistance, clients like Mr. Elwin are free to choose whether they prefer to dine in their rooms when staff is available for supervision and emergency assistance or to make the trek to the dining room. Mr. Elwin's need for supervision during mealtime has not been documented in the vignette. Emergencies are always anticipated in such a setting, but pinning his call button to his clothing should minimize even the remote risk that he will aspirate and choke on his food. Mr. Elwin should be able to choose between communal dining at his convenience and private dining at hours when sufficient staff are available to respond in case of an emergency. Mr. Elwin's exercise of choice should then not create undue burdens on staff or on other clients requiring feeding. He would be making his own choice, but it would be within the constraints of institutional parameters not unlike those found at a commercial restaurant. Within these parameters, client selection of a dining arrangement can have positive consequences for client morale while avoiding negative consequences to those clients whose choices are limited by physical condition and to staff who might otherwise be overworked.

CONCLUSION

By arranging its physical plant so that choices of different sizes of tables are available, by adopting a system of limited reservations and as-available dining, and by limiting the hours at which private dining is available, nursing homes can satisfy Mrs. Frank and Mr. Elwin, those who are concerned with rights and those who are concerned with costs as well. Positive effects on residents' morale of making autonomous dining choices can be achieved while negative effects to other residents, to staff, and to the institution's costs and efficient function are minimized. The individual rights of clients and staff—rights to autonomy, respect, care and concern, and justice—can be protected without trampling the corporate rights of a commercial nursing care facility. And that's something to chew on.

REFERENCES

American Psychiatric Association. (1980). *Diagnostic and statistical manual of mental disorders* (3rd ed.). Washington, DC: Author.

Brooks A. (1974). *Law, psychiatry and the mental health system.* Boston: Little, Brown.

Brooks A. (1980). *Law, psychiatry and the mental health system: 1980 supplement.* Boston and Toronto: Little, Brown.

Chang, B. L. (1978a). Generalized expectancy, situational perception of control and morale among institutionalized aged. *Nursing Research, 27*, 316–324.

Chang, B. L. (1978b). Perceived situational control of daily activities: A new tool. *Research in Nursing and Health, 1*, 181–186.

Collopy, B. J. (1988). Autonomy in long term care: Some crucial distinctions. *The Gerontologist, 28* (Suppl.), 10–17.

Dworkin, G. (1976). Autonomy and behavioral control, *The Hastings Center Report, 6*, 1–23.

Faden, R. & Beauchamp, T. (1986). *A history and theory of informed consent.* New York and Oxford: Oxford University Press.

Mill, J. S. (1961). *Utilitarianism* and *On liberty,* In *The utilitarians,* Garden City, NY: Doubleday, 401–600.

Rawls, J. (1971). *A theory of justice.* Cambridge, MA: Harvard University Press.

Ryden, M. (1984). Morale and perceived control in institutionalized elderly. *Nursing Research, 33*, 130–137.

Sartorius, R. (1988). *Paternalism* (2nd ed.). Minneapolis: University of Minnesota Press.

Waithe, M. (1982). *Acting for others: Towards a theory of paternalism.* Unpublished doctoral dissertation. University of Minnesota: Minneapolis.

Waithe, M. (1982). Why Mill was for paternalism. *International Journal of Law and Psychiatry, 5*, 4.

Waithe, M. (1988). Bibliography of paternalism. In R. Sartorius (Ed.), *Paternalism* (2nd ed.). Minneapolis: University of Minnesota Press, 275–278.

FOR FURTHER DISCUSSION: EDITORS' QUESTIONS

1. What principle should be used in arranging dining times and combinations? Is any kind of segregation appropriate?

2. In Mrs. Frank's situation, what would be in her best interests? What is in the best interests of Mr. Elwin?

3. Do residents have the right to complain about how other residents affect the aesthetics of meals?

4. What moral significance can be imputed to meals in nursing homes? Do meals have a special moral significance in a nursing home? Why or why not?

5. Should persons with senile dementia and persons with intact mental facilities be forced to mingle at meals or other activities?

6. Do nursing home employees have an obligation to tell the truth to residents? Can a "white lie" ever be justified? Was the lie to Mrs. Frank justified?

7. What moral norms ought to govern the allocation of meal places, times, and table arrangements from the viewpoint of nursing staff? Should the same norms govern residents and their families?

8. How much autonomy should residents be asked to yield or cede in the interests of the efficient operation of the home? How much autonomy, if any, can they be expected to voluntarily waive in the interests of efficient operation?

Chapter 11

PHONE PRIVILEGES

Mrs. Allison does not like living at Pleasantville. She didn't want to go there, and she keeps reminding her family on every visit that they said it would be only "temporary." Her adjustment has not proceeded very well from anyone's point of view.

Mrs. Allison telephones each of her four children at least daily to discuss how things have gone that day, to give them a list of things to bring on their next visit, and to continue her general campaign to get out of the facility. She makes these calls from the coin phone in the hall near the entrance to the dayroom. Because her fingers are arthritic, she needs help from the nurses to dial the numbers.

Mrs. Allison's oldest son and daughter, representing the children, went to see the administrator to request that the staff not help their mother use the telephone. They perceive her calls as a nuisance. Each call is just the same old thing. The calls are also somewhat upsetting to several of the grandchildren. One 10-year-old girl has taken to having bad dreams about her grandmother being locked away.

The staff are in a quandary. They do not know if it is their right to protect the family against Mrs. Allison and to cut off Mrs. Allison's main way of communication. The social worker suggested that maybe they should tell family members that it is their problem and that there is always the solution of an unlisted phone number. The director of nursing thought that it was not the facility's place even to put that idea in the family's head—and besides, both sons were in business and needed their numbers listed.

CASE COMMENTARY

Laurence B. McCullough

This case involves the following issues: the right of communication of nursing home residents, the obligations of family members to frail elderly relatives who are nursing home residents, the burden on family members that may occur when nursing home residents exercise their rights, the obligations of older persons (whether nursing home residents or not) to their family members, and the proper role of nursing homes in negotiating conflicts between residents and their families.

The immediate question at hand is whether nursing home staff should give Mrs. Allison the physical help needed to telephone her family members, or should they capitulate to family requests that they stop aiding and abetting Mrs. Allison in making what the family perceives as annoying calls. The staff is caught in the middle. To address this question, a theoretical framework for geriatric ethics is necessary. Although the framework that follows may seem an elaborate route to answering a knotty but straightforward question, the general approach to problem solving that is derived from this analysis can be applied to a wide range of similar problems. It will lead to a recognition that the staff cannot make decisions for any party to this dispute but must, in fact, undertake a process to help the participants achieve a resolution.

A THEORETICAL FRAMEWORK
FOR GERIATRIC ETHICS

Respect for autonomy is an important ethical principle in a theoretical framework for geriatric ethics, but it needs to be supplemented by the principles of beneficence and family responsibility (McCullough & Lipson, 1988). In my view, each is equally weighted in theory and none should take precedence or be considered weightier than any other.

The Principle of Respect for Autonomy

The principle of respect for autonomy is rooted in the recognition that all competent geriatrics patients have a perspective on their own best interests that is shaped by their values and beliefs. Those values and beliefs have many sources, and some are consciously created by the individuals themselves. Together they form a distinctive, more or less well-organized collection that defines each of us as a unique person. On the basis of our values and beliefs we assess alternatives that are available to us, arrive at a preference for one of the alternatives, and try to implement that preference, either on our own or with assistance of others as necessary.

To exercise autonomy, three related behaviors are necessary:

1. Identifying the values and beliefs relevant to judging available alternatives.
2. Arriving at a value-based preferences.
3. Implementing that preference, by oneself or with the assistance of others.

Clinical experience teaches forcefully that health care patients, especially frail elderly patients, have varying abilities to undertake these three tasks and frequently require help with one or more of them. Therefore, the clinician's responsibilities to the geriatric patient generated by the principle of respect for autonomy are as follows:

1. To recognize and acknowledge the validity of the values and beliefs of the older person, especially when those values and beliefs differ from those of the clinician.
2. To assist the older person to identify relevant values and beliefs.
3. To assist the older person to arrive at a value-based preference.
4. To refrain from interfering with the implementation of that preference by the older person or to assist with its implementation as necessary, given physical limitations on the older person's ability to do so.

It follows that two distinct senses of autonomy can be identified: choice-autonomy, which is the expression of a value-based preference, and resolution-autonomy, which is the implementation of that preference (Agree, Lipson, McCullough & Soldo, 1988); (McCullough & Lipson, 1988). Respect for choice autonomy (other chapters in this book call this distinction decisional versus executional demands the first three responsibilities listed above, whereas respect for resolution autonomy demands the fourth. In this analysis, respect for autonomy is a procedural principle.

Neither its substantive content nor the results of its application in actual circumstances and cases can be identified in advance. Respect for autonomy is measured by the process that occurs.

Respect for choice autonomy can always occur for competent patients, where competent means the ability to participate in the specific tasks described on page 7. Respect for resolution autonomy, however, can sometimes be justifiably overlooked because of conflict(s) with overriding obligations based on other ethical principles, namely beneficence and family responsibility.

The Principle of Beneficence

The principle of beneficence focuses the moral attention of the clinician on the consequences of actions. This is an entirely appropriate ethical consideration in health care because health care is a process very much concerned with and directed toward what clinicians take to be good consequences for the patient, for example, maintaining health. The obligation generated by the principle of beneficence in health care is to act in such a way as to produce the greater amount of good over harm for the patient.

The beneficence obligation is exercised in two phases: (1) the identification of relevant goods and harms and (2) a judgment about how they should be balanced when both goods and harms are involved, as they almost always are in geriatric care. The first is substantive and the second, procedural.

Substantive Dimension

The substantive dimension of beneficence in health care requires the specification of the goods that health care seeks on behalf of the patient and the harms that health care attempts to avoid. The basis for this specification is the peculiar claim of the health care professions to know what is in the best interests of patients without having to consult their particular values and beliefs, as required by the principle of respect for (choice-) autonomy. That is, in some spheres, the health care professions claim to know what goods should be sought for patients and what harms should be avoided. Their clinical knowledge and experience, however, affords a limited competence in matters of human goods and harms. Not all goods and harms fall within the scope of beneficence and health care, a feature of the principle of beneficence and health care that sometimes goes unappreciated in analyses of paternalism in health care such as that of Veatch (1981).

The goods that health care seeks for us can be defined in the following terms (Beauchamp & McCullough, 1984):

1. The prevention of untimely or premature death.
2. The prevention, elimination, or at least amelioration of disease, injury, handicap, and unnecessary physical pain and suffering. (Pain and suffering become unnecessary when they do not contribute to achieving the goods of beneficence in health care.)

Although health professionals in the three decades following World War II flirted with making prevention of death the primary good of health care, this flirtation was an aberration in the history of the principle of beneficence in health care. The qualifiers of preventing *untimely* or *premature* death added in (1) above represent a return to older ways of thinking after a turbulent exposure to the excesses of enthusiasm for critical care during its formative years.

The prevention, elimination, and amelioration of disease, injury, handicap, and unnecessary pain and suffering are especially relevant to geriatric health care because the health problems of the elderly are chronic in nature. This is not to say that frail elderly patients never experience acute episodes but only that such acute episodes usually occur in the context of chronic disease, injury, handicap, and perhaps unnecessary pain and suffering.

Procedural Dimension

In geriatric health care, the prevention of untimely death is not an absolute good. It must always be balanced against the other goods of health care. Indeed, as death becomes more imminent, the force of the good of preventing untimely death properly diminishes in favor of the other goods of health care. For elderly persons who are nursing home residents this is an especially important consideration, not only because of imminence of death but also because nursing home residents are likely to be at risk of physical pain and discomfort, not to mention myriad other personal and social losses. In the case of Mrs. Allison and her phone privileges, beneficence focuses us on the good of preventing the unnecessary suffering she might experience if her phone privileges are restricted, and it requires health professions to consider the consequences of such a restriction.

Second, beneficence-based judgments in geriatric health care are frequently and justifiably limited, first internally and then as a consequence of the principle of respect for autonomy (Christianson, 1974, 1978). Different clinicians can reasonably arrive at differing balancings of goods and harms involved in preventing further losses for geriatric patients with chronic conditions or long-term-care needs. Thus, the *outcome* of beneficence-based clinical judgment in geriatric health care is usually variable. Furthermore, personal, social, and other goods and harms unrelated to health care

are relevant for assessing such losses and the risk of their occurring. The specification of these goods and harms is beyond the scope of the principle of beneficence in health care because the health care profession's competence does not extend to all human goods and harms. Rather, they fall within the province of the autonomy of the elderly persons.

In the present case, the significance to Mrs. Allison of the personal and social goods of being in touch with her family, of needing to complain, of being needed, and whatever else she may find relevant and meaningful in her telephone calls—we don't know from the case description—is for Mrs. Allison to judge, not the health care professionals at Pleasantville Nursing Home. Respect for her choice autonomy and her resolution autonomy thus may override beneficence-based considerations, not because respect for autonomy is a more important principle than beneficence but because beneficence-based clinical judgments rarely should extend to social matters such as making telephone calls.

Finally, the principle of beneficence in health care applies not only to the patient but also to third parties to the patient-clinical relationship because these third parties can have their interests harmed by either the patient or the clinician. For example, nursing home policies and practices permitting residents to make phone calls at any time they want to (just like the rest of us "on the outside") can be harmful to the interests of Mrs. Allison's family members. Sometimes the goods and harms at stake for these third parties fall within the competence of beneficence-based judgments in health care, and sometimes they do not. The experience of Mrs. Allison's 10-year old granddaughter, who has bad dreams about her grandmother, seems to verge on an area of technical competence to make a beneficent judgment; whereas the stress, disruption, anger, and frustration of Mrs. Allison's children and children-in-law may be harms that fall outside the health care provider's purview.

In summary, competently made beneficence-based clinical judgments about the patient's best interests must be given theoretically equal weight with judgments based on respect for autonomy. However, beneficence-based judgments about matters unrelated to health care fall outside the scope of the moral authority of health care professionals to speak to human goods and harms, a significant limit that, in my judgment, geriatric health care professionals often fail to observe.

The Principle of Family Responsibility

Reference to families and to family responsibility must be included in any theoretical framework for geriatric ethics because of the heavy involvement of families in the "informal" care of elderly persons (Brody,

1977) and because health care decisions sometimes have adverse impact on the interests of involved family members. Family members confront a two-part ethical struggle when it comes to the care of frail parents or parents-in-law.

The first concerns their own sense of their obligation to support and care for parents and parents-in-law as a matter of reciprocal justice (McCullough & Lipson, 1988). Because the history of relationships between children and parents varies enormously and unpredictably (Callahan, 1987), one cannot specify a formula for reciprocal justice. The process becomes complicated and vexing when the different generations reach different judgments about those demands or when distrust is involved, as appears to be the case for Mrs. Allison.

The second part of the ethical struggle concerns how to balance one's obligations to parents against other obligations that one may have, for example, to spouse and children, and against legitimate self-interest. Ethically significant matters of self-interest might include pursuing a career, being able to rest or get away for a time from demanding long-term-care responsibilities, or living in as harmonious a household as the ordinary stresses of life permit. These are legitimately considered and weighed in the mix of responsibility to one's parents and other relatives. This mix is utterly variable and sometimes volatile.

Family responsibility is, like autonomy, an entirely procedural ethical principle. The obligations it generates for the clinician and nursing home administrator are those of the negotiator. The clinician or administrator should arrange to meet with family members to help them articulate their sense of responsibility to a parent, their other obligations, and their legitimate self-interests and to help them reach some reasonable balancing among the potentially conflicting demands in this mix. Family members should then meet with the resident so that both sides can reach a clear understanding of the reasoning processes and judgments of the other. The focus of these discussions should be on the basic values and beliefs of family members regarding the nursing home resident, which creates a potential common ground. The initial and continuing focus should not be on the decisions that have been made prior to the conflict but on the values and beliefs that led to those decisions. If the decisions themselves are the main focus, conflict will most likely be exacerbated. It is important to underscore that negotiation does not, and need not, always result in resolution of conflict. But it can always result in mutual understanding of why there was a conflict about particular decisions in the first place and why conflict may persist (Agree et al., 1988). In the case of Mrs. Allison, the role of the clinicians and administrator of the Pleasantville Nursing Home is not to impose a solution but to have procedures in place that will facilitate negotiation.

MRS. ALLISON'S CASE

The first thing that needs to be said about this case is that Pleasantville Nursing Home—and the local phone company—should be scolded for unnecessarily compounding physical, personal, and social losses of residents of the home by having a dial pay phone on the premises. A push-button phone should be installed forthwith so that patients like Mrs. Allison with mobility impairment of the hands can more easily place calls.

There is an additional ethically significant reason for doing so. It is clear from the case description that an implicit, but not articulated, part of the staff's problem is that Mrs. Allison's phone calls tax the limited resources of staff time and goodwill. One suspects that this factor contributes to staff frustration and anger. The administration of the home is ethically obligated to prevent unnecessary drains on such central resources in the moral life of a nursing home, and they should be faulted for failing to prevent an underlying but significant dimension of the case.

However, the main point of the case is the quandary in which the staff say they find themselves. The alternatives articulated by the staff seem to be three: (1) protecting Mrs. Allison's family, (2) cutting or limiting Mrs. Allison's communication with her family, and (3) telling the family that this is "their problem." This formulation indicates clearly that the staff has failed to understand their ethical obligations to Mrs. Allison and her family. They are operating without a theoretical framework within which they could negotiate ethical conflicts of the sort posed by Mrs. Allison's behavior and her family's response to it. The theoretical framework presented in the first half of this chapter becomes essential for addressing the particular issues in this case.

The first issue concerns whether or not Mrs. Allison was, in fact, deceived by her family into thinking that her placement at Pleasantville was temporary. If she was, then both respect for her autonomy and beneficence obligate the staff to inform her of the deception. If the staff was a party to the deception, Mrs. Allison should be told that as well. The principle of respect for autonomy obligates the staff to provide Mrs. Allison with information relevant to her decisions about calling her children, and information about actual deception is surely relevant to such decisions. In addition, as even a small amount of clinical experience teaches, in the long run deception incurs a higher risk of harmful consequences than of beneficial ones for the person deceived, as well as for staff members who must "remember the story" and hide their own misgivings from Mrs. Allison. It may be painful for the staff to disclose this information, but the ethical obligation to do so is not defeated by personal discomfort. After all, we have many ethical obligations that require us to act in ways that make us feel—temporarily, usually—uncomfortable.

If deception is not involved and Mrs. Allison's complaint expresses frustration or a sharp reaction to the change in her living environment, then a more nuanced approach is required. The first step is for the staff to appreciate that the conflict here is between Mrs. Allison's exercise of her autonomy and her children's, and presumably their spouses' (if there are any), judgments about family responsibility. (Beneficence, with its emphasis on preventing unnecessary suffering within the limited scope of the health care provider's competence, supports the autonomy of Mrs. Allison, as explained above.) As noted, both autonomy and family responsibility are entirely procedural in nature. Thus, for the staff to articulate their quandary in such substantive terms as a right to protect the family and the right to cut off Mrs. Allison's use of the pay phone is a serious conceptual error. In addition, to consider dumping the problem in the family's lap reflects a failure to understand the clinician's and administrator's roles in negotiation of conflicts between respect for autonomy and family responsibility. The situation is made worse by the staff having everyone, including themselves, focus on the actual decisions of Mrs. Allison and her children, rather than on the values and beliefs that underlie the behavior.

The second step is to implement the appropriate response to ethical conflicts based on procedural ethical principles, namely, putting procedures into place to permit the parties to the conflict to negotiate their different decisions. Staff and administration can facilitate this process in a number of significant ways.

First, the negotiating process should begin with all parties articulating their values and beliefs about their own interests, their obligations to others in the family, and their obligations and interests of others. I suspect that Mrs. Allison and her family would quickly discover the common ground that had eluded them, a problem compounded by the unreflective response of the staff and the virtual absence from the case of the senior administration of the home. That common ground would probably include the following: (1) all of the parties value regular communication; (2) all of Mrs. Allison's children would acknowledge the importance to her of being able to stay in touch and of continuing in some way to be their mother, an authority figure in their lives and not someone who has been put out of sight and therefore out of mind; and (3) the children could help Mrs. Allison appreciate the sometimes burdensome nature of her behavior.

The psychological stress of the one grandchild is, from my limited experience, probably due to the failure of her parents to explain convincingly why her grandmother is in the home and to their own distressed reactions to her grandmother's constant phone calls. This child's parents need some support and counseling about how to explain nursing home placement to children, including counseling about their own guilt about the decision to institutionalize Mrs. Allison.

The staff should keep in mind the list of ethical issues identified at the beginning of this commentary as a way for them to interpret the negotiating process and to be sure that the parties have addressed all of the issues. Complete consideration of the relevant issues is certainly one criterion for a successful negotiating process, even though complete agreement about their resolution is not always possible.

If Mrs. Allison were mentally confused or otherwise mentally impaired, the strategy would change. The first step would be a thorough workup of her mental impairment to determine as thoroughly as possible its causes and to identify strategies for its amelioration. Such impairment, for example, may be due to new medications or a temporary disorientation from being in new, unfamiliar surroundings and among strangers.

If such measures persistently fail to improve Mrs. Allison's mental status, then matters become significantly more complicated because the case now involves a patient with irreversibly and perhaps significantly reduced autonomy. Notice "reduced", not "absent" autonomy (Beauchamp & McCullough, 1984). Enough autonomy will remain that Mrs. Allison is likely to notice and resent limitations on behavior that she values, but she may be insufficiently able to appreciate the impact of that behavior on others. Some restrictions on access to the phone may therefore be reasonable. This should be discussed in the negotiating process, to the extent that Mrs. Allison can participate in it. This process should begin by her family being asked to appreciate the impact on Mrs. Allison of a threat to cut her off completely from her family. That alternative should be ruled out at the beginning. Thus, all parties can see that staying in touch is valued, something that elderly persons with any degree of mental impairment may well be able to appreciate. It should certainly not be assumed, without testing, that they are unable to appreciate this or the need for reasonable limits. Mrs. Allison's family is not saying that they want no communication; they are saying that they are getting too much. They should also be invited to think about the meaning of their remark that Mrs. Allison always talks about "the same old thing." Does she really? And if she does, perhaps this is a diagnostic sign of the need for more variety in her new setting or of incipient depression that could be successfully treated. In other words, sometimes the things we—not just the elderly in nursing homes—say in frustration are not simply psychological phenomena. Both the staff and Mrs. Allison's children apparently underinterpreted the message.

SUMMARY

In summary, the response to cases like this one, involving phone privileges, should be procedural in nature because the two ethical principles at the heart of the conflict in such cases—respect for autonomy (buttressed by beneficence) and family responsibility—are procedural ethical principles. Nursing home staff and administrators need to appreciate that *all* of the ethical conflicts between residents and their families will have a procedural dimension, even when substantive beneficence-based judgments about the resident's best interests are part of the conflict. Thus, resolution strategies should focus on the processes of negotiation. These processes should be quickly implemented in such cases.

One final comment. Nether the staff nor the administration of the home were thinking in terms of "preventive ethics" (McCullough & Lipson, 1988). There were surely warning signs about stress and frustration on the part of Mrs. Allison's children. Had they been heeded by staff and the negotiating process begun earlier, a very stressful and turbulent situation could have been prevented. In this light, it should be clear that all parties in a case like this have equal claim to the staff's obligation to encourage and support the negotiating process described above. A preventive rather than a reactive approach can reduce the time and other demands on staff of such a negotiating process. For example, the initial intake interview could include discussion with all parties about the importance they attached to staying in touch and, for Mrs. Allison's children, the importance that they properly attached to other obligations in their lives.

There is no evidence from the case description to think that Mrs. Allison could not appreciate and respond appropriately to such legitimate concerns on the part of her children. The goal of this process is to have Mrs. Allison and her children reach an accommodation that they agree to and enforce. It is therefore incorrect to think of this case in terms of restricting Mrs. Allison's autonomy without her consent; rather, one should think in terms of Mrs. Allison and her family mutually agreeing to limits of autonomy all around. In this way, nobody is labeled the problem, and nobody is labeled the victim. As with all preventive approaches, there are no doubt significant advantages in terms of staff morale and staff-resident relationship that could accrue from preventive ethics as part of the policies and practices of nursing home care.

REFERENCES

Agree, E.A., Lipson, S., McCullough, L.B. and Soldo, B. (1988). Long-term care decision making. In W. Reichel (Ed.), *Clinical aspects of aging* (3rd ed.) Baltimore: Williams and Wilkins.

Beauchamp, T.L. & McCullough, L.B. (1984). *Medical ethics: The moral responsibilities of physicians.* Englewood Cliffs, NJ: Prentice-Hall.

Brody, E.M. (1977). *Long-term care of older people: A practical guide.* New York: Human Services Press.

Callahan, D. (1987). What do children owe elderly parents? *Hastings Center Report, 15,* 31–37.

Christiansen, D. (1974). Dignity in aging. *Hastings Center Report, 4,* 6–8.

Christiansen, D. (1978). Dignity in aging: Notes on geriatric ethics. *Journal of Humanistic Psychology, 18,* 41–54.

McCullough, L.B. & Lipson, S. (1988). A framework for geriatric ethics. In W. Reichel (Ed.), *Clinical aspects of aging* (3rd ed.). Baltimore: Williams and Wilkins.

Veatch, R.M. (1981). *A theory of medical ethics.* New York: Basic Books.

FOR FURTHER DISCUSSION: EDITOR'S QUESTIONS

1. Is communication a fundamental right that the facility must permit its residents?
2. To whom does the facility owe its allegiance in this and similar situations? Do the demands of the resident take priority over those of the family?
3. Would the obligations here differ if the relatives outside the nursing home were not the children of the resident? Is the parent-child relationship of special ethical significance?
4. If the facility staff tries to deflect the telephone calls, are they improperly limiting Mrs. Allison's autonomy?
5. Would the situation be different if Mrs. Allison were mentally confused?
6. Does Mrs. Allison have an obligation to be more thoughtful of her family?
7. What are the limits of the family's obligations to respond to Mrs. Allison?
8. If Mrs. Allison's family is paying the nursing home bill, does this alter the relative obligation of the nursing home to both parties?
9. What is the foundation for an argument that facility staff should mediate between a resident and family members?
10. Does the staff have any obligation to be beneficent to Mrs. Allison's family?

Chapter 12

GUARDIAN ANGLES

GREG BLANKENSCHIFFT SEEKS GUARDIANSHIP

Mr. Blankenschifft is a 79-year-old resident of East-West Convalescent Center. He moved there almost 10 years ago, after his wife died. He entered a minimal-care unit because his health was really quite good. His son Greg lives in the same city, and his son Simon lives out of state. Of late, Mr. Blankenschifft has suffered some memory lapses and *once* was found wandering around outside at 2 A.M. clad only in his bathrobe.

His son Greg has started worrying about his father and his father's ability to manage his own affairs, and he wants to become his father's legal guardian. Greg has approached East-West's social worker, and she is glad to see Greg is planning ahead for his father's future. She chatted to the administrator when they were having lunch together, and the administrator said she wished that more relatives had Greg's sense of responsibility. Both social worker and administrator are ready to testify on behalf of Greg's guardianship.

When the social worker mentions to the home's director of nursing (DON) that Greg Blankenschifft is seeking legal guardianship for his father, the DON asks why. Other than the one incident, she says Mr. Blankenschifft had seemed fine in the last couple of weeks. On her own, the DON checks with Mr. Blankenschifft's floor nurse and the aides on his floor. They all concur that since the one incident when he was found outside he has been just fine—coherent, communicative, and taking part in social functions.

ALAN ABBOTT HOLDS GUARDIANSHIP

Mary Abbott is also 79. When she entered East-West, her youngest son was already her legal guardian. Mrs. Abbott had a stroke, which left her with some paralysis, very poor speech, and mild aphasia. She didn't want to cope with managing financial affairs and indicated that she preferred to have her son handle the money.

The social worker is unhappy with Mr. Abbott as guardian. A difficult part of her job in any event is making requests of guardians that they release more funds on behalf of the resident. In the case of the Abbotts, she has to plead with Alan Abbott before he will spend a cent of his mother's money for things that would give her pleasure: new clothes, a color television, or even the new wheelchair she needs. And Alan Abbott refuses to pay for physical therapy for his mother because he says, "The nursing home is getting $1600 a month; it should provide physical therapy." It is true that many of the families do misunderstand what is covered in the daily rate, and the social worker herself is a little embarrassed that physical therapy is not covered. But the younger Mr. Abbott's attitude makes her think he is more worried about conserving the estate than his mother's well-being.

The social worker always feels particularly helpless when a legal guardian makes a decision she considers against the residents' interests. "It is ironical," she says, "that some of these residents are almost worse off than people on Medicaid. At least we can get some services to the Medicaid recipients, but in cases like the Abbotts, the residents can't get access to their own money, and they aren't eligible for public programs. Still, I have to tread carefully. The home is always open to charges of conflict of interest,and why would a judge listen to a nursing home rather than the resident's own family?"

WORST CASE EXAMPLE

The worst situation that the social worker has encountered with family surrogates was that of Mr. Cohen. Mr. Cohen was a confused but garrulous and entertaining old man. The staff liked him a lot, and he seemed to enjoy his life. His son served as guardian, but the whole family was cohesive and presented a common front. When Mr. Cohen needed to have his pacemaker replaced, the family refused the operation. They were sure, they said, at age 87 their father would not want this procedure. In vain, the staff tried to explain the almost routine nature of the process. The family was obdurate. In disgust, the social worker said, "It's like throwing away the car because the battery is dead."

CASE COMMENTARY

Robert Schwartz

These three cases—the Abbott case, the Blankenschifft case, and the "Worst Case Example"—demonstrate the potential for abuse of the legal remedy of guardianship. Guardianship was designed and developed by the courts for limited use during a time when extended family structure and other social institutions made long-term-care facilities unknown and unnecessary. A guardianship proceeding is a legal action in which a petitioner (usually the potential guardian) seeks to exercise the personal legal authority of another person, designated the "ward." An order granting a guardianship has the effect of giving the guardian responsibility for the "care, custody, and control" of the ward, thus transferring legally recognized personal authority from the ward, who possesses the authority naturally, to a guardian, who is required to act on behalf of the ward (Uniform Probate Code, 1969, Article V; Uniform Guardianship and Protective Proceedings Act, 1982).

A guardian may be appointed only when the proposed ward is incapable of exercising the authority that is the subject of the guardianship. A guardianship may be general (and transfer all authority legally vested in the ward to the guardian for an indefinite time) or limited (and transfer only some of that authority or transfer authority for a limited amount of time). Although a guardianship can be limited to any particular authority otherwise residing in the ward (the right to make a particular health care decision, for example, or the right to expend money betting on the Red Sox), the most common form of limited guardianship is one that transfers authority over financial matters (but not personal matters) from the ward to the guardian. This form of limited guardianship is often called a conservatorship. Limited guardianship is now so common that sometimes the term "guardianship" is used to describe the transfer of only personal, not financial, authority. When the terms are used this way, the transfer of all authority from the ward could be accomplished only by the appointment of a "guardian and conservator" (Uniform Probate Code, 1969).

Like many traditional common law actions (and like kryptonite, the word processor, and the microwave oven), the guardianship process can be used for good or evil; it can be used to preserve autonomy or to overcome autonomy. These three cases are examples of the unrestrained general application of this legal doctrine, a doctrine that could be applied less anachronistically and with greater flexibility and creativity than the guardians (or proposed guardian, in the Blankenschifft case) thought possible.

Despite the fact that legal regulation of the substantive requirements for a guardianship and the procedures for obtaining one vary from state to state, the development of the Uniform Probate Code in 1969 and the subsequent Uniform Guardianship and Protective Proceedings Act of 1982 has generated a fairly narrow range of alternative state laws. Although these uniform laws are nothing more than recommendations to state legislatures, lawmakers have tended not to stray too far from them. The original Uniform Probate Code has been especially influential, whereas the Uniform Guardianship and Protective Proceedings Act, which was meant to serve as either an independent statute or an amendment to the Uniform Probate Code, has not yet had much effect. As a matter of general course, state laws provide plenary authority for the appointing judge to limit or condition the appointment of the guardian or conservator, and the cases are usually classified as probate cases. Probate courts grew out of the English ecclesiastical courts (not the courts of law), and the process thus employed is governed by a history that is different from that applied in most other cases.

Probate cases are often heard by judges who are used to ex parte (unopposed and uncontested) summary proceedings in which the good faith of the attorney appearing before the judge to seek the guardianship is the primary guarantee of the integrity of the process. A lawyer untrained in the unwritten and generally unreported flexibility available in guardianship proceedings can hardly be expected to avoid abuse of the process. A general guardianship requires less of an explanation to the judge than does a limited guardianship and thus is easier to obtain than any alternative. The lawyer for the petitioner generally seeks the general guardianship, and as the three cases illustrate, the appointment of general guardians where limited guardians would be appropriate inevitably poses a danger to the preservation of the autonomy of the ward.

GUARDIANSHIP AND AUTONOMY

The basic practical consequences of the possession of autonomy are clear: autonomy encompasses the right and opportunity to control one's own destiny, to rule one's own life, to be true to the values one has accepted through life. Whether we depend on Dworkin's (1987) seven different meanings of moral independence, Thomasma's (1984) five different types of freedom, Collopy's (1988) six polarities of autonomy, or any other description of what it means to be true to one's soul, it is clear that the guardianship process has the potential to destroy autonomy and the potential to preserve it.

The risk to autonomy through a process that transfers personal authority from one person to another is obvious, as is the potential for enhancing autonomy. When the guardianship process is used to express and execute the interests and values of a person who cannot otherwise express or execute them, it serves the interest of autonomy. When the process is used to veto those interests and values, it undermines autonomy. Does it serve or undermine autonomy in the Blankenschifft, Abbott, and "Worst" cases?

To determine how a guardianship can serve, rather than undercut, autonomy, we ought to investigate (1) when a guardianship is appropriate, (2) what process ought to be applied to provide for a guardianship, and (3) who ought to serve as guardians. Because of the nature of the cases presented, this chapter does not include an analysis of whether a person unable to express his or her own values, interests, and choices ought to be entitled to a guardian as a matter of right.

WHEN IS A GUARDIANSHIP APPROPRIATE?

Defining Incapacity

A guardianship appropriately serves the underlying value of autonomy only when it transfers authority from a ward who cannot exercise that authority to one who can exercise it on behalf of the ward to preserve the interests and values of the ward. Traditionally, the law has defined the ward's "incompetence" as the substantively necessary and sufficient grounds for a guardianship (Uniform Probate Code, 1969, Article V, original version), although more recently most proposed legislation has referred to the ward's "incapacity" (Uniform Guardianship and Protective Proceedings Act, 1982). The law has rarely formally defined incompetence or incapacity, preferring to finesse this essential policy issue for physicians to resolve by accepting (and usually requiring) medical testimony on the competence or capacity of the patient. In fact, medical testimony is generally dispositive of the issue. Determinations of competency for guardianship purposes are treated as legally analogous to determinations of competency to exercise informed consent to (or refusal of) medical care, and, not surprisingly, much of the law of competency now applied in guardianship cases arose in cases involving the informed consent to medical treatment.

Courts' attempts to test for competency have fallen into three categories: (1) tests that ask whether the proposed ward is acting the way other reasonable people (the judge and the doctor, most commonly) would act, (2) tests that ask whether the proposed ward falls into any predetermined categories that are defined by formal measurements of physical or mental health, and (3) tests that focus on the process employed by a proposed ward in making decisions. The first two kinds of tests are now routinely rejected; the first because it poses too great a threat to autonomy by permitting the substitution of the court's values for those of the proposed ward (Office of Technology Assessment, 1987; President's Commission, 1982) and the second because it has proved impossible to define appropriate competency pigeonholes (Stanley, Stanley, Guido, and Garvin, 1988).

If the goal of the guardianship process is to honor the values of the proposed ward, the court should find some functional incapacity before allowing for a surrogate decision maker. In 1982 the President's Commission identified three elements of "decisional capacity," a term that has come to replace "competency" as the description of the relevant characteristic of someone able to make decisions on his or her own behalf.

To possess decisional capacity a person must possess "a set of values and goals," "the ability to communicate and understand information," and "the ability to reason and deliberate about one's choices." (President's Commission, 1982). Because courts are uncomfortable evaluating the first and third of these elements, they therefore concentrate on the medical testimony relevant to the second element; but there is no question that any notion of autonomy would require all three. In fact, the greatest threat to autonomy may come out of the risk that courts will use medical evidence of a proposed ward's ability to understand or act rationally to camouflage a determination that a proposed ward's values are inappropriate.

The Presumption of the Limited Guardianship

If the three-part President's Commission test for decisional capacity is applied with the slightest rigor to the wide range of decisions that are made every day, it becomes apparent that few nursing home residents lack capacity to make every kind of decision. A person may lack the ability to make medical decisions but possess the capacity to make determinations about meals; a person may lack the capacity to manage the finances of a large corporation but still be perfectly capable of deciding what kind of exercise is appropriate, what kind of clothing he or she should wear, and with whom he or she wishes to associate. To the extent that we wish to honor a person's autonomy, that person should be subject to a guardianship only over those subjects in which he or she lacks decisional capacity. The application of this principle would permit the appointment of a general guardian with plenary and unrestricted authority to make decisions for the ward in the rarest of circumstances—it is hard to identify one other than the case of the comatose ward. Thus, guardianships should be limited to those particular kinds of decisions for which wards have been proven incapacitated. Indeed, this was the primary purpose for the promulgation of the Uniform Guardianship and Protective Proceedings Act in 1982. That proposed uniform act provides as follows:

> The Court shall exercise the authority [to appoint a guardian] conferred in this part so as to encourage the development of maximum self reliance and independence of the incapacitated person and make appointive and other orders only to the extent necessitated by the incapacitated person's mental and adaptive limitations or other conditions warranting the procedure. [Sec. 2-206(a)]

Since its promulgation in 1982 only two jurisdictions—the District of Columbia (effective 1987) and Alabama (effective 1988)—have adopted this uniform act, put forth as an improvement on the more widely adopted Uniform Probate Code. Most states retain some traditional form of guardianship process, although a few that have rejected the new uniform act appear to have been substantially affected by its purposes. Nothing would do more to protect the autonomy of nursing home residents than the death of the general guardianship, which is the current mode in guardianship proceedings, and the presumption of a limited guardianship.

"Delegated Autonomy" and Guardians for Those Not Incapacitated

But what of those people who believe that they cannot make wise decisions and, although they are not incompetent, wish to delegate their decision making authority to others? Of course, those people ought to be able to consult with anyone they wish to before making any decision on any issue, and those they consult—family members, for example— may define the universe of practical alternatives and real choices available to them (Dubler, 1988). A person cannot decide to be discharged to a family that will not take him anymore than that person can decide to be discharged to Buckingham Palace. However, the law should not participate with those who lack confidence in their own capacity for wisdom by allowing them to strip themselves of the ultimate authority to make decisions. "Delegated autonomy" (Collopy, 1988) is simply not autonomy, just as the newly popular notion of "negotiated consent" (Moody, 1988) is not voluntary consent. Both delegated autonomy and negotiated consent may serve as appropriate balances between beneficence and autonomy, and they may be socially valuable (and legally appropriate) doctrines, but they weaken rather than strengthen autonomy and thus ought to be suspect in institutions, like nursing homes, that may already limit autonomy.

The Cases

Given this brief analysis, the problems posed by the case studies are really quite easy. Mr. Blankenschifft does not appear to be decisionally incapacitated in any way. Absent some additional evidence that his conduct will place his life or health at risk, and that he wishes to avoid that risk, no judge should grant a general or limited guardianship over Mr. Blankenschifft. Given the standard that must be applied to preserve autonomy, it is hard to imagine what testimony the social worker and administrator could give that would be found relevant by a thoughtful judge.

Similarly, Mrs. Abbott does not appear to lack decisional capacity over the issues in dispute. To the extent the guardianship given to her son is a general guardianship, it would seem to violate the essential principle that one cannot award a general guardianship without proof of universal decisional incapacity. The fact that Mrs. Abbott wanted to have her son handle her money is irrelevant. If she is still capable of deciding whether a color television, a new wheelchair, or physical therapy are appropriate (and worth the cost), autonomy demands that they be her choices, not those of her son. Of course, she may consult her son, but one suspects his advice on selling General Motors is more likely to be accepted than his advice on buying a new television. In any case, both decisions ultimately ought to be his mother's.

The "worst case example" presents the most difficult case for the determination of whether a guardian (of some limited sort) is necessary. We simply do not have the information to determine if Mr. Cohen has the capacity to make a decision on the replacement of his pacemaker. Even if he does not, and a guardian is available to make that decision, it might be appropriate for that guardian to be someone other than the family member who, as guardian for other purposes, has decided where Mr. Cohen should live and what his daily routine ought to be. The matter of who should serve as guardian is discussed below.

In any event, these cases might present the same problem for nursing homes whether or not guardians are formally appointed. Although the nursing home should defer to the patients' own decisions in the absence the appointment of guardians, the institution may depend, de facto if not de jure, on the patients' families as decision makers. Where this is appropriately done—and it is probably substantially overdone now—the institutions ought to deal with the family members the way they would deal with formally appointed guardians. The informal use of family members as surrogate decision makers poses the same potential risks and benefits to the recognition of patient autonomy as does the use of legally appointed guardians—but without the procedural protections attendant upon the appointment of guardians.

WHAT PROCESS OUGHT BE APPLIED WHEN A GUARDIAN IS APPOINTED?

A guardianship process will be more likely to serve the interests of autonomy if the process is designed to recognize the potential risks and benefits that are the inevitable concomitants of a guardianship. Regular abuse of the guardianship process could be avoided by a more formalized and scrupulously followed judicial appointment and review procedure.

As studies indicate (Iris, 1988) and all lawyers know, a typical guardianship case is a procedural horror. Judges routinely engage in ex parte conduct that would be grounds for judicial discipline in cases that are taken seriously (Iris, 1988), and petitioning lawyers generally know how to get exactly what they want from the court—although the tricks of the guardianship counsel trade may vary from state to state. It is not hard to identify ways in which a procedure that is often based on a blink of the eye could be improved. Of course, the procedural suggestions made here should not be taken as evidence of universal disregard for procedural safeguards in guardianship cases. Many of these suggestions are employed by many courts, and some are even formally required (even if generally avoidable) under the Uniform Probate Code—at least in its current form, modified by the Uniform Guardianship and Protective Proceedings Act.

Judges should take guardianship cases seriously and recognize that they may result in the substantial limitation of a person's freedom to act on his own behalf, a limitation analogous to that involved in a civil commitment or criminal case. Judges who impose guardianships should be required to find that a proposed ward does not have decisional capacity to make the kinds of decisions to be granted to the guardian. A general finding of incompetence resulting in a general guardianship should be permitted, if at all, only when the proposed ward is comatose. A procedure that requires a judge to list the powers of the guardian and presumes that those not designated remain in the ward is thus preferable to a procedure that presumes a guardianship is general and plenary unless specifically limited by the judge.

In order to make the kinds of factual findings necessary to impose a guardianship properly, a judge will need better evidence than a physician's affidavit that the patient is incompetent. At the least, any medical evidence on which a judge relies ought to declare the nature and extent of the medical examination, the precise diagnosis and prognosis, and the medical consequences of those findings. The functional disability—the substantive basis for the finding of decisional incapacity—ought to be a conclusion for the judge, not for the expert medical witness. These findings of functional disability ought to be made with precision (and in writing) by any judge who imposes any guardianships. Judges should be as accountable for their orders in guardianship cases as in any others.

For the expert medical evidence to be meaningful, it ought to be presented under oath in open court, not merely by affidavit. No civil commitment proceeding could be conducted without the presence of the expert physician; the history of abuse of that process has demonstrated that the doctor has to be present to ensure the integrity of the process. The history of abuse of the guardianship process may require no less.

Further, for the presence of the testifying physician to be meaningful, there must be an adequate opportunity to examine and cross-examine that witness. This requires a guardian *ad litem* who seriously pursues the articulated interest of the proposed ward. Under most current processes the guardian *ad litem* acts as a court visitor and as a general investigator for the judge, not as an advocate for the expressed wishes of the proposed ward. Although a person's articulated desires may be "inauthentic" (Collopy, 1988), that is precisely what the judge is expected to determine. It short-circuits the process to have this determined, without argument, before the formal judicial process. There is nothing inherently troubling about requiring someone—the guardian *ad litem* seems like the obvious choice—to represent the articulated wishes of the proposed ward. Of course, the judge should also be anxious to hear from all of those likely to have information relevant to the values of the proposed ward, the ability of the proposed ward to understand and communicate information, and the ability of the proposed ward to deliberate and act rationally. This class of potential witness would surely include family, friends, and, for those who have spent substantial time in a nursing home, the nursing home administrators, nurses, and aides. Each of these potential witnesses ought to be given notice of the pending guardianship proceeding.

The guardianship proceeding should not end with the appointment of a guardian. The court maintains jurisdiction to modify the guardianship whenever any interested party requests it, and the judge should require regular review of each case under guardianship, in open court, with all of those with a potential interest in the case notified of the hearing. These review hearings ought to occur regularly, perhaps 30 or 60 days after an appointment of a guardian and every 6 months or so thereafter.

Judges have power to require virtually all of this process now, but they rarely do. Would it be a great imposition on an already overburdened state judiciary? Would it also be a heavy burden on petitioning lawyers, testifying physicians, and nursing homes? It would be, of course, but it would be worth it if we take the value of autonomy seriously. The guardianship process is analogous to the civil commitment process in that each is designed to remove decision-making authority from a person in order to serve, ultimately, that person's autonomy interest.

Conceptually, it is hard to distinguish a judge's order committing a person to a mental hospital from a judge's order appointing a guardian to consent to a person's maintenance at a nursing home. They involve identical intrusions upon a person's constitutionally protected liberty.

Virtually every procedural safeguard described here is now required in civil commitment cases, along with a few others (like a "clear and convincing evidence" standard of proof). Except for legal sloth (lawyers call it "lack of resources"), every safeguard could be offered to proposed wards as well. The legal requirement that these processes be afforded to those who may be civilly committed has given rise to forms of hearings (including special masters and in-hospital hearings) that could be adapted to make guardianship proceedings less burdensome. Although these procedural safeguards do not assure that a guardian will advance the autonomy interests of a person in an appropriate case, they make it less likely that a guardian will effectively veto such interests in a case that is not appropriate for a guardianship.

The consequences of these procedures on the three cases are quite obvious. No adequate procedure would permit Mr. Blankenschifft to become the ward of his son (or anyone else). Similarly, no adequate procedure would have granted Mrs. Abbott's son a plenary guardianship. Further, an adequate process not only would have permitted but would have encouraged (and perhaps required) the nursing home or its representative to be present at guardianship review hearings that could have resulted in the modification of the original guardianship order. Just the threat of the revelation of the son's activities might change his conduct. The "worst case example" would be appropriately handled by a nursing home petition to the court that granted the original guardianship. That petition could seek a modification of any order that would allow the guardian to deny permission for the pacemaker implant. This process is currently available; it is hard to imagine a court that would not take such a petition seriously. Indeed, the failure of the nursing home to bring this abuse of guardianship to the attention of the court might itself be considered abuse of the nursing home resident.

WHO SHOULD BE A GUARDIAN?

When it is appropriate to appoint a guardian, the value of autonomy can be served only if the guardian applies the principles of substituted judgment (not the best-interest standard) whenever possible to make the decisions that the ward, if competent, would make. The entire purpose of the guardianship is to assure that it is the ward's values, not those of the rest of the community, that determine the ward's fate. Thus, the guardian should be the person most likely to understand the values, interests, goals, and wishes of the ward. The guardian should also be a person with no interests that may conflict with the ward's interests. The presumption that family members are appropriate guardians arises out of the assumption that their conflict with the ward (they are often the ward's heirs and have an interest in preserving the estate) is insignificant in comparison with their likely understanding of the values and interests of the ward. Obviously, that assumption sometimes is incorrect, and others (including the nursing home staff in the Abbott and "worst case" examples) should have a chance to prove that.

There is often no family or close friend willing or able to serve as guardian. Ideally, the community should create a pool of altruistic potential guardians who are trained in determining the values and interests of their wards and acting on their findings (Gibson, 1988). It is not easy to discover the lifelong values of a nursing home resident who no longer maintains contact with any friends or family, but it is not impossible either. Trained guardians could learn how to prepare a values history for their wards by researching the interests, background, religious activity, social activity, and similar aspects of the ward's life. These potential guardians could then be appointed and directed to serve the autonomy interests of their wards. In fact, state guardians, state offices on aging, and nonprofit agencies now serve this function in many communities.

Having determined that guardianship is probably inappropriate in the Blankenschifft and Abbott cases, it makes little sense to speculate upon who would be appropriate guardians. Mr. Abbott's financial conflict with the apparent well-being of his mother makes him a suspect candidate though, and there is no evidence that the Blankenschifft son, the Abbott son, and the "worst case" guardian have given any systematic and careful thought to how they might apply substituted judgment to make decisions on behalf of their parents. This absence of any formal analysis of how their guardianships should be carried out is hardly surprising, but it is remediable. Nursing homes or their associations, state agencies, or other institutions could provide some formal training on discovering and applying the values of a ward. This training ought to be available to volunteer guardians unrelated to their wards as well as to family members who wish to understand better how they can apply the doctrine of substituted judgment. Courts tend to prefer trained accountants in complicated conservatorship cases; they ought to prefer trained guardians (or at the very least, guardians willing to be trained) in difficult guardianship cases. Of course, such preferences are likely to remain unfulfilled until guardian training programs are generally available.

PLANNING FOR INCAPACITY

A person foreseeing incapacity may wish to plan for that incapacity. This can be accomplished in different ways, but each requires the selection of a trusted decision maker and the education of that decision maker about the values, interests, beliefs, and desires of the likely incapacitated person (Alexander, 1979). We assume that a lifetime of intimate concern provides that education, and so we assume that family members are generally appropriately educated decision makers for the incapacitated. Of course, individuals may reject particular family members (or all family members) as potential decision makers. Others can be selected to act as surrogates. Ultimately, what is most important is that a person who is likely to become incapacitated inform those likely to be present when important decisions are to be made (other family members, doctors, nursing home administrators, business partners) as to who is to make which decisions and what the substantive bases of those decisions ought to be.

This advance selection may not require a legal component; those affected may feel bound by a clearly and competently articulated desire that some person have decision-making authority upon the incapacity of the one making the statement. In addition, such a statement is likely to be admitted as highly persuasive evidence at a subsequent guardianship proceeding; any judge wishing to use the guardianship process to preserve autonomy would appoint a guardian most likely to exercise substituted judgment for the ward, and thus there often would be a strong presumption in favor of someone previously nominated, formally or informally, by the ward (Uniform Guardianship and Protective Proceedings Act, 1982).

There will be times when a proposed ward will desire that a person with a potential conflict (a child and heir, e.g.) be appointed guardian or that decisions be made serving others' interests (like an heir's interest in the estate) even though it means denying something of apparent value (like nursing home amenities) to the proposed ward. If the desires are competently expressed at the time the guardianship is sought, the expression ought to give rise to careful scrutiny of the need for any guardian at all.

In any case, the doctrine of substituted judgment requires that the court appoint as guardian the person most able to carry out the wishes of the ward. Someone with an apparent conflict may still be better able to serve as guardian than any other potential guardian, but the conflict ought to be one factor in determining the propriety of the appointment. Thus, although the ward's designation will be relevant and persuasive, making it more likely that the court will find that the designee is best able to exercise the decision-making authority of the ward, the proposed ward's designation of a desired guardian will not be dispositive of the issue.

A ward's sincere statement that she would prefer parsimony in expenditures for her benefit in favor of her family members' realization of a larger estate similarly ought to be relevant evidence of how she would act if she were competent to act on her own behalf. It ought to be considered and respected by the guardian, whether a family member or someone else, for what it is worth. Applying the principle of substituted judgment, a guardian for a ward who led a particularly altruistic life ought to make the decision a particularly altruistic person would make.

Finally, a person who is concerned about impending incapacity may execute a durable power of attorney, which appoints an agent (called an attorney-in-fact and bearing no relationship to an attorney-at-law) to act on the principal's behalf. A power of attorney is an especially powerful document because it can include any limitations or conditions on the agent thought appropriate. The agent could be required to consult with particular friends, doctors, or nurses before making a decision or to refrain from making certain kinds of decisions or particular decisions (e.g., "The agent is not authorized to permit or allow my admission to Happytime Long Term Care Facility under any circumstances.")

Traditionally, powers of attorney have expired upon incapacity of the principal. The Uniform Probate Code now allows them to survive incapacity if their language unambiguously provides that (Article V, Sec. 5). Unfortunately, no one knows the limits of the kinds of decisions that can be delegated by a durable power of attorney. Traditionally, they have been used for transactions involving property. At least one court has suggested that they can be used for making health care decisions, and a few state legislatures have promulgated statutes that explicitly provide for such a use of durable powers. They are preferable to guardianships because they are executed while the principal is competent, and they require very little formal process. They are more worrisome than guardianships for just the same reason: there is little process to protect a principal easily coerced in the privacy of a nursing home room.

Mr. Blankenschifft may wish to execute a durable power of attorney or otherwise indicate his wishes and desires while he has the capacity to do so. A discussion of the potential options existing among Mr. Blankenschifft, his son, the social worker, the administrator, the floor nurse, and the DON may result in a well-thought-out and carefully limited durable power or, at the very least, a well-understood sense of how Mr. Blankenschifft wishes to be treated upon his incapacity. Mrs. Abbott would have benefited from the same discussion sometime earlier, whether it resulted in a durable power or merely her public statements about her expectations and desires. Mr. Cohen might have benefited from such a discussion too, especially because the eventual need to replace his pacemaker would have been known long ago and could have been discussed before his incapacity. Ultimately, nursing home residents, families, nursing homes, and medical professionals are better off if the society (perhaps through its long-term-care facilities) encourages (or requires) such general discussions, which are made difficult by the American medical and cultural tradition that permits only talk of recovery and increasing autonomy, not talk of impending deterioration and loss of autonomy (Callahan, 1987).

NURSING HOMES AND THE PRACTICALITIES OF DEALING WITH GUARDIANS

Given the recent development of the law of nursing home administration and the rather rapidly changing law of guardianship, it is not surprising that nursing home administrators and health care workers remain uncertain about the consequences of the appointment of a guardian for a resident and the relationship the health care providers should maintain with a resident-ward and the legally appointed guardian. Nursing home administrators probably do not realize that most lawyers and judges are also uncertain about the complete consequences of the appointment and that this is one of many areas of law where strong minded lawyers may govern through their invocation of the fear that arises from the ambiguity of the law. Despite this, there are some questions to which consensus answers have developed.

Stanley, B., Stanley, M., Guido, J., & Garvin, L. (1988). The functional capacity of elderly at risk. *The Gerontologist, 28* Suppl., 53–58.

Thomasma, D. (1984). Freedom, dependency, and the care of the very old. *Journal of the American Geriatrics Society, 32,* 906–914.

FOR FURTHER DISCUSSION:
EDITORS' QUESTIONS

1. It is conservatively estimated that over half of nursing home residents have some degree of cognitive impairment. However, in most nursing homes, relatively few residents have official guardians or conservators, although they may have an understanding that some relative is managing their affairs. Would it be better if regularized, legal arrangements were organized as a matter of course? For whom would it be better, and why?

2. When is the right time for a legal guardianship or conservatorship to be arranged? Are other options possible? What are the indications for seeking legally approved surrogates, and when might it be premature?

3. Does the facility have an obligation to determine a prospective guardian's motives? When should the client be notified, and how? If the resident agrees to a guardianship, does the facility have any right to raise questions, either at the time or later?

4. What should staff do when they think a guardian, or even a representative payer, is overly reluctant to buy things for the resident? Is the issue different if the purchases are medical rather than social (such as clothing and television)?

5. What should facility staff do if they think the guardian has an inadequate basis for making a decision? When, if ever, should a nursing home initiate reconsideration of the guardianship?

6. Is there any way that people can be better prepared to assume guardianship? Is a test of capability of a guardian feasible?

Chapter 13

LEAVING HOMES: Residents on Their Own Recognizance

GOING TO THE TAVERN

Mr. Birkennen has been at Springsteen Home for 7 months. He carries the diagnosis of alcohol dependency with severe bouts of depression and some history of violence (though the latter has never been exhibited at Springsteen Home). He is also a wheelchair-bound paraplegic who needs help in dressing. At age 67 he is younger than most residents, but the Veterans Administration (VA) social worker who referred him said that he is incapable of living on his own. He divorced his wife when his two children were babies, and during his career in the military they almost never heard from him. His adult children are now not prepared to take him in, though they have an interest in his well-being. The VA pays for Mr. Birkennen's care. Though some of the aides describe him as "owlie" (vernacular for crabby), he doesn't cause much trouble. "He keeps pretty much his own company" is the way nurse's aides describe him.

The one problem with Mr. Birkennen is that he likes to wheel himself on walks around the home's neighborhood. Unfortunately, his walks usually end at the local tavern. When he comes back, there are unmistakable signs on his breath that he has been drinking, although his limited income puts curbs on his consumption. The home has been called several times to retrieve Mr. Birkennen when the bartender believes he cannot go home safely. The administrator, director of nursing, and social worker are becoming concerned that the home will be held liable if Mr. Birkennen should be hurt or if he gets belligerent and hurts others.

Mr. Birkennen's children are firmly against any type of physical restraint. They believe him to be of sound mind and feel that physical restraints would only agitate him.

After discussions with Mr. Birkennen's family and the nursing home staff, the physician has hit on what he considers a wonderful solution to Mr. Birkennen's tavern travels. He noted on the medical chart that Mr. Birkennen should be kept in pajamas and bathrobe all day and that his clothes should be removed from his room. The physician believed that being in a bathrobe would deter Mr. Birkennen from going outside and thus to the tavern. The family does not object because this is not a use of conventional restraints. A staff member who is uncomfortable about this practice anonymously calls the nursing home ombudsman to ask about it.

GOING TO THE COFFEE SHOP

Mr. Olsen also lives at Springsteen Home. He is now 91 years old and has been a resident almost 20 years. He is "spry and witty." He is a favorite with all of the nurses and aides because he is always willing to lend a hand or ear to fellow residents with problems. Ever since his admission, Mr. Olsen has liked to take a daily walk to the small business district four blocks away; he usually ends up at the neighborhood's small coffee shop, the Northstar. In fact, he is considered a regular fixture at the Northstar, where he is well liked.

Over the years Mr. Olsen has become generally more frail. He walks extremely slowly. Lately, too, his eyesight has begun to fail. Even with new glasses, he has major problems with his peripheral and depth vision. Watching him from the nursing home window, the director of nurses has noticed that he sometimes has trouble at the traffic light in front of the home. Either he starts out when it is red, or it is red before he gets across. For all she knows, he may be having problems with other lights, too. She doubts he is capable of distinguishing red from green when the sun glares off the lights. Although no accidents have occurred on his trips to the Northstar, she is beginning to worry about the home's liability if he should be hit by a car. She can't spare personnel to escort him to the Northstar and back and wonders if an order is needed that restricts him to the home. Yet she hates to deprive him of daily excursions that give him so much pleasure. She wonders if it is her obligation to keep him safe. She is also planning to ask the home's lawyer whether warning Mr. Olsen of the danger and having him sign a waiver of liability would get the home off the hook. She is reminded of the solution used in Mr. Birkennen's case, but somehow that just doesn't seem right for Mr. Olsen.

CASE COMMENTARY

Reinhard Priester

The responsibilities of nursing homes include providing nursing care and such personal services as might be required for the health, safety, good grooming, and well-being of the residents. As these two cases illustrate, it may sometimes be necessary for the nursing home to institute rules and regulations or make decisions that restrict residents' freedom and independence in order to protect them—as well as to protect the institution's interests. Springsteen Home is worried about its liability should Mr. Birkennen or Mr. Olsen injure himself or others while on trips outside the home. It is also concerned—more so in Mr. Olsen's case—about making a decision respectful of residents' freedom. A review of the ethical and legal issues raised will illuminate what would be appropriate responses to Mr. Birkennen's and Mr. Olsen's disquieting sojourns. Since the home has already reached a decision for Mr. Birkennen, his case will be the primary focus of this commentary.

DECIDING THE CASES

Since his arrival at Springsteen Home, Mr. Birkennen has frequently wheeled himself to the local tavern and has harmed no one on these excursions. Nor has he exhibited any violence since coming to the home, despite a record of such behavior. Is the home then correct, out of concern for its liability, to stop Mr. Birkennen from visiting the tavern by confining him to the home in his pajamas and bathrobe and hiding his clothes? Clearly, no: This is the wrong decision, for the wrong reasons, using the wrong process.

The Wrong Decision

Entering a nursing home strips an individual of much personal autonomy (Jameton, 1988). Residents are bound to follow a set of institutional rules and customs; they frequently need assistance with activities of daily living and are generally dependent on the staff. A complete restoration of their mental and physical abilities is often no longer possible; thus, nonmedical goals, such as maintaining independence, become more important. As the "Appropriate Autonomy in Everyday Life in Nursing Homes" project demonstrates, everyday events—not the dramatic medical decisions such as terminating life-sustaining treatment—comprise the majority of residents' concerns about autonomy. Furthermore, for the elderly, particularly those with physical limitations, the outward reaches of autonomy shrink: shaping long-range goals becomes less important than managing the short-term or day-to-day aspects of life (Collopy, 1988).

Residents are entitled to the maximum self-determination and dignity possible. Springsteen Home's "wonderful solution to Mr. Birkennen's tavern travels" clearly does not maximize his self-determination; rather, it severely and unnecessarily restricts his freedom to determine how he will spend his days. An alternative, less restrictive of Mr. Birkennen's autonomy, may provide a better balance between his interests and the home's. The doctrine of "least restrictive alternative" has been used by American courts in a number of branches of the law, including recent application to the law dealing with the rights of the mentally handicapped. For the care of the mentally ill, the doctrine requires that, to the extent possible, those providing care must not unnecessarily infringe on their patients' liberty. Deprivations of liberty solely because of dangers to the ill persons themselves must not be beyond what is necessary for their protection.

In general, the doctrine of least restrictive alternative offers a means to reconcile the conflicting interests at stake. Although the doctrine does not dictate any particular response, it directs the decision maker to make decisions that are least restrictive of individual freedom and most appropriate under the circumstance.

For Mr. Birkennen and Mr. Olsen, least restrictive alternative analysis requires balancing the home's interests in minimizing its potential for liability versus the residents' interests in maximizing their autonomy. The decision made must be least restrictive of Mr. Birkennen's and Mr. Olsen's freedom and independence. Confining the men to the home is an extreme option. Many other alternatives exist; for example, the home could restrict their excursions to days when a staff member of volunteer from the community could accompany them. Or there may be other residents, less frail than Mr. Olsen and more responsible than Mr. Birkennen, who could accompany them. Solitary excursions could then be denied. Or the home could make an agreement with Mr. Birkennen and the tavern regarding the number of drinks served on an outing. To maximize Mr. Birkennen's and Mr. Olsen's autonomy and yet minimize its risk of liability, the home should explore these and other less restrictive alternatives.

Similarly, Springsteen Home and the residents, through a process of give-and-take discussion, could work toward a compromise, that is, "a position that more or less 'splits the difference' between two opposing positions" (see Benjamin, this volume). Searching for either a compromise or least restrictive alternative would not necessarily lead to the same decision, but both procedures require the nursing home to achieve decisions respectful of the resident's autonomy.

The home's special dress order for Mr. Birkennen exhibits a marked disrespect for his dignity. Forcing an ambulatory resident to remain in his pajamas and bathrobe all day is insulting, degrading, and embarrassing—to the resident and to others. It also unfairly preys on Mr. Birkennen's inability to dress himself. Furthermore, clothes are an important statement of individuality; they provide identity and help define a person. Hiding Mr. Birkennen's clothing robs him of this expression of individuality.

Finally, the dress order is not a decision without risks of harm to the resident. It imposes the sick role on Mr. Birkennen and may be expected to result in depression, greater passivity, and adverse effects on his health. These risks must be considered in a decision regarding Mr. Birkennen's care.

The Wrong Reasons

The primary goal of health care, whether in an acute-, ambulatory-, or long-term-care facility, is to benefit the patient. Decisions regarding care of nursing home residents should be guided by the residents' needs, not the home's interests. Springsteen Home's concern about its liability is an invalid reason for restricting Mr. Birkennen to the home. However, restriction might be appropriate if the probability of significant harm is much greater than in Mr. Birkennen's case. The risk of harm under present circumstances is extremely vague.

The home's concern for Mr. Birkennen's safety is an alternative justification for restricting him to the home. But this would be tantamount to the home deciding the restriction is in Mr. Birkennen's best interest. Ordinarily, an individual is assumed to be the best judge of his or her own interests. For someone who lacks the capacity to determine his or her own interests, parents, physicians, or some other decision maker must decide that person's interests. Unless Mr. Birkennen is shown to lack such capacity, the principle of autonomy requires his—not the home's—determination of his interests to take precedence (Buchanen, 1981). The home's concern for his safety, however well intentioned, would therefore also be an invalid reason for restricting him to the home.

Treating Mr. Birkennen's alcoholism may, however, be a more legitimate reason for confining him to the home. Insofar as possible, a nursing home should provide for a resident's health care needs. If the home
is treating Mr. Birkennen for his alcohol dependency and restricting
him to the home is part of the treatment regimen, then confinement to
the home is perhaps appropriate, although the "special dress order"
would remain an inappropriate means. Encouraging, cajoling, or per-
suading Mr. Birkennen to stop his trips to the tavern out of fear of the
home's liability for injuries rests on shakier ethical ground than confinement to the home as a necessary part of his alcoholism treatment.
Of course, Mr. Birkennen retains the right to refuse this and any other
form of medical treatment.

The Wrong Process

The decision to limit Mr. Birkennen's mobility, and the contemplated
decisions, clearly concern his health and safety. Thus, the decision-
making process should be the same as for other medical care decisions.
From this perspective, the home's decision-making process was flawed
because it excluded Mr. Birkennen. Respecting individual autonomy in a
nursing home—that is, protecting a resident against unwanted restrictions on liberty and permitting self-determination—requires that the
resident be involved in and give consent to decisions regarding care. The
physician consulted with the family and the nursing staff before deciding on the special dress order. (It may be argued that Mr. Birkennen's
family enabled his alcoholism, and therefore their role in his treatment
should be appropriately circumscribed.) But the physician failed to involve Mr. Birkennen in the decision or obtain his consent, thus violating
his autonomy. And the physician's continued failure to inform him of
the reasons for the special dress order compounds this violation.

The physician's obligation to include the resident could be overridden
if the resident were incompetent. Although Mr. Birkennen is an alcoholic
with a history of severe bouts of depression, he is not incompetent. All
individuals are presumed competent to make decisions affecting their
health as well as other aspects of their lives until proven otherwise. To
overcome this presumption requires a clear showing of the individual's
lack of decision-making ability. In a medical context, an individual is
incompetent if he or she lacks the capacity to understand and appreciate
the information needed to give informed consent or informed refusal to
the treatment or care under consideration. Since there is no indication
that Mr. Birkennen currently lacks such capacity, he should have been
included in the decision confining him to the home.

Similarly, if the home seeks to restrict Mr. Olsen's walks, he must be included in the decision-making process. Though physically frail, Mr. Olsen remains spry and witty, with no indication that he lacks the capacity to make decisions regarding his health.

APPLICABLE LAW

In addition to these ethical considerations, the obligations of a nursing home to provide for the safety of its residents are also determined by applicable law. As a general rule, a nursing home has the duty to exercise reasonable care toward residents and third parties and may be negligent for failure to do so (Protecting, 1985). A nursing home may be liable for damages if (1) the nursing home owed a duty of care to the plaintiff, (2) the nursing home failed to fulfill this duty, (3) the plaintiff was injured, and (4) the nursing home's failure to fulfill its duty was the proximate cause of the plaintiff's injuries.

The courts have emphasized that a nursing home, although not an insurer, has a duty to exercise for the benefit of its patients such reasonable care for and attention to their safety as their mental and physical conditions, if known, may require, to the extent that such physical or mental ailments render them unable to look after their own safety (83 ALR 3d 871). Thus, the duty of a nursing home to exercise reasonable care varies in proportion to residents' ability to look after their own safety. The nursing home must guard only against hazards that a reasonable person would foresee.

These common law duties of a nursing home may be affected by statute, ordinance, or regulations. Rules and regulations of a state's department of health relating to nursing homes, for example, may articulate a standard of reasonable care that should be adhered to. Similarly, if a nursing home participates in Medicare and Medicaid, as the majority do, or accepts VA patients (as in this situation), it is subject to federal regulations governing virtually all aspects of nursing home activity.

Three cases in which nursing homes were found liable for failure to adequately supervise or observe residents help clarify the applicable standard of care. In *Junke v. Evangelical Lutheran Good Samaritan Hospital*[1] one resident—known to frequently "wander around the nursing home and in the rooms of other residents, pushing, tripping, and hurting others" and generally to be very belligerent—pushed another resident and caused her serious injuries. In finding the nursing home liable, the court

[1] 634 P 2d 1132 (Kan. App. 1981).

noted that the resident was injured while at the nursing home and, more important, that the nursing home knew of the propensity of the other resident to be belligerent and violent.

In *Golden Villa Nursing Home, Inc. v. Smith*[2] a resident wandered off the grounds through an unlocked gate, darted onto the highway adjacent to the nursing home, and collided with a motorcycle. A long-time resident, 68 years old, she had been diagnosed as suffering from an "increasing state of confusion and an increased tendency to wander." In finding the nursing home liable for injuries sustained by both the resident and the motorcyclist, the court similarly stressed the home's knowledge of the resident's tendency to wander.

Finally, in *Bezark v. Kostner Manor Inc.*[3] a nursing home was found liable when it failed to protect a resident against assault by a fellow resident, who was known to have been frequently intoxicated on the premises and to have been quarrelsome when intoxicated.

These cases indicate that Springsteen Home is justifiably concerned about possible liability for harm Mr. Birkennen or Mr. Olsen may suffer or cause to another person. The home is aware that both Mr. Birkennen and Mr. Olsen habitually take trips into the home's surrounding neighborhood. The home's staff has personally witnessed Mr. Olsen's difficulty in crossing busy streets and has retrieved Mr. Birkennen from the tavern when it was feared he could not come home safely. In light of their particular mental and physical conditions—and the home's knowledge of their tendency to wander—the home must exercise a higher level of care.

The potential for harm is easily foreseen. Mr. Birkennen, 67 years old, alcohol dependent, and confined to a wheelchair, is in danger of harm when he must negotiate his way back to the nursing home alone after drinking at the local tavern, a danger clearly foreseen by the bartender. Similarly, Mr. Olsen, 91 years old and physically frail, must cross several busy streets on his daily walk to the coffee shop. That Mr. Olsen may be hit by a car or suffer some other accident can reasonably be foreseen, as indicated by the director of nurses' concern. To reduce the risk of liability, therefore, the home should take steps to assure Mr. Birkennen's and Mr. Olsen's safety.

The home is also exploring whether a "a waiver of liability" signed by Mr. Olsen would "get [it] off the hook." A waiver in this circumstance amounts to an assumption of risk by Mr. Olsen, which the home could then raise as a defense if Mr. Olsen is injured and sues the home for negligence. An assumption of risk requires that the plaintiff understand

[2] 674 SW 2d 343 (Tex. App. 14 Dist. 1984).
[3] 172 NE 2d 424, 29 III App. 2d 106 (1961).

the nature of the risk and voluntarily choose to subject himself to the risk. It may be difficult for the home to assure Mr. Olsen's understanding and voluntariness in this situation. Moreover, even if Mr. Olsen's assumption of risk is proven, it may only diminish his recovery, not absolve the home from liability altogether.

CONCLUSION

Springsteen Home is faced with difficult decisions in the care of Mr. Birkennen and Mr. Olsen. The excursions fulfill a number of the residents' social, emotional, and psychological needs. Equally valued alternatives may be difficult to find. However, to assure the health and safety of its residents, the home must take appropriate action, guided by legal and ethical considerations. Although law and ethics in this situation do not conflict, they exhibit a tension that must be reconciled. The law related to nursing home liability for injuries suffered by its residents clearly suggests that Springsteen Home should take action to restrict Mr. Birkennen's and Mr. Olsen's mobility. On the other hand, ethical considerations require their autonomy to be maximized, with due recognition of competing goals such as the residents' safety and best medical interests. As suggested, the legal doctrine of least restrictive alternatives should be used to reconcile this tension. The doctrine requires balancing the competing interests of the home and the residents and formulating a decision least restrictive of the residents' individual freedom. And regardless of the ultimate decision reached, unless Mr. Birkennen and Mr. Olsen are deemed incompetent, they must be included in the decision-making process.

REFERENCES

Buchanen, A. E. (1981). Medical paternalism. In M. Cohen, T. Nagel, & T. Scanlon (Eds.), *Medicine and moral philosophy.* Princeton, NJ; Princeton University Press.

Collopy, B. J. (1988). Autonomy in long-term care: Some crucial distinctions. *The Gerontologist, 28* (Suppl.), 10–18.

Jameton, A. (1988). In the borderlands of autonomy: Responsibility in long term care facilities. *The Gerontologist, 28* (Suppl.), 18–24.

Patient tort liability of rest, convalescent, or nursing homes, 83 ALR3d 871.

Protecting nursing home patients. (1985). *Trial, 21,* 54.

FOR MOTHER'S OWN PROTECTION

Restraints have recently been prescribed for Mrs. Harper. Her balance is so poor that she needs them to sit safely in her wheelchair. She begs the nurse's aide not to apply them. The nurse's aide doesn't much like using restraints herself. She thinks they are justified for safety "when they are for the patient's own good" (such as in the case of Mrs. Harper) but not when they are just to make it easier for staff to get their work done. Mrs. Harper says she would rather take the chance and fall than be tied up, but her family does not feel this way. They want Mother to be protected and have said so.

OVER A DAUGHTER'S OBJECTIONS

The situation is almost the opposite with Mrs. Jackson and her daughter. The daughter comes and reads the riot act whenever her mother is tied. Mrs. Jackson is somewhat confused, and her balance is poor. Mrs. Jackson's daughter is aware that her mother could fall and hurt herself but can't bear to see her restrained. She thinks her mother would prefer to take her chances. So far, the facility has allowed the daughter to call the shots.

THE HOUDINI

Mr. Ellwood, an obstreperous man with fairly advanced dementia, is restrained in bed at night. He wears mitts so that he will not scratch himself, and he is tied into the bed. He is almost a "Houdini" in his ability to worm out of the restraints, which he clearly does not like. The nurses justify this to themselves by saying, "What are we to do? He really isn't safe. Would it be better to medicate him?"

THE LIBERATOR

Mr. Andrews is a nice gentleman, somewhat confused but really almost no trouble at all, except for one personal quirk. He wanders around releasing the restraints on other people. As the DON says, with a wry smile,

"He's our regular liberator." Mr. Andrews seems upset to see people tied up, especially if they are begging to be released. Although everyone likes Mr. Andrews, the problem is getting severe. The staff are considering whether Mr. Andrews should himself be in a Geri-chair.

CASE COMMENTARY

Andrew Jameton

In discussing this series of cases on physical restraints, it is best to begin with what we know. The main thing we are sure of is that there is and should be a strong ethical presumption against using restraints. Nevertheless, this presumption can be overridden; good reasons for using restraints can be offered. Since avoiding restraints is ethically important, the reasons for using them must be well defined, limited, and serious enough to outweigh our initial presumption.

Why should we make this initial judgment against restraints? First, we favor a basic liberty of action. People want their hands free and their feet unbound; they want to be able to stand up and sit down at will. Almost anyone who experiences such limitations finds them eventually burdensome; those who prefer being physically restrained for long periods without reasons are subject to the label of mental illness. We are talking here of elemental liberty. We are not talking of liberty of social choice or the exercise of personal judgment. The phrase "least restrictive alternative" used in nursing homes does not fully convey this sense of basic bodily choice.

The activities restricted by physical restraints are so basic that we cannot easily distinguish between (a) the ability to engage in the activities and (b) the ability to make choices about engaging in them. Normally, the former is treated more as a matter of physical competence; the latter, of mental competence. But in regard to activities like walking, sitting, standing, and stooping, the two competencies merge. To be physically restrained is to be both incompetent and unable to make choices.

Second, bonds increase a person's vulnerability to neglect, harm, and exploitation. Since bonds restrict an important dimension of activity, they restrict the ability of residents to protect themselves; indeed, restraints occasionally strangle residents. For these reasons, my grandfather advised me many years ago when I played cowboys and Indians, "Never let anybody tie you up." Mr. Meineki's case describes an incident where his confinement to a wheelchair provided an opportunity for abuse: "Mrs. Meineki comes for her usual daily visit, finds her husband's chair, along with two other chairs, tied to a railing near the nurses' station."

Last, physical restraint is one method among many that may deal more or less well with the problem at hand in comparison to alternatives. Simple changes in the structure of the environment might obviate a problem attributed wrongly to the resident. One example of environmental change to resolve a problem is that of a resident who tended to wander into other rooms when walking to the bathroom at night; he also was in danger of falling. Restraints were considered, but instead, the supervising nurse made several changes: She lowered the bed, installed a nightlight, placed a commode by the bed, and arranged teaching on how to get in and out of bed safely.

A resident in danger is often in danger due to the environment. In many cases of a perceived need for restraints, corresponding environmental changes can be found to obviate the problem. Architectural ingenuity is thus called for in designing homes, rooms, hallways, and equipment to reduce the need for restraints.

The possibility of using restraints ethically arises partly from the ambiguities of personal power and partly from the multidimensional nature of human liberty. For instance, it is by no means impossible for a person who suffers physical limitations to exercise unrestricted personal or social power; Franklin Roosevelt stands as an excellent symbol for this. Similarly, restraints can support an individual's interests and thereby support personal autonomy. Seat belts make a good comparison to restraints. Although they hinder motion in a car, this hindrance actually serves choices to protect life and health. To consider another example, sane mountain climbers prefer being bound to one another for safety on steep faces. Insofar as restraints actually increase the opportunity of a person to be involved in activities, they can serve personal liberty and mature choices.

Dimensions of personal choice are involved in the decision to begin using restraints and in decisions to put them on and take them off. Because people in cars can put their belts on and take them off at will, their restraints are more clearly voluntary than in the Ulysses situation, where a person chooses to be bound but cannot choose at will to be unbound again. And the Ulysses situation involves more autonomy than that of the resident who has no choices at all.

Consider a nursing home example. Residents sometimes sit in Geri-chairs. These chairs act as restraints because of the table across the lap. However, residents sometimes slump so badly in these chairs that it would be helpful to tie a restraint at their waists to keep them from sliding down in the chair. A legal view of this second restraint would see it as a double restraint and therefore much more restrictive. But it could be argued that the restraint would be a comfort and convenience to the resident as well as to staff. Such a device would thus extend liberty.

Aides and nurses in nursing homes have characterized some restraints as reminders to residents to call for help or to use support in walking, rather than as a means of preventing moving about. If this is indeed the case, restraints should be more often designed like seat belts so that they can be removed by the resident without assistance. Franklin Roosevelt doubtless had ready help available when he needed assistance; if such assistance were as readily available to nursing home residents, physical restraints would be barely restrictive at all.

In a nursing home it is often difficult to sort out the level of voluntariness involved in residents' decisions. This is in part because of the background of involuntary admission, physical and mental limitations of residents, and professional domination over the rules and activities of life in the home. Paralysis from polio restrains without human choice or purpose. Socially imposed restraints constitute an intermediate range between purely voluntary and totally involuntary, meaningless restraints.

The degree of voluntariness experienced with socially imposed physical restraints may vary. A resident may negotiate with nurses and physicians to choose a restraint he or she can control. Or the resident may be tied down against his or her will and struggle ceaselessly for release, like Mr. Ellwood, who "is almost like a 'Houdini' in his ability to worm out of the restraints." A key question, then, is whether a particular use of restraints supports the resident's choices, wishes to engage in activity, and participation in the social life of the nursing home or represents a further restriction, even if necessary, of the resident's desired modes of daily living.

Bonds chafe, need adjustment, and create work and inconvenience for staff. A resident who previously could walk up and down the hall, use the bathroom, or get in and out of bed unattended will now need to use a call button. Although the nurse in Mrs. Harper's case suggests that "They . . . make it easier for staff to get their work done," restraints save time only when the staff neglects prompt attention to residents' needs while they are tied up. The trouble that the staff suffers in avoiding restraints is the trouble primarily of ingenuity rather than raw time and labor. Restraints sometimes ease staff work by easing neglect of residents. Thus, assistance to staff is a poor justification for the use of restraints.

It can be argued that restraints can save time by helping aides use time efficiently, as in the case of residents tied during the morning breakfast rush and then tended to during less busy hours. But if we take the ethical presumption against restraints seriously, this is not a good enough reason for using restraints. Restraints should be confined to cases of dangerousness to self or others; homes where restraints are needed to get daily jobs done are understaffed homes.

Careful problem analysis is needed to make the judgment to use restraints. Moreover, use of restraints takes place over time and is subject to
constant reassessment. A decision to spurn restraints is open to the use of
restraints later; the use of restraints is an occasion to learn from their
effects and to consider revisions.

FACTORS IN DECIDING TO RESTRAIN

The ongoing judgment to use or avoid restraints thus involves a number
of factors balanced against the background of the presumption against
using them. The following are major factors to consider:

1. Danger to others, its frequency and intensity.
2. Danger to self, its frequency and intensity.
3. Wishes of the resident.
4. Mental competence of the resident.
5. Comfort of the resident with the restraints.
6. Wishes of the family.

Danger to Others

Ordinarily, ethical decisions in the nursing home should be modeled on
similar decisions made in the world at large. In that model, restrictions on
liberty are severely limited and often require judicial procedures; indeed,
the government limits and regulates the use of restraints in nursing homes.
The reasons for using restraints are also similar to those in the outside
world. Danger to others is the major accepted ground for involuntary limitations on activity. Danger needs definition, however. When Mr. Meineki
is described as "belligerent" and "abusive," we don't know if he is actually
dangerous; but when he is described as "strik[ing] out at other residents
with his hands and with his cane," we become concerned with the safety
of others. We will also want to ask how often this occurs; one spectacular
incident can be turned, like legend, into a permanent character trait.

If we believe the story, he can use a lighter cane, and he may still be
dangerous. He can be confined to his room, but he then faces prison-like
restrictions. He cannot be told not to strike at others or be meaningfully
punished because he is demented. In daily life, if a person is dangerous to
others, we do not require that they consent to restrictions; we are entitled
to demand restrictions without consent. There may well be other ways to
cope with the problem (what sets him off?), but if we cannot solve the
problem with less imposition on him, his consent is not ordinarily needed

and the justification for restraints is of the right kind. Danger to others is thus the most important reason for considering restraints.

Danger to Self

This is the second classic justification for restrictions on the activities of people. This is the issue in the cases of Mrs. Harper, Mrs. Jackson, and Mr. Ellwood. The first two have poor balance; Mr. Ellwood scratches himself. Because people reside in nursing homes partly for their protection and because nurses and aides have a justified responsibility to protect residents, danger to self is a good reason for considering restraints. At the same time, it is the reason most likely to run amok.

It is important to distinguish those cases in which the protectiveness of restraints actually serves a resident's autonomy and aids a resident in getting about the home from those cases in which restraints involve significant additional sacrifices. It would be perfectly reasonable to permit a level of risk in order to maintain significant liberties for a patient, just as we permit people in every walk of life to take risks in order to conduct activities they regard as worthwhile.

What the staff often believes to be the law—that they are required to protect residents—is best seen as a construct of their own consciences: They would feel responsible if one of the residents fell down. They would have trouble facing the family and telling them they did not protect this vulnerable person. If it happens on their turf and on their shift, it is their responsibility. This view may indeed represent an overextension of the concept of professional responsibility, but the nursing home environment is sufficiently restrictive that it can be rightly said that the staff maintains substantial control over their residents' lives. Whatever choices residents make, the staff retains some responsibility for the safety of residents. The problem of judgment is to draw the line between too much responsibility and too little in the nursing home context.

As in the case of danger to others, we must be concerned with the concrete story: How bad are Mrs. Harper's and Mrs. Jackson's problems of balance? Why are Mr. Ellwood's fingernails not being kept well trimmed? Danger to self is the second legitimate reason for using restraints, depending on the seriousness of the risk, alternatives, effectiveness, drawbacks, and so on.

Wishes of the Resident

Since protection of residents is an important function of nursing homes, nursing homes are essentially paternalistic in their purpose. We must sooner or later come to the key issue of the conflict between the resident's wishes and staff perception of their safety or the safety of others.

The nursing home is a context in which a strong antipaternalist philosophical line sounds specious; it must be understood how the closeness of life there makes it difficult to distinguish self-protection from protection of others and how difficult it is to see a physically and mentally vulnerable resident as someone fully capable of clear choices on these issues.

The resolution of disagreement does not lie in determining who is to decide nor in negotiating exchanges regarding other matters (e.g., "We will let you smoke if you wear this restraint"); instead, it requires a careful examination of the reasons on both sides. The party to a dispute with the soundest position should carry the day. Since Mrs. Harper is able to refuse restraints, she may also be able to discuss their pros and cons. If she cannot address the matter fully, a careful analysis of her activities and needs, her ability to balance, and the actual availability of assistance can help in making a judgment. If the question is one of danger to self rather than danger to others, residents should have more scope for choice, because residents have more responsibility not to harm other residents than not to harm themselves. It is important to remember that safety is not the only or paramount value. If restraints greatly hinder activities important to the resident, safety can be sacrificed to protect other values.

If a resident requested the use of restraints in a situation in which the staff felt they were not needed for safety, should they be used? In the introductory discussion we considered cases in which the use of restraints actually extended a person's activities. If the resident is correct and restraints would help in this way, this would be a good reason for considering restraints.

Mental Competence

The mental competence of the resident seems to be the most common problem around which questions of residents' wishes revolve in a nursing home. Even though most residents are seen as being deficient in mental competency, no extensive efforts are made to maintain competency or to assist residents in making considered decisions. The wishes of residents who appear mentally deficient receive less serious consideration, although specific incompetencies would affect different decisions differently. It is difficult in nursing homes to sort out the legitimate from the illegitimate judgments in this continuum of human deterioration.

Mrs. Harper has poor balance but is able to express her wishes clearly. Mrs. Jackson is described as "somewhat confused," a condition that may affect both her ability to make decisions about restraints and to keep her balance. Mr. Ellwood suffers from advanced dementia but is still described as "an obstreperous man," as though it were a character trait. Indeed, character traits of residents are often swept into linguistic corners of the diminutive and disrespectful, which also diminish the power of residents to engage according to their wishes. Mr. Andrews, for instance, is described as "a nice gentleman" with a "quirk" of releasing residents from restraints; at 40, he might have been described as "a warm man dedicated to human liberty."

Declining mental competence combines with other untoward physical changes associated with aging to decrease respect for the resident in the eyes of others, thus opening residents to the risk being degraded by restraints. Let us make it clear: Lack of mental competence is never by itself a reason for use of restraints, and the specific need of restraints should be sorted out from any general demeaning of residents. Restraint *is* a relevant consideration if lack of mental competence and lack of balance synergistically combine to increase risk; if mental competence so affects judgment that a resident, perfectly capable of walking, may wander off into the horizon and danger; or if the resident refuses restraints but appears not to appreciate the risks because of mental confusion. Indeed, the nature of restraints is such that they are more appropriate when the resident cannot be educated, persuaded, or reminded by more rational means.

Mr. Andrews is an important case in point. He is the "liberator" of restrained residents. Despite the demeaning description of his character, he appears to be mentally competent. If the residents he liberates actually need restraints, his judgment is poor. He appears to me to be precisely the nursing home model of the criminal in the outer world. His conduct, as behavior deliberately risky to others, requires treatment by persuasion, authority, punishment, or firing from the home. We do not tie up people because they misbehave but because in their helplessness they may do harm that they would not wish to do were they able to avoid it.

The quickness of the home to respond to Mr. Andrews with restraints indicates the extent to which the concept of responsibility has been medicalized in nursing homes. Decisions to restrain are made by the physician with the advice of nursing staff, aides, residents, and families. These decisions place the physician—not a judge, administrator, or jury —in the position of making decisions to limit liberty. Such decisions make sense where liberty is being restricted because the impetus for the problem is medical in nature and the response to it is also appropriately medical. However, restraints exist in a gray zone between issues of medicine and issues of social liberty. Mr. Andrews's behavior, as described, has not been diagnosed as illness; it is perhaps antisocial, perhaps political rebellion, perhaps the humane act of a deeply committed man. Although his problems may ultimately be medical, we should not classify them immediately as such, nor should all problem conduct in a nursing home be viewed through medical spectacles.

Decisions to restrain a resident for a significant period ought involve a review by a committee process that mixes professional and resident representatives. Such committees should work under policies making the sorts of distinctions about responsibility and dignity that I am struggling to express here. Such committees would provide the opportunity to regulate the tension between collective governance of the institution and the medical services that residents receive.

Resident Comfort

Nothing is more pitiful than to see a person struggling helplessly against bonds that are seen as necessary. Indeed, discomfort is a good reason for not using restraints and considering other alternatives. Mr. Ellwood's case is a good one; he struggles in his restraints every night and often manages to worm out of them, with the result that they both cause him discomfort and do not work; indeed, the nurses are considering medication as an option. Moreover, Mr. Ellwood is too demented to express his wishes verbally. A useful maxim is that the greater the mental deficiency, the more important observed comfort is in considering the use of restraints. A person who is competent and says she does not want the restraints, even though she appears comfortable, must be taken seriously; and an uncomfortable, competent person who says that she wants restraints must also be taken seriously. In the absence of expressed wishes, observed discomfort is key.

"Chemical restraints" is a misnomer, because medications are global in their effects and act in so many different ways. Some medications improve functioning, and others cause it to deteriorate, depending on the resident and the medication. Recent reports indicate excessive use of sedation to simplify management in nursing homes; therefore, they should be approached with extreme caution. Careful observation of the resident's overall condition is thus important in the use of both medication and physical restraints.

The Wishes of the Family

The role of family wishes depends on how we view the relationship of the family to the resident. The autonomy model sees the family primarily as the agent of the resident. We want to know what the family believes to be the resident's wishes and interest; the family's wishes and interests are clearly secondary. This model is operative in Mrs. Jackson's case.

Mrs. Jackson is confused, and we want to know what she would want. Her daughter can tell us something of her wishes: "[My] mother," says the daughter, "would prefer to take her chances." This model contrasts with the view of many nursing homes, especially those where families pay the bill: The resident is being kept in the home on behalf of the family; it provides care for the resident in the place of the family and acts primarily as the family's agent.

In its extreme form, the latter model might be termed a "veterinary" model because the resident has little standing as a person. The function of the home may be to assuage the conscience of the family and to reduce inconvenience to them; as a bonus, it can provide a parent, spouse, or sibling in good enough shape to be entertaining during brief visits.

Unfortunately, the autonomy model also has its defects in its extreme; families share mutual responsibilities and interpretations of life that require mutual consideration. Insofar as possible, decisions should involve both residents and their families. Thus, families are entitled to participate in the decision process: Mrs. Meineki, for instance, "feels that it [restraining her husband] is wrong, but doesn't know what choices she may have." It should be made clear to her that she is needed in the decision process. Mrs. Harper's family "wants mother to be protected" although Mrs. Harper "begs the nurse's aide not to apply them." The family and resident thus disagree; it would be appropriate for the staff to support family and resident in coming to an agreement on the issue. In the absence of agreement, the staff still has much room in which to exercise their own judgment. If the most reasonable position cannot be mutually discovered, the bottom line should be to follow the recent philosophy of the rights of the individual and to rely on the resident's wishes over those of the family.

WEIGHING THE FACTORS

These factors all interrelate in the process of judgment. Each factor by itself identifies a topic for discussion. By discussing each topic, one learns what weight to give to each factor in making judgments. No case or factor stands alone; instead, the range of cases studied shapes our estimate of the relevant considerations. The decisions we make on a range of cases indicates which factors we regard as more important and tell us how we see them as interrelated. We are engaged here in the moral enterprise termed "casuistry," the study of cases.

There are limitations to casuistry, however. The range of cases appears to cover those that were perceived by nursing home staff as genuinely problematic. In the first place, it would also be productive to obtain cases from others: from residents, families, and the observer collecting cases: What did the observer, from an outside perspective, perceive as problematic?

In the second place, no nonproblematic cases were offered. For clarification of concepts, it is also helpful to study cases in which the moral judgment to restrain the resident is clearly correct.

Also missing are cases problematic in another sense: the sorry tales of corruption and mishandling that inspired regulations restricting the use of restraints a decade ago. Have such abuses ceased? Do the problematic cases before us represent genuine moral confusion or borderline cases of practices that verge on the corrupt? Also missing are the cases that function as moral lessons or illustrations: the story of the old woman left unbound who wandered out into the street and was struck by a passing truck, or the contrasting parable of the old man strangled by his bonds when he slipped out of bed in spite of his restraints.

Missing too are the philosophical cases, the cases that press the conceptual analysis into the margins of the impossible: What if we had a drug without side effects that would paralyze the arms of Mr. Ellwood, who scratched himself at night? What if we could install a small telecommunications port residents so that their walking paths could be programmed from the nursing station? What if we had a mind-reading machine so that we could tell, by placing it against the head, what the resident really wants even when he or she is demented? What if Mr. Meineki, now restrained, can be expected to live 100 more years and thus may be kept in bonds a century? Such cases can be generated to stretch and test the moral conceptions being used to analyze the cases. Some of these speculations also may suggest useful technological innovations for limiting dangerous activity in safer, more focused ways that do not hinder resident autonomy as much as do older techniques. Most important, such cases and ideas should not be considered only to resolve ethics puzzles; they should also aid in establishing more dignified and humane forms of care for older adults with debilitating conditions.

FOR FURTHER DISCUSSION:
EDITORS' QUESTIONS

1. What procedures should be developed for the use of restraints in a nursing home?

2. What informed consent procedures should prevail?
3. When may a resident refuse restraints?
4. How should competency determinations influence resident consent procedures?
5. Does the patient's surrogate have the right to refuse or consent? In general, what role should family or surrogates have in decisions about restraints?
6. What is the proper role of other residents?
7. Once a restraint is initiated, what should be the considerations to terminate that restraint?
8. What is the moral justification for restraints? How do the expressed justifications in these cases measure up—protecting other residents from Mr. Meineki, protecting Mrs. Harper and Mrs. Jackson from injury, keeping Mr. Andrews from interfering with the treatment plans of others, making it possible for the staff to get some work done?
9. Can an atmosphere that is respectful to residents prevail when restraints are used? What role, if any, should appearances play in the decision to initiate restraints and choose the form of restraints?
10. What considerations arise regarding various forms of restraints —for example, physical ties of various kinds, the Geri-chair, chemical restraints, locked doors, constant surveillance? Are any forms more worrisome from an ethical standpoint than others?

Chapter 15

BATHING: On the Boundaries of Health Treatment

Marilyn Forsythe, a nurse's aide, is troubled about the care of Mr. Hill, a long-term resident. Ms. Forsythe tells the story like this:

"Until a few months weeks ago Mr. Hill was a cheerful, active, 90-year-old man. He moved here 8 years ago, and as long as I've been here, he's been the kind of person you could trust with extra privileges. Sometimes he ran the elevator, and he usually volunteered to take the nursing home dog for an evening walk. He chaired the Residents' Council and liked to work in his 'garden.' The garden is really two dozen plants that he and his roommate tend carefully. Mr. Hill is a severe diabetic, but has always administered his own insulin.

"A few months ago Mr. Hill slipped and almost fell in the shower. Since that time he has become belligerent at bathtime. He's now extremely fearful and refuses to take a shower even though we always help and watch. He demands that the aides bathe him, and he spends an increasing time in bed or resting in his room. Occasionally, he is incontinent, and he sometimes seems a bit confused. When we try to get him to make an effort, he says, 'I have my rights.' He sometimes reminds us that he's been a 'good citizen' of the home for years and that he pays to receive at least a decent amount of care. He says he hasn't needed much care before, but now he does, and *that* is *that.*

"The other aide and I are overworked. The residents being admitted these days are getting sicker and sicker. One of the other floors is a bit better staffed, but there is no bed available for Mr. Hill there. Besides, he wouldn't want to move—he's been in that room with the garden for so long. But things are getting tough here. An aide quit this month, saying she was 'burned out,' and nobody has been hired yet to replace her. Even if it was *right* to give in to Mr. Hill's demands, we haven't time to give him unnecessary bed baths.

"Anyway, we are worried about the changes in his behavior. He says he is going to resign as president of the council, and sometimes he even asks us to water the plants. If we give in to his insistence on bed baths and keep coddling him in other ways, we will contribute to his dependence, and he will just fail even more. All our in-service training sessions say that the purpose of good nursing is to encourage independence. That's the philosophy around here—we should get residents to do for themselves, even if it takes them longer.

"Mr. Hill gives us an argument on that. He says good nurses are supposed to help residents and give them the care they need. He says all of this talk of his independence is an excuse for not spending the time to help him. He's even turned a bit nasty. The other day, he practically accused me of wanting to neglect his care.

"Our nursing supervisor tells us to be more forceful and to *make* him shower regularly. She suggests we humor him with the bed bath for awhile but never forget that our long-range goal is to get him to the shower. The nurse says someone with diabetes needs to be particularly clean to prevent skin breakdown. The other aide and I don't want to force residents into doing something they really don't want to do, but we know you can't get a resident as clean with a bed bath as you can with a shower.

"Mr. Hill's occasional incontinence, his sometimes shabby appearance, and, most of all, his general attitude have made his roommate complain that Mr. Hill has become 'a smelly old man who just wants to sit around all day.' We don't know if he really means it, but his roommate says if this keeps up, he may request a room transfer.

"Mr. Hill's son came from out of state for one of his visits and was appalled by his father's decline. He said it was fine with him if we forced his dad to shower since 'that's what's good for him.' Of course, it's easy for his son to say that—he isn't on the scene, hearing Mr. Hill beg that we not take him to that shower. We still don't like to go against Mr. Hill's wishes. At least, he is still eating and administering his own insulin."

CASE COMMENTARY

Mila Ann Aroskar

The general understanding in our society is that bathing and good hygiene are healthful practices and enhance our aesthetic values. Mr. Hill's situation raises the question as to whether bathing might in some instances be considered a medical treatment. To grapple with this case, let us imagine that Marilyn Forsythe's supervisor has taken the time to consider the issues together with Marilyn and has provided her with reading matter and helped her interpret it. Their ongoing discussions are presented below in the voice of the nursing supervisor speaking to Marilyn.

THE SITUATION

Imagine for a moment that you are Mr. Hill. You feel that you aren't as "sharp" as you used to be. When you slipped in the shower a few months ago, you suddenly remembered your neighbor who slipped and fell in the shower, broke his hip, and died in the operating room. You are terrified that this will happen to you if you ever take a shower again. No one is aware of your great fear because you don't want anyone to consider you a "sissy." You know that the aides are overworked. At the same time, you feel that they owe you some special consideration because you have always been cooperative and required little help.

Imagine now that you are an aide on Mr. Hill's unit. You have often helped Mr. Hill water his plants and appreciate that he has always been very cooperative in the past. You know that bathing and good hygiene are essential for his well-being because he is a severe diabetic. You also feel that the demands made on the aides on your unit are unreasonable. Residents are often sicker than they were a year ago. You often feel inadequately prepared to care for them, and they require more aide time for care.

Mr. Hill's refusal to shower independently is just one more burden for you. You wonder if there are other ways to resolve this issue than a lengthy battle with Mr. Hill whenever bathing is mentioned to him. You also realize that in many instances assisting a resident with a shower or tub bath takes more time than a bed bath.

A friend shared some information from an ethics conference that you think would be helpful because you know that ethics has something to do with making decisions about how we treat people. You've also heard rumors that an "ethics committee" may be started by the director of nursing. You decide to take some time on your day off and look at this material because you are very concerned that Mr. Hill is not being treated respectfully nor are the aides. Then you will discuss the situation with your supervisor.

IMPORTANCE OF PROCESS: ENHANCING AUTONOMY

As you start reading the materials, you note that there is a great emphasis on how decisions are made as well as what decisions are made when ethical problems occur. The process for making decisions before acting is very important from an ethical perspective. Various components in the process require attention in order to arrive at an ethically sound decision. Components include identification of "facts": who is involved in the situation and how they view it, what ethical values are at stake or in conflict, and what help there might be in looking at ethical principles. It also requires making a decision, acting on it, and evaluating the action and the decision-making process.

As you read further, you find that there is a great deal of discussion about individual autonomy—what it is and is not. First of all, individual autonomy does not mean that a person can do whatever he or she wants to do regardless of the consequences to self or to others. Bruce Miller's (1981) perspectives on autonomy provide some ways of looking at autonomy that seem important for you to consider as you attempt to find a more compassionate way to deal with Mr. Hill and issues around his bathing.

Miller first discusses autonomy as free action, which indicates an action that is voluntary, intentional, and uncoerced. Treatments require permission from the person to be treated in order to enhance free action. Miller's second sense of autonomy is autonomy as authenticity. The autonomous person is self-directed according to a consistent set of his or her own beliefs, desires, and actions over time. Criteria to consider would be the conformity or lack of conformity of Mr. Hill's current decisions and actions with his beliefs, desires, and actions over time and whether Mr. Hill has given informed or implied consent. Mr. Hill's present fear of and refusal to shower do not seem to reflect his beliefs and attitudes over time, to your knowledge, and you worry that Mr. Hill's actions may not be completely voluntary.

Miller discusses autonomy in a third sense as effective deliberation, which indicates that Mr. Hill must have the capacity to know that a decision is required. Mr. Hill must be able to deliberate about the decision and the available alternatives, evaluate the alternatives, and make a choice about the action he wishes to take. This might be viewed as the capacity to exercise freedom of choice. If Mr. Hill is unable to do this, he lacks autonomy. His fears may well be impeding his autonomy in this sense. The legal doctrine of informed consent is generally understood to come out of this sense of autonomy as effective deliberation.

We seldom think about any requirement of informed consent for procedures such as bathing and would probably incorporate bathing as an example of implied consent that is understood upon entrance into the nursing home. However, one should be sensitive to the fact that a caregiver does need consent in a broad sense for touching another person. This is problematic if Mr. Hill resists bathing and attempts are made to force him to take a shower, involving touching to which he did not consent. This aspect of autonomy seems crucial in Mr. Hill's situation because there may be a question as to whether or not he is able to deliberate about the decision on showering.

At the same time, just because Mr. Hill makes a decision that does not agree with the aides or with his son does not mean automatically that he is incapable of making such decisions. His circumstances might justify some paternalism on the part of the nurse, the aides, or his son because Mr. Hill may lack the capacity at times to make decisions that are in his best interests and that reflect his beliefs, attitudes, positions, and values about his health over time. In the absence of bathing and adequate hygiene, there is the potential for harm to Mr. Hill's health. According to James Childress (1981), justified paternalism involves intervention as a last resort when it is necessary to prevent harm and the person's choices are not fully voluntary because of some internal or external constraints. This does not mean that Mr. Hill can justifiably be forced or "made" to take a shower without looking at alternatives.

Other aspects of the decision-making process must also be considered, such as identification of modifications of or alternatives to using the shower. Options for Mr. Hill (and other residents) might be a seating arrangement in the shower stall, installation of an antiskid shower floor, a tub bath, a bed bath, a sponge bath, alternating a bed bath with a shower, or no bath. The last alternative does not seem viable primarily for medical reasons (i.e., Mr. Hill's severe diabetes) and secondarily for aesthetic reasons. Although bathing is not usually regarded as a medical treatment, an argument could be made that Mr. Hill's bath does have some medically related purposes and consequences for his health.

This seemingly makes the case that for Mr. Hill bathing is akin to a medical treatment. If this is the case, he could still legally refuse the bath as a medical treatment as long as he is able to deliberate about and evaluate the consequences of refusal. He has not been declared legally incompetent, so the nursing home staff is responsible for assessment of his capability to make this decision or, at least, to participate in making the decision. The staff should be sensitive to the fact that his decision-making capacity may be compromised at the times when he is confused, but this does not mean that he is always in a compromised state with regard to making decisions. Even if a physician were to write an order for a shower or bath, implementing physician orders is generally a nursing responsibility and would most likely be resolved by actions of the aides alone or in consultation with the supervising nurse.

Each of the alternatives would require discussion with Mr. Hill as to their feasibility and desirability from his perspective and the perspective of the staff. Their purposes and potential consequences should be discussed. Such a discussion demonstrates respect for Mr. Hill's dignity and worth as a person and for his autonomy. A purpose of the discussion would be to discover Mr. Hill's reasons for refusing to take a shower. This process, carried out in a gentle, skillful way, would also be respectful of the dignity and worth of the aides as persons, as such discussion also serves as a place for different perspectives to be heard and taken seriously.

CONFLICTING VALUES: AUTONOMY AND AVOIDANCE OF HARM

For you as the aide, there is conflict between enhancing Mr. Hill's autonomy, your desire (and that of the nursing home) to avoid immediate and long-term harm to Mr. Hill's safety and well-being, and the most efficient use of your time and energy given the circumstances of understaffing and sicker residents on your unit. Clearly, you can see that a reasoned process of decision making also requires time, which is a scarce resource in your nursing home. The trade-offs of not taking time to determine a better way to make decisions with Mr. Hill are use of further staff time and energy in what is turning into an increasingly adversarial situation with great frustration on both sides.

You can see that there are different kinds of situations involving residents and aides, in which resident autonomy and the aide's goal of avoiding harm are in conflict. You are convinced that a clear process for making reasoned decisions would be helpful when there is serious disagreement or conflicting values. The values in conflict may be moral values, such as autonomy, or other types of values, such as efficiency. If a nursing home has a mechanism for dealing with such conflicts, this could be viewed as practicing a type of "preventive ethic," which could be used even before there is serious disagreement. There would be an expectation by nursing and the home's administration of assessing a situation and getting input from residents and staff *prior* to escalation into energy- and time-consuming adversarialism. Some functions of a Residents' Council or an ethics committee can be viewed in this light.

RESIDENTS' RIGHTS: AIDES' OBLIGATIONS?

You continue to think about the issue of respecting Mr. Hill's autonomy when it seems that his capacity for decision making in his best interests is at times somewhat diminished. You feel that "making" Mr. Hill shower as suggested by the nurse is not ethically acceptable if it means negating Mr. Hill's decision-making autonomy or not taking it seriously in decisions made by others. At the same time, you are troubled about his demands for a bed bath. You are concerned that along with the allocation of scarce time and energy of aides there is more at stake here than simply agreeing to go along with Mr. Hill's demands, particularly since he stated that a bed bath is owed to him as his "right." If Mr. Hill is stating that he has the right to a bed bath in what he sees as a justified claim, who has the obligation to satisfy this claim? One could argue that this is an obligation of the aides, the nurses, or the administration of the nursing home, or some combination of these individuals. However, not everyone would agree that this is Mr. Hill's right. It may be an expectation, a hope, or a demand. It is not automatically a right as a justified claim or as an individual resident's possession, particularly if the claim is based on past "good" behavior as defined by a resident. Care provided by staff is founded on respect for the person and enhancing well-being. It is not dependent on a resident's behavior, good or bad.

You remember from your orientation classes that there is no specific "right to a bed bath" mentioned in the Residents' Bill of Rights. You also realize that if all of the residents on your unit demand a bed bath as a "right," this is untenable even if it meets the moral criterion of universalizability (i.e., everyone in the same or similar situations being treated similarly). No other activities or goals could be accomplished because most of the aides' time would be spent in bathing residents and helping those who are incontinent to remain clean and dry. What would happen to other important functions of the aides, such as getting residents to activities, assisting residents at mealtime, or helping those to the bathroom who need assistance? A bed bath for everyone is not realistic. It is also not desirable from a health perspective for some residents who wish to have a bed bath. More active participation in bathing is possible, and bathing may be therapeutic in the sense of not contributing to further dependence but enhancing and encouraging independence and resident autonomy if this is a goal in the nursing home. Nursing homes often increase resident dependency based on the value of efficiency.

CONFLICTING VALUES: AUTONOMY AND FAIR DISTRIBUTION OF RESOURCES

The nursing home administration is legally and morally responsible if residents do not have aides readily available for needed assistance. Aides bear the burdens in stress and exhaustion but do not allocate overall resources within the nursing home. Aides might think that only administrators and supervisors have to worry about distributive justice issues because they have the legal and moral responsibility for securing adequate staff to meet resident needs. However, aides also have distributive issues with which to contend on a daily basis. Aides are and have to be concerned about a fair distribution of their time and energy. These are important distribution decisions about finite human resources.

There is no overall consensus on how to resolve issues of distributive justice in our society. Various ideas exist as to what constitutes justice with a goal of treating people fairly and equitably. The following ideas serve as a basis for distributing burdens and benefits in society generally and in health care specifically: treating individuals according to need, treating individuals according to effort or merit, treating individuals according to their social worth and contributions, and making sure that the least advantaged or most vulnerable also benefit when there are benefits for the most advantaged. We can also consider some combination of these ideas, such as treating individuals according to need and making sure that if an individual is a member of a disadvantaged group (being poor or ill) that he or she will also benefit from policy decisions if the wealthy are benefited by those decisions.

One of the challenges for the aides in working with Mr. Hill, if need is a basis for decisions about allocating their time and energy for care, is to decide what Mr. Hill "needs." If they are paying attention to enhancing his autonomy, it would be morally inadequate for them to decide alone what he needs with regard to bathing unless he has been judged legally incompetent. Although he is confused at times, you and other aides who work with Mr. Hill are convinced that he is still able to make most decisions for himself, as he continues to administer his own insulin, generally takes care of his "garden," and has not talked about resigning as chair of the Residents' Council for the last two weeks. His son's most recent visit had a positive effect on Mr. Hill, who is taking better care of himself in all respects other than still refusing to shower. Even his room-mate has commented on the improvement. Decisions should be made about the shower in discussion with Mr. Hill, using some form of shared decision making.

Making the case that this decision should be made for Mr. Hill by someone else without his input would be difficult if not impossible. The aides could discuss their position (again) with Mr. Hill with regard to some of the realities of the unit. Everyone involved in Mr. Hill's care, including the nurse, could participate. Mr. Hill's son could also be present if Mr. Hill wishes. This would also be an appropriate forum to clarify the Residents' Bill of Rights in nursing homes.

OBLIGATIONS AND THE NOTION OF COMMUNITY

The nature of the nursing home as a community has not been clearly decided. An argument could be made that Mr. Hill is living in a situation comparable to a family or a neighborhood, where there is an obligation to consider the welfare of all individuals as there is some sense of shared citizenship. In reality, Mr. Hill cannot have all of his demands met auto-matically whether he lives in a family or lives by himself in a neighbor-hood or a nursing home. Providing for the welfare of all individuals living and working in the nursing home must be balanced with meeting the needs of each individual. These two aspects will often be in tension for aides, as they are for administrators. Aides often must seek to meet the needs of each individual at the same time that they must consider all of the individuals assigned to them for care when they make decisions about allocation of their time and energy.

Another issue of distributive justice that aides are involved with is the allocation of scarce material resources in the nursing home, such as use of the television set and use of phones if residents do not have their own. Most do not and must depend on the resources that are available for all of the residents. Again, enhancement of autonomy would suggest that these decisions require some mutual discussion when residents are able to par-ticipate in the process of decision making about allocation of these re-sources. Most often the aides negotiate this process and decide whether or not it will occur in a participatory way or whether decisions will be made in a more arbitrary manner. Given the serious understaffing that occurs on units, the arbitrary mode may be viewed as the most efficient way to make allocation decisions. Such arbitrary decision making may be viewed as a trade-off between the value of resident autonomy and the value of efficiency, at least for the short term. There may be long-term costs, as the process by which allocation decisions are made will undoubtedly continue to be an issue. Both aides and residents will probably experience dissatisfaction if these decisions are viewed only from the short-term perspective.

Nursing homes do have both a moral and a legal obligation to provide adequate staffing to meet resident needs. This is a difficult obligation to meet given the severe shortage of staff in most of the nursing homes in the United States, which results from variables such as low wages, the nature and stress of the work, and the disvalue placed on the work by our society. This is a challenge that cannot be resolved by nursing home administrators alone; it requires social and political decisions and actions.

Mr. Hill cannot ethically be forced or "made" to take a shower. There are alternatives. Furthermore, the aides should not be put in a position that leaves them with few or no alternatives other than coercively using their power over residents. Taking the position that bathing is a medical treatment would not be a compelling argument for the nursing assistants to use with Mr. Hill. He has the right to make choices about medical treatments and to accept or refuse them. The potential consequences of not bathing to his health and well-being may justify some degree of paternalism and require a clear and compassionate process for his involvement in the everyday decisions that affect him. This will benefit Mr. Hill, his roommate, and the nursing home staff, both short-term and long-term, by providing a model that is respectful of all of the individuals involved. If Mr. Hill absolutely refused any hygienic measures with actual detrimental consequences to his health, or if he became a serious burden to others in his immediate environment due to intolerable odor, then arrangements for his care elsewhere might have to be made with his son as a last resort. Such action could also be justified if dealing with Mr. Hill's care requirements put the welfare of other residents at demonstrable risk.

AIDES AS MORAL AGENTS AND DECISION MAKERS

The claim has been made that aides in nursing homes do not make decisions but only do as they are told. At best, their caring and decision making are almost invisible. According to the data gathered for the study of everyday autonomy in nursing homes on which this case study is based, aides

Chapter 16

CARING ON DEMAND: How Responsive Is Responsive Enough?

Mrs. Smith is an 82-year old woman whose single room is decorated with cheerful curtains and numerous family pictures. A spectacular quilt covers her bed. She is a tiny woman with obvious arthritis and contractures. During our visit she is sitting in a wheelchair. She tells us she is unable to get out of bed without help and can walk only a few steps alone. She offers us chocolates from a box on her night table and apologizes because she has no tea or coffee to serve before we start our interview.

MRS. SMITH'S FEAR OF "ACCIDENTS"

Mrs. Smith has lived in the facility for 2 years. "It is not home, but I try not to complain." She knows that it is better than many other nursing homes, including the place she first went when she left the hospital. "My children wouldn't let me stay there." This nursing home also has the advantage of being close to both her son and her daughter.

Mrs. Smith's biggest complaint is that the nurses take such a long time to answer the call button. She has a particular horror that she might wet the bed, an accident that has happened to her three times so far. "I am old, and my bladder doesn't work the way it used to. I can't wait very long for help." Mrs. Smith says it always takes 15 minutes, and sometimes it takes more than half an hour for the call button to be answered. Moreover, once when she asked an aide to take her to the bathroom, the aide said, "I already took you an hour ago, and I don't have time now." Mrs. Smith knows the aides are busy and tries to be considerate. "Anyone with a brain here tries to make it easier for the girls." She is reconciled to waiting half an hour or so for other things—being put down for a nap, getting a glass of juice, or getting someone to reach for a magazine, but she considers getting to the bathroom an emergency. She doesn't think that help going to the toilet should be limited to a certain number of times a shift.

Once Mrs. Smith confided in her favorite aide about her great fear that she might have an accident in her bed. Trying to reassure her, the aide cheerfully said that Mrs. Smith shouldn't worry. "If an accident happens when I'm on duty, I'll have you clean and comfortable in no time." Mrs. Smith thought the aide missed the point.

NURSE'S AIDES VIEWS

At this facility, nurse's aides are assigned about 15 residents for the day and evening shifts. (At night each aide gets at least twice as many residents.) The aides vary in how responsive they are to special requests. One aide told us that she makes a special effort to answer bells quickly and to do things that the resident wants. Usually, she can be flexible about evening routines, "though it sure is easier to let people stay up later than usual than to help them get to bed just exactly when they want." This aide prides herself that she can comply with most requests "at least within an hour." She knows some people feel even a half an hour is too long to wait, but "when you are the arms and legs for 15 people, things can get out of hand." Another aide told us that it is frustrating to have to "redo my tasks" when she thinks she has things finished. Examples of redoing included putting someone back down for a nap a second time and taking someone to the toilet again when they had just gone. The aide usually could tolerate considerable double work but resented those people who call out all day asking for help. She recognized that Mrs. Smith usually knows when she needs to go to the bathroom and seldom just "cries wolf," but others just want to get attention and really don't know what they need. "You should spend a shift here, and you'd see how people call out constantly as we go up and down the hall—nurse, get me this, get me that. Don't we have rights too?"

CASE COMMENTARY

Sara T. Fry

In the case of Mrs. Smith, a mentally competent 82-year old woman expresses her needs to feel comfortable, to be free of urinary accidents, and to have her dignity intact. Having lived in the nursing home for over 2 years, Mrs. Smith has slowly come to regard the nursing home as her residence. Although the nursing home is probably not like the home she once maintained, it is, for all practical purposes, her "home" and more than likely will her permanent residence for the remainder of her life. Although a son and daughter live nearby and visit her, there is no denying that Mrs. Smith lives her life within the nursing home environment. Whatever autonomy she can exercise can be realized only within the scope of the nursing home's capacities to recognize her autonomy.

Like many elderly women, Mrs. Smith has limited mobility because of arthritis and other changes of the aging process. She also has urinary urgency and lives in near constant fear that she might not make it to the bathroom to empty her bladder. Because of her limited mobility she is dependent on the nursing home staff to help her out of bed and to the bathroom for this not-to-be-denied function of her body. She can make choices and even decide when and where certain functions of her body will be exercised. But she cannot follow through with her choices and actions without the assistance of another person.

Under ideal conditions, a person meets personal needs (such as bladder emptying) individually and autonomously. Under conditions of physical impairment, however, these needs can be met only with the assistance of another person. A mentally competent individual can express these needs verbally and even select or choose the actions that will satisfy them. Another person, however, must physically assist the individual in such actions or carry out the actions for them.

In recent years it has become fashionable to advocate a greater amount of autonomy for the elderly. If more options, more resources, more public assistance, and the like were available, then the elderly would, presumably have more autonomy and the majority of their needs would be adequately satisfied. Autonomy, that treasured moral value of a libertarian society, is being advocated for the elderly in much the same way that autonomy is seemingly advocated for everyone through whatever is more and better. Autonomy is proposed as a right that may be claimed by the elderly, and conversely, respect for elder autonomy is a duty that must be fulfilled on the part of society, especially those who provide daily care and attention in nursing homes.

But how much autonomy is really possible where the elderly, especially those confined to nursing homes, are concerned? How can one be autonomous when hampered by decreasing physical and mental abilities and decreased social support networks? It seems to be an undisputed fact that the amount of autonomy an elderly person enjoys is extremely limited with the passing of years, a fact that affects life-style, happiness, and even how and when one dies. Although we ideally might want to promote the autonomy of the elderly as much as possible, the reality of what it means to be elderly makes us realize that the human value of self-determination must be supported by the value of well-being in the daily care of the elderly. Recognition of the role of other values in matters of particular significance to the elderly—specifically, the value of well-being in matters such as living comfortably, providing for bodily functions, and living with human dignity intact—simply cannot be overlooked when the care of an elderly individual is being considered.

SELF-DETERMINATION

Self-determination is an important value in our society. We tend to protect self-determination both because of its instrumental value in enhancing a person's sense of well-being and its intrinsic value as an element of personal worth and integrity (President's Commission, 1983).

Like many elderly individuals, Mrs. Smith has decisional autonomy (in the sense of the freedom to *make* choices) but little executional autonomy in the sense of the freedom to execute choices (Collopy, 1988). The scope of her autonomy is therefore limited. It creates a situation in which decisional autonomy is easily eroded once the elderly person's executional autonomy diminishes or is eventually lost. In such situations the value of self-determination is endangered. The potential for this type of situation is readily evident in the case of Mrs. Smith.

The nursing assistants who respond to Mrs. Smith's call button indicate that they respect her decisional autonomy. The call button functions as an indicator that Mrs. Smith has made a decision ("My bladder is full and I want to go to the bathroom."). When they respond promptly, their response indicates recognition that her executional autonomy is diminished and that they must act for her. When they take a long time to respond to the call button, this indicates disrespect for her total autonomy because Mrs. Smith's decisional autonomy can be satisfied only by assisted executional autonomy.

If the nursing assistant does not arrive at her room in time to assist her to the bathroom, her decision to empty her bladder becomes a null-and-void decision—in other words, her decisional autonomy has been rendered meaningless where this particular bodily function is concerned. The nursing aide who cheerfully reassured Mrs. Smith that she would quickly clean her up if she had an urinary accident in bed demonstrates how decisional autonomy is easily eroded when an elderly person's executional autonomy becomes diminished or lost. The result is a devaluing of self-determination.

In the best of all worlds every assistant in a nursing home would respect the full autonomy (decisional and executional) of every resident. Unfortunately, a nursing home environment is not conducive to this type of respect for autonomy. A nursing assistant's acknowledgment of individual choice or action is always made against background recognition of every other nursing home resident's exercise of individual autonomy. Hence, the nursing assistant's decision to facilitate Mrs. Smith's efforts to empty her bladder in the bathroom is made against all competing requests for assistance with daily living from other residents in the home. To facilitate her choice to empty her bladder *now rather than later* requires more than simple respect for autonomy. It requires respect for the importance of the value of well-being.

WELL-BEING

Well-being is also an important value in our society. Well-being is what is experienced by individuals when their subjective interests are or have been fulfilled. We tend to protect well-being in our society because it is essential to one's sense of individuality and enjoyment of human dignity. Indeed, the maximization of well-being is regarded as "the primary goal of health care" (President's Commission, 1983, p. 26). For this reason alone, perhaps it should be given more consideration than it currently has in discussions of health care ethics. Certainly, the correlation of well-being with the value of self-determination is fundamentally important to discussions of autonomy among nursing home residents.

The need for consideration of the value of well-being is readily evident in Mrs. Smith's situation. Although anyone who cares for a nursing home resident must respect the resident's choices of actions (or decisional autonomy), the caregiver has less obligation to compensate for the resident's lack of executional autonomy apart from some sense of obligation to enhance the residents well-being. In other words, when executional autonomy is diminished or even lost, decisional autonomy is abrogated *unless* the obligation to promote and enhance well-being becomes the value of prime importance. Hence, in the case of Mrs.

Smith, whatever degree of importance the nursing assistant accords to Mrs. Smith's sense of well-being will become the decisional factor in deciding to respond to her call button *now rather than later.*

It is only because of a sense of obligation to protect Mrs. Smith's well-being that the nursing assistant will respond in a timely fashion to assist her execution of her decision to empty her bladder. By responding now rather than later, the nursing assistant's actions not only protect Mrs. Smith's self-determination but her well-being as well. The protection of both values is important to the realization of autonomy among nursing home residents, but the obligation to protect well-being seems to be the critical factor in maintaining decisional autonomy when executional autonomy is diminished or lost. It is that factor that links autonomy to a person's human individuality and dignity.

What might be proposed to enhance staff attitudes and efforts to care for nursing residents like Mrs. Smith? In particular, what type of moral framework might be proposed to increase staff obligations to enhance nursing home residents' well-being when their executional autonomy is diminished?

A MODEL OF CARING

It is proposed that a "model of caring" might provide an appropriate framework for the consideration of staff obligations and residents' self-determination and well-being. Such a model focuses on the relationship between caregiver and care receiver and promises to enhance the carrying out of moral obligations to vulnerable individuals in the health care system (Fry, 1989).

Four senses of care are essential to this model. As described by Pellegrino (1985), these senses of care are as follows:

1. Compassion or being concerned for another person.
2. Doing for others what they cannot do for themselves.
3. Amelioration of the medical problem experienced by a patient.
4. Carrying out necessary procedures (personal and technical) with attention to detail and perfection.

The above senses of care are not separable and comprise what is called "integral care" (Pellegrino, 1985). Such care is a moral obligation and is not an option that can be exercised or interpreted within the health care system according to idiosyncratic professional interpretations of responsibility. As Pellegrino points out, the moral obligation to care in this manner is created by the special human relationship that brings together the one who needs assistance (or is ill) and the one who offers to help. It also requires an ethic that attends to the concept of care in the broad sense and that makes caring a strong moral obligation between care receiver and caregiver.

Applying a Model of Caring to the Case Situation

Viewing the care of Mrs. Smith from a model of caring broadens the significance and meaning of nursing home assistants' interactions with residents. First, the purpose of assistants' actions will be to care for residents and *not* simply to respond to their requests for help. To care will mean to acknowledge the values that are important to the resident. In the case of Mrs. Smith, caring for her entails acknowledgment of her self-determination as well as her sense of well-being.

Second, caring for Mrs. Smith will indicate compassion on the part of the helping individual. Nursing assistants in nursing homes are not often recognized and rewarded for the high amount of compassion they extend toward elderly residents who depend on them for daily care and nurturance. It is very hard to care for the same individuals day after day with an attitude of compassion or a sense of concern for those individuals. Yet nursing assistants do provide care for residents on a daily basis, and many do so with compassion. In the case of Mrs. Smith, acting with compassion when she presses the call button provides for the values of self-determination and well-being as she has defined them. When these values are respected, then we might say that Mrs. Smith has truly been cared for.

Third, a model of caring will support the recognition of Mrs. Smith's physical problem (urinary urgency), which requires the type of skill that the nursing assistant, more than anyone else, provides best. To expend this skill in Mrs. Smith's physical care means that her particular physical problem is of concern to the nursing staff and that she is entitled to a certain level of care as a result. However, Mrs. Smith is entitled to *care*, not merely technical assistance for physical problems.

Last, a model of caring will enable nursing assistants to view their work with the elderly in nursing homes as entailing a certain type of moral excellence. Anyone may provide technical assistance to an elderly resident, but only someone who operates from a moral obligation of caring will respond to residents' needs as they define them within a framework of values of importance to them. To care for residents in this manner is to do morally worthy actions on behalf of those who cannot do for themselves. Despite the care of many elderly residents and the performance of many unpleasant tasks, nursing assistants need to view their work as more than mere tasks and functions. To care for Mrs. Smith from a model of caring is to do more than simply respond to her call button when she calls. It means to respond to her morally and to acknowledge the values (self-determination and well-being) that are important to her.

CONCLUSIONS

If obligations to care for elderly individuals in the nursing home environment can be discussed within the framework of a model of caring, there is reason to believe that elderly autonomy can be enhanced and protected. The model of caring discussed here promises to protect the values of self-determination and well-being that are especially vulnerable under conditions of diminished autonomy because of decreasing ability to execute individual choices and actions during the aging process. It is only within a framework of moral obligation that significant and important human values find protection. For nursing assistants who care for elderly nursing home residents, such a model of caring supports and enhances the various roles and actions that they daily expend on any resident's behalf.

REFERENCES

Callahan, D. (1985). What do children owe elderly parents? *Hastings Center Report, 15*(2), 32–37.

Collopy, B. J. (1988). Autonomy in long term care: Some crucial distinctions. *The Gerontologist, 28,* (Suppl.), 10–17.

Fry, S. T. (1989). The philosophical foundations of caring. In M. Leininger (ed.), *Ethical care in context: Current issues.* Detroit: Wayne State University Press.

Fuchs, V. R. (1984). Though much is taken: Reflecting on aging, health, and medical care. *Milbank Memorial Quarterly, 62*(2), 160.

May, W. F. Who cares for the elderly? *Hastings Center Report, 12*(6), 31–37.

Pellegrino, E. D. (1985). The caring ethic: The relation of physician to patient. In A. H. Bishop & J. R. Scudder (eds.). *Caring, curing, coping: Nurse, physician, patient relationships* Birmingham, AL: University of Alabama Press, 8–30.

President's Commission for the Study of Ethical Problems in Medicine and Biomedical and Behavioral Research. (1983). *Deciding to forego life sustaining treatment.* Washington, DC: U.S. Government Printing Office.

FOR FURTHER DISCUSSION: EDITORS' QUESTIONS

1. How much effort and resources need to be expended to fulfill requests of nursing home residents for attention and care? Is there an ethical obligation to prevent Mrs. Smith from having urinary accidents in her bed?
2. Does Mrs. Smith have a prior claim to this attention because she is cognitively intact, compared to others who seem not to mind when they have urinary accidents?
3. What priority should be given to prevention of urinary accidents compared to other matters?
4. What constitutes reasonable efforts and expenditures to fulfill the requests of residents?
5. How should an adequate ratio of staff to residents be determined?
6. How should staff balance the multiple requests they receive for variations from routines, for getting people things they want, for making people more comfortable?
7. What staff attitude toward their work and the residents would be most conducive to maintaining the autonomy of the residents?
8. What principles of fairness should govern the allocation of staff time, and are these the same from the perspective of staff, management, and residents?
9. Do you agree with Dr. Fry that nursing home personnel have a moral obligation to act according to a "model of caring" that includes technically competent health care, help with functioning, compassion, and attention to detail?
10. Do you ground the obligation to deliver care with compassion and to treat the resident with dignity in a principle of beneficence (i.e., respect for well-being) or a principle of autonomy? Make a case for each position.

Chapter 17

BEYOND THE CALL OF DUTY:
A Nurse's Aide Uses Her Judgment

Kim Clark is an experienced nurse's aide who has worked for 15 years in the nursing home industry. She quit high school "as soon as it was legal," and immediately took her first nurse's aide job. She has worked in six facilities all told, changing jobs for a variety of practical reasons. She has been working at her present job on the evening shift at Pine Tree Convalescent Home for 8 years. She likes this facility quite well and has no plans to change. She now earns $4.25 an hour.

AN UNAUTHORIZED SMOKE

Kim describes herself as someone who "thinks for myself." On the evening shift, "when there aren't many nurses around to run to, you have to make some decisions." Kim has come to know "my residents" very well. She tries to keep them cheerful, and she chats with the "night owls" who have trouble sleeping. A few months ago, a feisty 87-year-old lady with congestive heart failure was admitted with a doctor's order that she was not to smoke. The resident was willing to comply in general with the recommendation but wanted one cigarette each night. Kim lowers her voice and says, "This interview won't get back to the facility, will it?" On being reassured, she told the interviewer that she gives the resident one cigarette a night, and they have their smoke together during Kim's late break. Kim no doubt feels that she is handling this situation properly. She expresses contempt for the doctor's order. "At age 87, really!" Kim did not perceive this as a difficult decision, though she remains discreet about her involvement in doling out the cigarettes.

A DRUG INTERVENTION

Other decisions give Kim more pause. The most difficult decision she has ever made as a nurse's aide involved Miss Emma McComb, a resident who was being "turned into a zombie" because of the amount of medicine she was receiving. The aide repeatedly told her supervisor, the licensed practical nurse (LPN) who distributed medicines on the evening shift, that "instead of calming Emma down, the meds were zonking Emma out." She wanted her supervisor to report this through channels so that the day shift could follow up on the issue. Three months passed and nothing changed.

Kim finally went "over the boss's head" and talked to Emma's sister, who visited most evenings after supper. "Her sister just sat on the chair and looked at Emma and shook her head over her condition." Kim told Emma's sister that in her opinion Emma was getting the wrong medicine and suggested the family should check into it. In fact, the family did take the hint and called the doctor. Subsequently, Emma McComb's prescriptions were changed, and the dose of one major drug was reduced. Kim Clark noticed that Emma became much more responsive than she had been before. Kim felt justified in speaking up, even though "I don't know anything about medicines and I sure am not a doctor." She admitted she was nervous about the situation because "I could have got into trouble."

CASE COMMENTARY

Diane K. Kjervik

The central question posed by the actions of Kim Clark, the nurse's aide, is whether her judgments jeopardized the autonomy of the two nursing home residents. Autonomy means self-will, including the freedom to think about one's values and beliefs about a given situation, to identify one's feelings about the situation, to make choices among alternative responses, and to act on those choices. Autonomy does not mean isolation from other persons or elements of the environment. Information from outside oneself is imperative to knowing and understanding options, and sometimes one's autonomous action requires the helpful actions of others.

A breach of autonomy exists when information is provided but the interpretation of the information or the choice stemming from the information is imposed from the outside. In terms of actions, autonomy is violated when, instead of acting on behalf of a person by using the person's values to guide one's action, one acts in place of the person by using one's own values.

In the two case scenarios, the unauthorized smoke and the drug intervention, there is a temptation to focus on the nurse's aide's rights: whether she had the right to decide independently to alter the cardiovascular treatment plan and whether she had the right to deviate from professional channels to bring about a change in a prescribed drug. I prefer to analyze the responsibilities she has as a nonprofessional health care worker, as one who performs her role without the state authority and obligation granted by licensure, without a professional code of ethics to mandate and guide her actions, and without professional standards of practice generated by a professional organization and enforced in courts of law. In this context, I focus on the resident's autonomy and whether Kim Clark's actions either enhanced or reduced the autonomy.

The overriding responsibility of a nurse's aide is loyalty to his or her employer, that is, to carry out the duties assigned by the employer. Of course, the assignment of duties must be in harmony with whatever collective bargaining agreement exists, if there is one, but many nurse's aides are "at will" employees who can be discharged at the will of the employer subject to certain state and federal law restrictions such as antidiscrimination laws. Some nurse's aides carry out their duties with serious consideration given to the personal ethical standards they hold, such as whether it is right or wrong to let an elderly person do things that contradict the treatment plan. In this sense, the nurse's aide is a moral agent, and actions taken or not taken reflect personal values. But these are personal standards, measured against the aide's own yardstick, as opposed to, for instance, expectations of a registered nurse, whose value choices in the patient care situation are analyzed in relation to the nurses' professional code of ethics as well as the legal standard of care.

A nurse's aide may have more discretion in the patient care situation than registered nurses or social workers. The latter are employees of the nursing home and owe it the duty of loyalty, but they also owe another, sometimes conflicting duty to the professional standards of care established by experts in their fields (Gorlin, 1986). However, in reality, the nurse's aide who uses a personal judgment that runs counter to the established treatment plan has virtually no fallback position from the duty of loyalty to the employer. The nurse's aides functions are ministerial, whereas the professional is accorded considerable latitude for professional judgment. The professional is expected to use judgment and discretion and is, in fact, hired to do so. The nurse's aide must rely on discretion allowed by the employer and guidance from her own conscience. If the nurse's aide's judgment as a moral agent deviates from the employer's expectations, she should be cognizant of the risks so that the risks taken are truly taken knowingly.

One problem encountered at times, and possibly existing in the cases examined here, is the bright, experienced, and independent-thinking nurse's aide who personally does not support the treatment plan. Although Kim Clark was not well educated formally, some aides hold baccalaureate degrees in psychology and other fields, giving them scientific insights on which to base independent opinions. Also, nurse's aides are often the only health care providers on duty, which puts them in the position of feeling free and sometimes feeling obligated to exercise independent judgment. In addition to feeling the sense of heavy responsibility with little authority, they are very poorly paid, which leads to feelings of dissatisfaction, frustration, and burnout. These factors put residents in nursing homes at risk of receiving poor and possibly abusive care.

THE UNAUTHORIZED SMOKE

Kim Clark decided that the resident with congestive heart failure could have one cigarette at night despite the doctor's order to the contrary. Her judgment appears to be based on her own attitude about the age of the patient—that is, an 87-year-old patient will die soon anyway. However, in terms of maintaining the resident's autonomy, the nurse's aide had several questions to consider. Did the resident request the cigarette based on adequate information about its potentially lethal effect? A person's choice needs to be informed, or else it is not truly consensual. And was the resident's decision made voluntarily, or was subtle manipulation and coercion involved? How vulnerable was the resident feeling in relation to the nurse's aide and thus more subject to the suggestion of a cigarette?

A question of power differences arises here that Kim Clark perhaps did not consider. Was the resident competent to make the decision about smoking? If she was seriously confused and had a recent history of harmful self-neglect, a substitute decision maker, such as a guardian or conservator, may have been needed to consider and decide options for her. However, patients have the right to make foolish and even harmful decisions about their care if they are competent and act voluntarily upon adequate information. The principles of autonomy and self-determination protect this right (Kjervik & Grove, 1988).

The question of whether a nursing home resident's smoking should be a matter of medical or nursing intervention can also be raised. It can be argued that the no-smoking order should not have been written because to dictate personal habits jeopardizes the resident's autonomy and turns a personal, everyday decision into a medical one. However, everyday decisions such as the time for eating, the dietary menu, and the time for dressing are part of nursing interventions for persons in need of health care. Health means more than attending to the ill foot or the confused mind. In the nursing home it means structuring a milieu for optimum health behaviors. Obviously, smoking is a health-related behavior and should be considered in the treatment approach both medically and from the nursing standpoint. However, this does not mean that mandates are necessary regarding these behaviors; a reasonable part of the health care plan can be a recommendation to the patient rather than a mandate.

The physician in this case could have noted in the chart that he or she had advised the patient not to smoke and what her verbal response was to this suggestion. Presumably, this would have adequately discharged the physician's duty to preserve the resident's health at its maximum level. However, the doctor chose to write an order prohibiting smoking, which possibly indicates that he or she felt very strongly that smoking would bring immediate harm to resident. Once the order was written, the nursing staff was obligated to follow it, and choosing to violate it would place their jobs and licenses at risk. Through her action as a moral agent, Kim Clark knowingly chose to violate the order, placing herself at risk of losing her job and her employer at risk of legal sanctions.

I believe nurse's aides must feel very removed from the professional decision-making process regarding their patients, including any consideration given to the patient's autonomy. Treatment care conferences should include the aides so that they can hear the rationales for various professional decisions and make suggestions that they find reasonable. Had Kim Clark been included in the care planning conference, she might have had a better understanding of the negative aspects of the cigarette smoking—not only that the smoking would jeopardize life itself but also that the 87-year-old woman's quality of remaining life would be diminished by smoking. Had she understood this, she might have been less likely to act in opposition to the doctor's order.

Also, had she been a respected participant in the care conference, she could have voiced her personal values about the smoking issue and the reasons for them. She might have been able to influence the opinions of others to allow an occasional smoke with the patient.

Kim Clark might also have been educated to the autonomy process by being in a care conference that included the patient (or patient's representative) and having an opportunity to listen and to help the patient voice the patient's values not only about smoking but also about quality of life, feelings about being 87 years old, and what choice the patient wanted to make when all the facts were discussed openly. Had she and the patient been included, she might have felt a commitment to the professional smoking decision as a member of a team, and the resident's autonomy would have been well served.

Whether to smoke on the sly with the resident was justified from the viewpoint of acceptable deception is also raised by the facts in this case. Human beings certainly keep secrets from one another, and in a society that values privacy, secrecy in some situations is justifiable. Personal points of view, actions, and feelings can be hidden from others. Nursing home staffs have numerous personal reactions to residents that they keep secret from the residents, and vice versa. But in this case the secret involved a conspiracy to break the rules of the nursing home, not solely by residents but by a resident and a staff member. Although it may be easy to argue away the hidden decision about a smoke, it would not be as easy to argue away a mutual decision to take illicit drugs or to plan to help other residents to "escape" from the nursing home. In other words, condoning secrets that staff choose to enter into with residents may create disorganization, jeopardy to other residents' safety, and a lack of predictability about rules of the nursing home.

If secrecy were allowed among residents and staff, staff members could use power differentials to manipulate or coerce the residents' behavior. In a situation of open communication, other staff or family members could support or speak on behalf of a resident, and coercion and manipulation would be less likely to occur. If there is a bad rule or staff decision, it should be challenged openly in a team meeting, a Residents' Council, or other appropriate forum where the democratic process can be used to solve the problem.

THE DRUG INTERVENTION

Under an "ends justify the means" analysis Kim Clark was justified in going to the family with her concern about Emma McComb's drug dose, but she was not justified in doing so in terms of the value of teamwork with staff and her duty of loyalty to her employer. Unlike the smoking example, there is no question of harm to the patient arising from Kim Clark's action, which was clearly directed at helping Emma McComb regain her lucidity. Without lucidity, Miss McComb could not be autonomous. By acting on Miss McComb's behalf, Kim Clark helped her to exercise her autonomy.

As part of her nurse's aide job description, Kim Clark typically would have been expected to report the patient's problem to her supervisor or to someone above her supervisor if nothing was done. Nurse's aides usually write notes in the charts each shift. Did Kim Clark write her observations in the chart? If so, the charge nurse (RN) should have picked up her comments even if the LPN overlooked them. If the RN, who is responsible for all nursing care given under her supervision, also missed the aide's concerns, Kim Clark had the obligation to her employer to go up the chain of command, to the head nurse, then the supervisor, and then the director of nursing. Kim Clark had the duty to her employer to use the designated channel of authority because going outside the usual channel put her employer at risk of a lawsuit on grounds of negligent treatment and negligent supervision. Also, she had some obligation to work as a member of a health care team to meet patient care goals. The ethic of caring as described by Carol Gilligan (1982; Fry, this volume) emphasizes the importance of interconnectedness among people and responsibility to others. Kim Clark jeopardized this ethic of teamwork and mutual trust among colleagues by going outside the employment channels.

In terms of power inequities or the concept of justice, Kim Clark's action empowered the patient by speaking for her during a time when she could not raise her voice. There was no evidence in this example that Miss McComb wanted to be heavily sedated, whereas in the smoking example, the feisty 87 year-old had expressed some desire to smoke. There is no evidence in this situation that Miss McComb was manipulated or coerced into anything. Rather, this was a clear-cut iatrogenic problem that, if left unattended, might have created serious problems for the patient.

PROCEDURAL RECOMMENDATIONS

Based on the two nurse's aide case examples, several recommendations emerge for addressing two general aspects of autonomy: uncoerced provision of information and choices and assistance given the resident to act on choices made.

Uncoerced Information and Choices

Both case examples point to the need for team care conferences that include both nurse's aides and residents with whom the aides are working. In these conferences, staff members (RNs, social workers, MDs, dietitians) could discuss treatment plans with the resident, including activities of daily living such as smoking, socializing, eating, and dressing. The resident would be encouraged to state his or her own values. It would be ideal if the resident's values could be written down for the benefit of staff who weren't in attendance at the meeting and also for future reference by those in attendance. If the resident was not able to clearly state his or her values, a primary caretaker or other close relative or friend would be asked to attend the care conference to give a statement of the resident's values as recalled. The conference could be used to clarify and resolve ethical dilemmas arising from the treatment plan.

In order to reduce one coercive aspect of the care conference, the resident or relative should be given some time between the conference and decision making. The resident or substitute decision maker should not be pressured by time. A time frame for decision making could be decided on during the conference. Use of a patient advocate for the resident or substitute would serve to empower the resident in relation to the expertise and strength of the staff.

Prior to these conferences, the head nurse would have to be careful to arrange staffing so that certain aides would be assigned consistently to certain residents, preferably residents whom the aides have expressed a preference to work with. The consistent assignments would increase the aide's involvement with these residents, including plans for their care.

In-service education programs for staff on how to maintain residents' autonomy would serve as a vehicle for discussion of the issue and joint problem solving by professional and nonprofessional staff. The staff could consider methods to empower residents, such as active listening and responsible assertiveness (Lange & Jakubowski, 1977).

Most important, nurse's aides' own values should be identified and respected by professional staff. Many aides have benevolent intentions, and these caring feelings for residents need to blended with information about the importance of the resident's autonomy; for example, that the resident cannot be helped without having control over some parts of the decision-making process. Power differences among staff members arising from racial, cultural, gender, or ethnic variations should be recognized and reduced as much as possible. Respect for nurse's aides' values may be passed on by the aide to the resident in parallel fashion in the form of increased respect for the resident's values and choices.

Assisting the Resident to Exercise Autonomy

A values specification process could help nurse's aides to separate their own values from those of the residents. This process should precede any efforts on the part of nurse's aides to act on behalf of or speak for the residents. As part of their supervisory responsibilities, registered nurses should look for evidence that this values analysis has occurred. In fact, the RN perhaps should specifically address this matter in a regular fashion, for example, through shift reports and performance reviews.

Staff members should be clearly informed by the employer about the channels of communication to follow if problems with patient care occur. Nurse's aides should be given permission to go above their immediate supervisor to the next level of authority if corrective action is not taken by the supervisor. It is in the employer's best interest to establish such norms among employees in that the employer must know about potential legal problems in order to take corrective action. This method of empowering supervisees would place pressure on supervisors to maintain good relations with their supervisees and be more responsive to their concerns. This is not to overlook the authority held by supervisors to make tough patient care decisions, but it is to recognize the importance of no one level of authority being above criticism. Without a norm of open debate and criticism, a spirit of teamwork cannot evolve. Empowering nurse's aides would have a positive effect on residents in that a more satisfied aide will provide better care for a resident, and having learned about the benefits of personal empowerment, the aide is more apt to respect, appreciate, and ultimately empower the resident.

SUMMARY

In analyzing these case examples, I chose to focus on the nurse's aide's responsibilities rather than on her rights. The autonomy of the patient seemed a more important issue to me than the independence of the aide. In the smoking example, the resident's autonomy was possibly violated by allowing and perhaps encouraging the resident to follow a self-destructive path without a clear understanding of the patient's values and no knowledge of prior staff discussion with the patient about the rationale for the decision. In the drug example, the possible violation of autonomy came in acting on behalf of the resident without knowledge of the patient's wishes or values, although one could reasonably presume the resident did not want to be overdosed with tranquilizers. The ethical problem in this example resided more in the relationship between the aide and the staff. In going around professional channels, she put her employer in legal jeopardy and did not act as a responsible member of a team.

REFERENCES

Gilligan, C. (1982). *In a different voice.* Cambridge, MA: Harvard University Press.

Gorlin, R. (Ed.) (1986). *Codes of professional responsibility.* Washington, DC: Bureau of National Affairs.

Kjervik, D. (1989). Ethics and law related to informed consent: Voluntariness and public policy issues, In *Proceedings of the First National Conference on Nursing Research and Clinical Management of Alzheimer's Disease.* Minneapolis: University of Minnesota.

Kjervik, D. & Grove, S. (1988). The legal meaning of consent in unequal power relationships. *Journal of Professional Nursing, 4*(3), 192–204.

Lange, A. & Jakubowski, P. (1977). *Responsible assertive behavior.* Champaign, IL: Research Press.

FOR FURTHER DISCUSSION: EDITORS' QUESTIONS

1. Was Kim Clark correct in going directly to the family in the matter of Emma McComb? Is this an example of an aide going appropriately beyond the call of duty or inappropriately beyond the scope of practice?
2. What outcomes would justify an aide's interventions to change a treatment plan?
3. What are the similarities and differences in the two interventions, the cigarette and the drug discussion with the relative?
4. What is the nature of responsibility inherent in Ms. Clark's role as a nurse's aide? What kind of relationship should exist between the paraprofessional caregiving staff and the resident, the nursing staff, the administrator, the medical director, the attending physician, the other health care personnel, and the residents' families?
5. Does a nursing home have a right to limit social behavior on matters such as smoking and diet given that similar patients living in their own homes are free to decide how far they will allow medical advice and pursuit of healthy life-styles?
6. Do you agree with Dr. Kjervik that "the overriding responsibility of a nurse's aide is loyalty to his or her employer?" What would be the arguments to justify this position? What other loyalties could be posited besides loyalty to employer?

Chapter 18

DEATH OF A RESIDENT

Alice Bennett had worked on the evening shift for 2 years at Green Terrace Convalescent Home. Over time she felt she had come to know the residents quite well. She learned about their past lives and met their families. In a more general way, she was aware of the residents' health problems from piecing together things said by the residents or the staff and by looking at their charts. "Nobody bothers to tell us about changes in the residents' condition, but we usually figure it out."

Both residents and family members like Alice and appreciate her energy and enthusiasm. She is a lively young woman who had grown up in the neighborhood of the facility and who attended college during the day. She was initially attracted to the position because of the convenient hours and a fondness for old people.

At Green Terrace, nurse's aides on the evening shift are assigned a group of 12 to 15 residents, for whom they have primary responsibility. They are responsible for getting their residents to the dining room and to activities, giving them any baths scheduled for that shift, and doing bedtime routines. The baths require cooperation from residents and from other aides (if two are needed to give the bath). A sign-up sheet is posted on the shower room door, and somehow "with everyone giving a little bit," it all works out. During dinner service the aides all go to the dining room and help out more generally with the meal service.

One day when Alice was passing the food and buttering bread for those who needed help, Marjorie Perkins, one of the residents assigned to another aide, told Alice that she was feeling weak and wanted to leave the dining room. As Alice tells the story:

> Mrs. Perkins said she felt like she was going to die. Her complaints were vague—she just felt weak all over. I reassured her that she would be fine and asked if she could wait to go to her room until her aide (who was in the kitchen) was free. Mrs. Perkins insisted that she needed to get back to her room. I looked around, couldn't see anyone to ask, and decided I had better go with her. Then she asked me to help her get into her nightclothes and into bed. She kept saying, "I am going to die," and I kept telling her, "Don't worry, I promise you, you are not going to die." I got her in bed and went back to the dining room. I told her aide that Mrs. Perkins felt sick and I had helped her to bed. Then I got so busy with the evening routines that I forgot all about it.
>
> At about 8:30, I heard some of the staff talking about what to do about "the body." It blew my mind when I realized that Marjorie Perkins had died. I must have been the last person who saw her. I can't think how many times I had promised her she wouldn't die. As far as anyone knew, Marjorie was in good shape, although generally frail. She was certainly not expected to die.
>
> For the rest of the shift I let my routine go. I guess the others felt sorry for me because nobody objected. Marjorie's two roommates were in the television room. I went back and told them. I wanted to make sure that they didn't wander into their room and get a shock. One of the roommates told me she really appreciated that I talked to her, that she didn't like it when people just disappeared and she didn't know what happened to them. The other didn't say much at all. I also had to speak to the resident's daughter. I guess I was the last person who saw her mother alive. I would never have left her alone if I had believed she would really die. Maybe I should have called the nurse from the other wing, or maybe I should just have stayed with her and forgot about the dining room. Shouldn't a nursing home make sure that residents don't die alone? I will never forget that day. It was the first time I ever saw a dead person, and I was very scared.

In the aftermath of the death of Mrs. Perkins, Alice began discussing the subject with other aides. She found she wasn't alone in worrying about death in the nursing home. Other staff members also had strong feelings and memorable incidents. Mildred, an older aide who had worked at the facility for years, said that several times dying residents had asked her to promise to do particular things. Mildred would usually agree "because it brings them some peace," yet she wondered if it was right to make promises haphazardly. Another aide was worried when the facility concealed a poor prognosis from the patients: "There's one lady now who thinks she's doing fine, but we know that her cancer's back and it's just a matter of time. Is it right to keep her in the dark?"

One male aide confided that he left a previous home because he became friendly with a resident who had a do-not-resuscitate order, and when the time came he thought "it stank" to have to let his friend die. Several aides told Alice that they would never go near a dead body, that they had made it clear when they started that they wouldn't prepare bodies. Alice even talked to someone—Janet—who had a less dramatic version of her own story. When she was working day shift, Janet had urged a resident to get up despite the latter's protests that she didn't feel well. The next day when Janet came to work, she learned the resident had died in the night. Many of the aides turned out to be quite unsure of how to handle an emergency and frightened that they might do the wrong thing. One aide recalled feeling desperately confused on several occasions about whether to remain with a resident in trouble or leave the resident to summon help.

The most surprising comment came from Olivia, a nurse's aide in her 30s whom Alice had regarded as not particularly sensitive or interested in her job. Olivia told Alice that she planned to find new work as soon as possible. For Olivia the most troublesome thing about being a nurse's aide was that "I don't cry anymore when people die—even people outside the nursing home."

After these discussions, Alice appreciated that the staff had an abundance of feelings about death in the nursing home, but she was more confused than ever about how it should be handled.

CASE COMMENTARY

Care of the Dying and the Newly Dead

Terrie Wetle

Wonders are many on earth, and the greatest of these / Is man . . .
For every ill he hath found its remedy / Save only death.
                                        SOPHOCLES (ANTIGONE)

Death is increasingly more likely to occur away from home and family, and in institutional settings attended by strangers. This shift in care of the dying away from family members and loved ones requires a reexamination of our moral obligations, formal rules, and informal practices regarding the dying and newly dead. There are many pathways—from living a life to being alive to actively dying to being dead—and the transitions among these stages are neither clearly demarcated nor easily predictable. For the purposes of this analysis, however, care of individuals in the following stages will be discussed: (1) the frail and concerned, (2) the actively dying, and (3) the newly dead.

It should be noted at the outset that there are distinct and conflicting individual beliefs and cultural mores regarding what is considered to be moral and appropriate behavior in caring for the dying and newly dead. These differing expectations lead to unclear obligations, resulting in confusion, anger, and guilt on the part of staff charged with this care. This is particularly true for situations in which scarce resources and limited personnel force staff to choose among competing demands. Moreover, as resources are increasingly restricted, the gap between what is ideal or desired and what is practical and feasible expands. Although it may be comforting or intellectually satisfying to discuss what constitutes exemplary behavior in ideal circumstances, an effort will be made in this analysis to examine the parameters of "good enough" ethics in the real world of constrained resources.

In the case at hand, Alice Bennett is a well-meaning, hardworking nursing home aide confronting the death of a resident for the first time. In her effort to care for Mrs. Perkins, a resident who expresses the feeling that she's going to die, Alice is confused regarding her obligations to Mrs. Perkins. When Mrs. Perkins does indeed die, Alice then reflects on her obligations to the family and to other residents. Let us begin with consideration of care of frail nursing home residents who are concerned with death.

FRAIL AND CONCERNED

Long-term-care residents constitute a population that, because of illness, frailty, and advanced age, is at increased risk of death. Although efforts have been made to improve the perception, nursing homes are viewed by most people as places where people go to die. It should be no surprise that individuals entering and living in nursing homes think about death and may be concerned about the process of dying. There is, however, a general conspiracy of silence among staff and residents on this important topic (Wetle, Levkoff, Cwikel, & Rosen, 1988). Discomfort with the topic, fear of being morbid, and concerns for the feelings of others all contribute to an ongoing charade that denies death as a common and expected event in this setting.

Conspiracy of Silence

Why are staff silent? Avoidance of the topic of death, particularly with elderly or terminally ill patients, has been well documented in the population at large and among health care professionals (Weisman, 1972). This discomfort in discussing death with individuals who, because of illness or advanced age, are believed to be close to death has been attributed to many factors. First, there is fear of causing pain or upset by pointing out or reminding an individual that his or her death is more or less imminent. Second, there continues to exist a relatively strong taboo regarding discussing the more personal aspects of death concerns (Kalish, 1976). Because of this general taboo, health care professionals have little experience, common language, or symbols with which to engage in such discussions.

Informal practices of the institution may reinforce the tendency toward silence on this important topic. Efforts to maintain a positive and cheerful atmosphere, for example, may preclude such discussions. Nursing home residents may themselves contribute to the silence by avoiding the topic of death with staff members, out of concern for the staff members' feelings or in reaction to verbal and nonverbal clues that this is a forbidden topic. Yet chronic disease and physical frailty bring death to mind, and for some, may in fact reduce fear of death (Peschel & Peschel, 1983). Moreover, the opportunity to talk about death and the dying process may reduce fear of death, whereas denial of the opportunity to discuss impending death may increase emotional pain and suffering.

Tolstoy (1980) described this process dramatically in *The Death of Ivan Ilych*, as the patient consulted one doctor after another, none of whom would admit he was dying:

> What tormented Ivan Ilych was that deception . . . their not wishing to admit what they all knew and what he knew, but wanting to lie to him concerning his terrible condition, and wishing and forcing him to participate in that lie (p. 423).

Not only was Ivan Ilych denied the opportunity to make peace with his death, the "falsity around him and within him did more than anything else to poison his last days" (p. 424).

Knowledge of Resident's Health and Prognosis

Another barrier to open discussion and appropriate response to death concerns among residents is limited knowledge among the staff regarding the health of and prognosis for individual residents. Although the nursing

staff may be provided such information, nurse's aides and other personnel are less likely to be adequately informed. Often there are concerns regarding the ability of such staff to understand and process
technical information, although with rather modest efforts to simplify
and clarify, adequate information can be communicated. Moreover, improved understanding of individual illnesses is likely to enhance patient care. For example, explaining that the slow response of an
individual with Parkinson's disease is a symptom of that disease, not
just a matter of stubbornness, is likely to increase both understanding
and tolerance on the part of the aide.

Resident information may also be withheld in an effort to protect the
privacy of residents. Instructions and guidelines regarding confidentiality of resident information should be provided to all nursing home staff,
with regular refresher in-service training to emphasize appropriate behavior. Despite concerns over patient privacy, institutions have an obligation to provide information required to perform job duties adequately.
Moreover, provision of accurate and timely information is likely to cur-
tail the spread of rumors and inappropriate information.

Nursing home staff members are sometimes asked by families or other
care providers to withhold health-related information from residents.
This places the staff in a particularly uncomfortable bind. Residents are
most likely to turn to providers of day-to-day care with questions and
concerns regarding health and prognosis. Instructions "not to tell" place
nurses and aides in the position of lying to the resident, either directly by
denial or indirectly by avoiding the topic. It should be noted that decisions to withhold information from residents regarding their own condition, particularly as regards life-threatening illness, are in direct conflict
with ethical values of individual autonomy and self-determination. Most
ethicists would agree that such actions are rarely justified and must be
carefully considered. Moreover, family members should be encouraged
to reconsider a decision not to tell, not only because such a decision
conflicts with concepts of individual autonomy but because it is likely to
interfere with their ongoing relationship with the resident. Efforts
should be made to avoid circumstances in which staff are asked to lie to
or withhold information from residents.

This is not to suggest that aides be charged with the responsibility for
detailed discussions of disease or prognosis but rather that they be provided guidelines for how to respond to such questions. Usually the most
appropriate response to the assertion "I feel like I'm going to die" is clarification of those feelings for more specificity regarding symptoms. A simple
response of "Why do you feel that way?" or "Tell me more about your
feelings" will elicit information regarding a specific complaint or symptom to which staff can make appropriate response.

In the case under discussion, it would have been preferable for Alice to avoid promises to Mrs. Perkins that she "was not going to die" or that she "would be fine" but rather to inquire in more detail about Mrs. Perkins's feelings as she assisted her to bed. Denial of such feelings is neither reassuring to the patient nor conducive to building trusting relationships and, as in this case, engenders guilt when the resident dies.

The timing of staff training on these issues is important. Ideally, such training would be provided on an ongoing basis beginning prior to patient care and continuing with regular in-service "refreshers." Given the staffing constraints in most facilities, time for training is a precious and limited commodity. Therefore, role modeling by more experienced staff takes on added importance, as do staff debriefings after an upsetting event such as the death of Mrs. Perkins. These debriefings need require relatively modest time investment but should encourage sharing of feelings and suggestions for alternative approaches in future situations.

Do Residents Know When They're Going To Die?

An important aspect of this case is Alice Bennett's concern that Mrs. Perkins knew that she was going to die and that Alice responded inappropriately. The first question is whether, indeed, individuals know when death is imminent. There is a relatively strong folk belief that we do sense when death is imminent. Unfortunately, there are few, if any, data to support such a belief. Certainly, we are all aware of anecdotal experiences in which a patient expresses such an awareness just prior to death, but there are innumerable counterbalancing experiences in which the patient expresses the feeling of impending death but does not die. This is partly because the statement "I feel like I'm going to die" is used commonly to express feelings of severe pain, depression, anxiety, or desire for attention. As described above, the staff should be provided guidance in reasonable responses to such statements. It should also be noted that appropriate response is, to some degree, determined by characteristics of individual residents. For some residents, such a statement is indicative of a serious and acute concern. For others, such statements are a rather routine part of conversation and have less to do with immediate feelings and more to do with accustomed interaction patterns.

A corollary question to whether residents know whether they are about to die, is whether the staff can know that a resident is about to die. In general, unless the resident is in the acute stress of serious illness, it is difficult to predict imminent death. In a nursing home setting, where a majority of patients carry rather serious burdens of disease and disability, distinguishing those individuals for whom death is imminent is often difficult. However, in some cases, imminent death is relatively probable. If we believe that death is imminent, how do we change our behavior?

CARE OF THE DYING

When we know or are fairly certain that death is imminent, what are our obligations? Expectations of appropriate behavior toward the dying are strongly culturally determined. Several common themes emerge: that the dying be treated with concern and respect, that to the degree possible their wishes be granted, and that death should occur in the company of others.

The Right of an "Accompanied" Death

Literary and cultural tradition indicates an ideal of an "accompanied" death, as opposed to the fear of dying alone and unattended. For some cultural groups, this translates into extended "deathbed watches" involving multiple members of the family sitting at the bedside in shifts. In some cases, these culturally determined behaviors may come into conflict with facility rules and the needs of other patients. For example, an acute-care nurse describes one family constellation as follows:

> He was the Gypsy king or something and had really bad congestive heart failure and emphysema. They brought him to our unit from the emergency room, and we only had a semiprivate bed left. People just kept coming in. They were sitting on his bed, in the hallways, and in the visitors' lounge. They were all real loud, smoking and eating food from the outside. We tried to tell them that visiting hours were over, but they wouldn't leave. Normally, when someone is so sick, we let one or two family stay as long as they want, but this must have been 30 people. They acted like it was some kind of party. I felt sorry for the other patients.

When we don't understand differences in cultural expectations, or when they compete with the interests of others, conflicts can arise. The resolution of these conflicts may be compounded when scarce resources make it impossible to fully accommodate competing interests or wishes. In the example just cited, the staff could have made efforts to find a private room or indicated space in which the extended family could congregate, other than the patient's bedside. At some point, however, the staff may be required to set limits on the number of family in attendance at any one time out of concern for the rights of other patients and the continued function of the unit.

The more likely circumstance in the nursing home setting, however, is that few family members or friends, if any, are available to attend the deaths of loved ones. This function therefore falls to the staff. Is the staff morally obligated to attend the death of a resident? The first question, of course, is whether the patient prefers or desires such attendance. Just as the obligation to "attend a death" is a matter of cultural practice, so too is the desire to have one's own death attended a matter of individual preference. Some residents are very clear about not wanting to "die alone." Unfortunately, even if the patient clearly expresses a wish to have a staff member or family present at the bedside, it may be difficult, if not impossible, to honor such a request because of competing demands.

In the current case, Alice Bennett acted in a caring and compassionate way by accompanying Mrs. Perkins to her room and helping her into her nightclothes and into bed. Was she then obligated to stay with Mrs. Perkins? Did Mrs. Perkins want Alice to stay with her, or was the reassurance that Alice or her assigned aide would check in on her later sufficient? If Mrs. Perkins did request that Alice stay, how could Alice balance this request with competing obligations for other patients?

Once again we are faced with the distinction between the ideal response and the practical reality. Ideally, patients who are in the process of dying should have companionship if they wish, preferably family and other loved ones. Unfortunately, several factors contribute to the likely absence of family members. First, there may be no family, or families may live too far away to be in regular attendance; families may have competing demands that limit their time at the bedside; families may be uncomfortable in the nursing home or with the death process; and finally, our uncertainty regarding when death is likely to occur may preclude the presence of family members even if they wished to be there.

Other alternatives are sometimes available, such as a friend who also resides in the home. The following comment was provided by a nursing home resident participating in a study of resident participation in health care decisions (Wetle et al., 1988). She describes the death of another resident in the facility.

> I spent a lot of time in her room that last two weeks. She was my friend . . . . We both lived at the center for more than three years, and I didn't want her to be alone. I knew she was pretty sick because she would fade in and out, but when she opened her eyes, I wanted her to see me. At first the nurses tried to keep me out, but then they mainly left me alone with her. Now that she's gone, I feel good that I did it, but wonder who will sit with me (quotation from unpublished data of author).

When family or friends are not available, the responsibility then falls to the staff. Given the staffing patterns of most long-term-care facilities, it is unlikely that staff members are conveniently available to sit at the bedside for long periods of time. Sometimes, it is sufficient reassurance to agree to sit with the patient for a few minutes or until the patient falls asleep. But staff may be faced with the difficult decision of leaving the bedside of a resident who clearly does not wish to be left alone. There is no absolute moral obligation to remain at the bedside of a dying patient; however, there is a clinical duty to make a patient in acute physical or emotional distress as comfortable as possible.

Nursing homes should develop and promulgate clear policy regarding staff obligations in this regard. The staff should be made aware of institutional policy and provided support in following these directives. Supervisors should regularly review care plans for patients thought to be near death, with clear guidelines regarding resuscitation efforts, responses to patient requests, and how to respond should a crisis occur. Staff debriefings following a resident's death are a good way to share feelings and concerns, reinforce appropriate behavior, and review institutional policy.

CARE OF THE NEWLY DEAD

In all cultures there are special obligations and expectations regarding care of the newly dead—in other words, the corpse. In general, the duty is to treat the body in a dignified and respectful manner. There are also legal duties pertaining to the newly dead. For example, depending on the circumstances of the death, there may be a legal responsibility to notify the police, the coroner, or other legal authority. There may be the responsibility not to move the body or alter the immediate area around the body. In some states the body may not be moved until officially pronounced dead. In other states there are statutory obligations for physician involvement. Obviously, the staff should be informed of these legal requirements and provided with clear policy and expectations regarding care of the newly dead. The staff should also be assisted in working through their feelings regarding the care of the dead body. Sensitivity to fears and apprehension are useful in the development of healthy attitudes and practical behaviors. Although facilities are not morally obligated to change the duties of a staff member who is uncomfortable in caring for the dead, good management practice would include efforts to address these concerns by additional educational experiences and role modeling by senior staff.

Informing Family, Residents, and Staff

Related to care of the newly dead is informing family, roommates, and other residents that the death has occurred (Creek, 1980; Robinson, 1981). Individual facilities have different policies regarding who is responsible for notifying families. Tolle and colleagues (1984) describe a trend toward the use of telephones rather than in-person notification; and for the death of a nursing home resident, a nurse or other staff member may replace the physician in notification of families. Respect for the feelings and concerns of other residents requires that they be notified when a fellow resident dies. Mrs. Perkins's roommate was very clear in expressing her gratitude for being informed and about her upset when residents just "disappear" without comment from staff. Not only is such a disappearance disturbing, but it may actually lead to fears among residents that their own deaths may go unnoticed and unmarked. The following comment from a nursing home resident interviewed in our own previously cited study (Wetle et al., 1988) expresses such a concern.

> Nobody ever comes right out and says "Mrs. Smith kicked the bucket." It's always, she was transferred to the hospital, or we moved her to the south wing. Well, we all know what "moved to the south wing means." . . . It means you're dead. They act like nothing happened. Well, something did happen. Someone died . . . . Will anyone say a word for me when I die or will I just disappear? (quotation from unpublished data of author).

To assume that the residents are unaware that a death has occurred is both naive and destructive to the development of trusting relationships. Moreover, this particular conspiracy of silence interferes with the grief process of residents, who may have had a relationship with the deceased, and it may lead to unnecessary fears or concerns for surviving residents.

Some facilities plan brief services or memorial meetings to which residents and staff are invited. Staff and residents report that such services provide closure and are actually reassuring, allowing the expression of grief or relief that suffering is over for the deceased. Again quoting from our own data (Wetle et al., 1988), we find such a memorial services described by a nursing home aide.

> We just gather in the day room and people are invited to just say something they remember about the person. You know, like "Jim sure liked his coffee, I remember how he always had a third cup, but he was real nice to help with the wheel chairs." Or "I'll miss Jim's stories about the old country." (quotation from unpublished data of author).

Staff Debriefing Following Death

The death of someone we know or provide care for can be an upsetting and disturbing event. Generally, training of nursing home personnel does not include analysis of feelings regarding dying or death. Many younger personnel enter the workplace having had no prior experience with death on a firsthand basis. Preparation for deaths of residents, including both information regarding what to do and discussion of feelings and personal concerns, is an important duty for the facility. After a death occurs, debriefing provides opportunity for sharing feelings and concerns, expressions of sadness or relief, and a sense of closure. These debriefings combined with the memorial services mentioned above are likely to improve the emotional response to death and improve care to the dying.

CONCLUSION

The development of an "ethical" organization requires attention to the fears, concerns, and expectations of both residents and staff at all levels. Although this may require additional investments of time and resources, in the long run rewards will be realized through enhanced care, improved staff satisfaction, and improved comfort for families and residents. Moreover, staff support of the type described above is likely to accrue savings via improved staff retention and employee satisfaction. Because our moral obligations in these matters are not clearcut but heavily dependent on cultural expectations, open dialogue takes on increased importance, as does the process of decision making. Attention to improving care of the dying and newly dead will improve quality of life for nursing home residents and those who provide their care.

REFERENCES

Creek, L. V. (1980). How to tell the family the patient has died. *Postgraduate Medicine, 68,* 207–209.

Kalish, R. A. (1976). Death and dying in a social context. In R. H. Binstock & E. Shanas (Eds.), *Handbook of aging and the social sciences.* New York: Van Nostrand Reinhold, pp. 483–503.

Peschel, R. E., & Peschel, E. R. (1983). The face of death: Case history, literary histories. *Perspectives in Biology and Medicine, 26,* (3), 394–410.

Robinson, M. A. (1981). Informing the family of sudden death. *American Family Physician, 23,* 115–118.

Tolstoy, L. (1980). The death of Ivan Ilych. In R. F. Weir (Ed.), *Death in literature.* New York: Columbia University Press, pp. 386–440.

Tolle, S. W., Elliot, D. L., Hickam, D. H. (1984). Physician attitudes and practices at the time of patient death. *Archives of Internal Medicine, 144,* 2389–2391.

Weisman, A. D. (1972). Denial and middle knowledge. In A. D. Weisman (Ed.) *On Dying and denying: A psychiatric study of terminality.* New York: Behavioral Publication (pp. 56–78).

Wetle, T., Levkoff, S., Cwikel, J., & Rosen, A. (1988). Nursing home resident participation in medical decisions: Perceptions and preferences. *The Gerontologist, 28,* (Suppl.), 32–38.

FOR FURTHER DISCUSSION: EDITORS' QUESTIONS

1. If a nursing home anticipates that a resident is near death, what are its obligations to a dying resident? Is the facility obliged to offer privacy? Constant attendance from staff? When in the dying processing do any of these obligations begin?

2. How does the cognitive state of the dying resident influence the facility's obligation?

3. What are the obligations of nurse's aides to care for dying residents? Must aides attend the dying, and must they care for the body?

4. How should aides handle requests of dying patients? Should they give comfort by making "deathbed promises" they are not sure they can keep?

5. What should they be taught to do when residents remark that they feel sick or think they are going to die soon?

6. How much information about a resident's condition should be given to paraprofessional nurse's aides (some of whom have not graduated from high school)? Without such information, aides may be unaware of the imminence of some predictable deaths.

7. Does the facility management have any obligation to assist nurse's aides in dealing emotionally with death among the residents? What are these obligations?

8. What is the facility's obligation to other residents in relation to death in a nursing home? Does the facility have any obligation to

inform other residents about the death? Or, on the contrary, does it have an obligation to protect other residents and preserve privacy for the deceased resident and the family?

9. From a moral standpoint, how should the nurse's aide and facility responses at the time of Marjorie Perkins's sudden death be evaluated?

Chapter 19

DRESSING FOR 'SUCCESS'

Clara Smith, a widow of 80, has lived at Vistaview Home for almost 6 years. Vistaview is a for-profit facility with 152 beds. Six years ago both of Clara's legs were amputated at the knees. She does not have weight-bearing prostheses.

Clara has always been attentive to her personal appearance. She has strong likes and dislikes, particularly in matters pertaining to her personal life. For that matter, she maintains strong opinions about things that go on around her. Last Halloween, when old, confused Mrs. McDougal was painted up and costumed like a clown, Clara complained to the administrator that it wasn't fair to make fun of poor Mrs. McDougal like that. The administrator told Clara that Mrs. McDougal was enjoying all the attention (and Clara knew that was true) and that no harm was done. Clara wasn't so sure; something about it struck her as disrespectful, but she did not pursue the complaint.

As for her own life, she has always had a "routine." She prides herself on her attractiveness and makes every effort to wear clothes and cosmetics that enhance her appearance.

Beth Festinger has worked at Vistaview as a nursing assistant for 2 years. Her mother, who had also worked there for many years, helped get her the job. Beth considers herself a conscientious and responsible aide. She enjoys her job and the floor she works on. She feels that the routines of the day are very important to making the operation of the nursing home go smoothly. She believes that the home has about the right number of staff members for the floor.

She is especially happy that she is able to get to know her patients. "I get to know them fairly well. They may not know me by name, but they all know me by face. Sometimes when I have extra time I will go into their rooms and talk. They love to hear about my personal life, and you can learn so much from them too. They have their favorite aides, and we have our favorite residents."

Clara is not one of Beth's favorites. Clara insists on wearing clothing that is not designed for someone with missing limbs. She wants to wear things she has always worn, including some dresses she brought with her to Vistaview.

Beth finds it very hard to give Clara a choice about what she will wear. "I try to give my residents as much choice as I can within the regulations. I know, myself, I have preferences about what I wear each day, and they should too." But Clara is very picky. She wants every accessory just so. She brought a large selection of scarves and costume jewelry, which is stored on her shelf and in her drawers. "She can't reach anything herself and you could spend a lot of time just looking for the earrings she wants." Besides, Beth adds, "Clara is very difficult to manage if she wears certain dresses. I cannot get her on the toilet easily, and it works out better if she wears some of her dresses backwards—then I can get the dress up at the same time I sit her on the toilet."

Clara hates the restrictions Beth has imposed on her wardrobe. She feels like a "fool walking around with my dress ass-backwards."

CASE COMMENTARY

Martin Benjamin

Our sense of ourselves as whole and particular persons is determined in part by our capacity to realize over the course of our lives a set of integrated and individuating personal choices and characteristics. Continuity with the past contributes to the integrity or wholeness of a human life. Distinctiveness contributes to its identity. In Clara Smith's case, retaining certain routines, especially those pertaining to dress and appearance, is both integrity- and identity-preserving. Wearing what she has worn in the past (including some dresses that predate the amputation of her legs) helps to preserve her wholeness, or integrity, and dressing as she chooses contributes to her identity as a particular person. The latter becomes especially important as advancing age and institutionalized living limit other ways of expressing individuality. Dressing as she pleases allows Clara to express herself and assert her own unique personality (see Battin, this volume). If Vistaview Home is to respect Clara's dignity and integrity as an individual, it must do what it can to accommodate her preferences on this and related matters.

DECISIONAL AND EXECUTIONAL AUTONOMY

Because she is disabled, Clara is not, by herself, fully autonomous with respect to dress and personal appearance. In her case there is a gap between what Collopy (1988) has identified as decisional autonomy and autonomy of execution. Clara Smith is fully capable of exercising decisional autonomy, but the loss of her legs severely restricts executional autonomy. She can decide what to wear, but she cannot dress herself. Unless her autonomous decisions about dress and personal appearance are executed by someone else, her overall integrity and identity will be considerably diminished. Yet help is not always forthcoming.

Conflicting Routines

The person designated to help Clara with her clothing is nursing assistant Beth Festinger. Like Clara, Beth is also wedded to certain routines. These routines, she feels, are very important in making the operation of the nursing home go smoothly. Clara's insistence on wearing clothing not designed for women without legs and having every accessory placed "just so" disrupts Beth's routines. Because, as Beth puts it, "Clara is very difficult to manage if she wears certain dresses," she finds it difficult to get Clara on the toilet easily. Thus, she has taken to putting some of Clara's dresses on backward, which, she says, enables her to get the dress up at the same time she seats Clara on the toilet.

Having to walk around with her "dress ass-backwards" is an affront to Clara's dignity. Not only are her autonomous decisions not executed, but she is made to feel like a "fool." Even if Clara has been reluctant to mention this to Beth directly, her previous complaint when Mrs. McDougal was dressed like a clown reveals how deeply she must feel the assault on her dignity.

Is Beth's conduct ethically justifiable? Given the details of the case, it seems that it is not. Vistaview Home in general and Beth Festinger in particular have a prima facie or basic obligation to preserve residents' autonomy and to help them to maintain their integrity and identity if they can do so without violating equally if not more important obligations to other residents. In this case, at least as it is presented, Beth is not justified in failing to fulfill this obligation to Clara.

First Things First

If the Vistaview Home were seriously understaffed, so that caregivers were able to provide patients only the most elemental care, one might readily justify Beth's preoccupation with efficiency at the expense of Clara's autonomy, integrity, and identity. Meeting other patients' more basic biological needs would be more important, if a choice needed to be made, than helping Clara express herself through a time-consuming concern with particular clothing. Although Clara would still have ethical grounds for complaint, the appropriate target would not be Beth, who would be trying to make the best of a bad situation, but rather the managers or the owners of the nursing home or perhaps society at large.

This is not, however, the situation described in the case. Beth believes that the home is adequately staffed and admits to having "extra time" to go into the rooms of her favorite residents and talk. They enjoy hearing about her personal life, and she enjoys their company as well. For Beth these conversations are often personally enriching.

That Beth does this is in itself unobjectionable. Indeed, getting to know one's patients and engaging them in friendly conversation is an important part of a caregiver's role. If a nursing assistant spends time chatting with residents after her more basic obligations have been fulfilled, there can be little ground for complaint, even if she does not do it with everyone alike. Genuine conversation of this sort requires a core of mutual interest, and not all people have the same interests. Indeed, some residents may enjoy talking with Beth, whereas others may find her company bothersome. But just as attending to patients' basic biological needs is prior condition to supporting their exercise of autonomy, so too is supporting patients' autonomy a prior obligation to engaging them in convivial conversation. Getting to know one's "favorite" patients better should not come at the expense of neglecting the rights or violating the dignity of other patients.

As written, the case suggests that Beth's routinely putting some of Clara's dresses on backward is designed in part to enable her to spend more time talking with her favorite residents. Clara is not one of Beth's favorites. Dressing and undressing her is burdensome, as is helping her with the toilet. Strong-minded, picky, and perhaps not all that interested in Beth's personal life, Clara is not the sort of resident with whom Beth cares to spend extra time. But this is beside the point. Patients need not be likable to have a right to have their autonomy, integrity, and identity accorded a certain measure of respect, especially when they are disabled, institutionalized, or both. As long as Clara's requests are not unreasonable or so time-consuming that satisfying them prevents Beth from attending to the similar requests of other residents, she must fulfill them if she is to help Clara execute her autonomous decisions and thereby sustain and express her sense of herself as a whole and particular person.

A MORE DIFFICULT SITUATION

Suppose now that the home is not so well staffed or that the time required to satisfy all of Clara's concerns about her personal appearance cuts into the time Beth has available to attend to the integrity- and identity-preserving autonomy of other residents. If this were the case, Beth would have no extra time to visit the rooms of her favorite residents and talk. Time not spent helping to realize *all* of Clara's preferences would be spent (let us assume) more or less equitably helping to realize similar preferences or satisfy more basic needs of other residents. In these circumstances Beth could, let us suppose, fully attend to Clara's concerns about her dress and appearance only at the expense of similar or more important needs and concerns of other residents.

Here the "routines of the day" adopted by Beth to make the operation of the nursing home go smoothly are grounded in a concern for making the most efficient and equitable use of a limited and extremely valuable resource—her time and energy. For her these routines are also integrity-preserving. Maintaining them and the values of justice and efficiency they help to secure contributes to Beth's conception of herself as a conscientious and responsible aide. Included among her routines, let us suppose, is (regrettably) restricting Clara's choice about what she will wear. Beth feels she cannot spend as much time as Clara would like searching for or adjusting her accessories, and she allows Clara to wear certain dresses (those that create time-consuming difficulties when seating her on the toilet) only if they are worn backward.

Once we suppose that Beth is motivated by a need to provide just and efficient care for an overly large patient population rather than by a dislike of Clara and/or a desire to spend more time chatting with and getting to know residents she finds more congenial, the case becomes more difficult. How much consideration should be given to matters of clothing and dress selection in such circumstances? Is it possible to work out some sort of compromise that would allow Clara to retain adequate dignity, integrity, identity, and autonomy without significantly compromising Beth's integrity or the rights and needs of other residents? I think so.

Compromise

A compromise, as understood here, is a position that more or less "splits the difference" between two opposing positions and that is arrived at through a process of give-and-take discussion involving mutual respect and mutual concession. The term "compromise" refers to both an *outcome* and a *process*. As outcome, it is *something reached*, and as process, *a way of reaching*.

A compromise position is importantly different from a middle-of-the-road or synthesis position. If, for example, two parties hold conflicting positions (*A* and *B*), and each comes to regard a third position, *S* (a synthesis that combines the strongest features of *A* and *B* while avoiding their drawbacks), as superior to both *A* and *B* and then embrace it, we do not have a compromise. There has been no compromise or concession by either party. In adopting *S*, each has abandoned what is now regarded as a less correct view (either *A* or *B*) for one (*S*) that is, on its own terms, much better. The result is one form of (rational) *resolution* of the initial conflict, not a compromise.

If, however, the party holding *A* and the party holding *B* remain wedded to their respective positions and find themselves in circumstances in which both cannot be realized, they may, after mutually respectful give-and-take discussion, agree to a compromise position, *C*, which somehow seems to split the difference between *A* and *B*. Each party will, in this event, make certain concessions to the other for the sake of agreement on a single course of action that seems to have some independent validity and to capture as much of the spirit of *A* as it does of *B*, and vice versa. The matter is not, however, fully settled; there is no closure, no final harmony. A compromise is not a rational resolution. It makes the best of what both parties to the disagreement regard as a bad situation; and each may continue to try to persuade the other (or some third party to whom each may try to appeal) of the superiority of either *A* or *B* or to see that the same situation does not arise in the future.

Consider the reconstructed conflict between Clara Smith and Beth Festinger. Might there be a well-grounded compromise position that more or less splits the difference between them? If, after a bit of mutually respectful discussion of the matter, Beth were to acknowledge (1) the importance of clothing and dress selection to an individual's identity and integrity (especially when other ways of maintaining wholeness and particularity are being eroded by the requirements of institutional living); (2) the distinction between decisional autonomy and autonomy of execution, together with the need of patients like Clara for someone to help with the latter; and (3) the importance of maintaining residents' dignity, she might then be more inclined to search for alternatives that would go at least partway in meeting Clara's demands. Correspondingly, if, after discussing the matter with Beth, Clara were to acknowledge (1) the unfortunate circumstances in which Beth finds herself, (2) the importance of Beth's maintaining her own integrity, and (3) the equal needs and rights of other residents to whom Beth is responsible, she may be then more inclined to moderate her demands so as to go at least partway in accommodating these conflicting considerations.

If Beth and Clara were to try to accommodate each other through compromise, the result might take several forms. Depending on how Beth could juggle or alter her routines, she might be able to allot more time to helping Clara with clothing on some days than on others. Perhaps this time could, by mutual agreement, be regularly scheduled so that Clara could be assured that on certain days she would be able to dress as she wished. She might also be given a choice as to whether she wants to wear dresses that are difficult to manage backward or not at all. Certain of these dresses, worn correctly, might be designated for special occasions, such as Clara's birthday, certain holidays, every Sunday, or the first Sunday of the month, and so on. As for Clara's jewelry and accessories, reorganizing them might make it easier for Beth to find them in the mornings; and perhaps another resident, if asked, would be happy to help Clara adjust them if Beth is unable to do more than place them in the generally correct area. At the same, time Beth and Clara might be able to join forces in trying to ameliorate the external circumstances that have forced them to compromise on this matter.

In a compromise of this sort, Clara and Beth would each obtain part, but not all, of what she wants. Clara's dignity would be intact, and she would have (perhaps only barely) enough choice, discretion, and autonomy with respect to dress and personal appearance to adequately preserve her integrity and her identity as a particular person. She would not, however, be able to dress exactly as she wants to whenever she wants to. Beth would retain a large part of her overall routine, but she would still be spending more time attending to Clara's concerns about clothing than she would like to; and she would do so at some inconvenience insofar as she must work out and implement their new agreement and perhaps reorganize Clara's jewelry and accessories.

Integrity

In addition to the use I have emphasized, the term "compromise" also has a well-known pejorative use. Talk of "compromising one's principles" or "compromising one's integrity" suggests that compromise is ethically dishonorable—a sign of moral weakness, hypocrisy, opportunism, and so on. Some go so far as to say that a person cannot embrace a compromise position on a matter of ethical importance without compromising (in the sense of betraying) his or her basic ethical convictions (Rand, 1964). But is this always so? Is it possible to hold a particular position, say either A or B, on a certain matter and at the same time agree on a certain compromise, C, without compromising one's integrity?

To see how a compromise of this sort may be integrity-preserving it is important, following a suggestion of Arthur Kuflik (1979), to distinguish (1) what one believes ought to be done in a particular case, leaving aside for the moment that there is a rationally irreconcilable conflict, from (2) what one judges ought to be done, *all things considered*, when among the things to be considered is the existence of such a conflict:

> When an issue is in dispute there is more to be considered than the issue itself—for example, the importance of peace, the presumption against settling matters by force, the intrinsic good of participating in a process in which each side must hear the other side out and try to see matters from the other's point of view, the extent to which the matter does admit reasonable differences of opinion and the significance of a settlement in which each party feels assured of the other's respect for its own seriousness and sincerity in the matter (p. 51).

These considerations of tolerance and mutual respect reflect values and principles that many of us hold dear and that partially determine who we are and what we stand for. If, for example, Clara Smith and Beth Festinger, in addition to their opposing positions in the case under consideration, also place a high value on toleration and mutual respect, agreeing to a plausible compromise may threaten the overall integrity of neither party. On the contrary, when they take into consideration all of their values and principles, together with the fact that they disagree and that there is something to be said for each position, the compromise position may be more integrity-preserving than any available alternative.

The main point is that, as most of us on reflection will acknowledge, our identity is constituted in part by a complex constellation of occasionally conflicting values and principles. In certain cases it will not be possible to act in accord with all of them. Beth may, for example, believe both that Clara is overly concerned about her personal appearance *and* in the values identified in the foregoing passage from Kuflik, especially the presumption against settling matters by force. In such cases of internal as well as external conflict we will often pursue that course of action that seems, on balance, to follow from the preponderance of our central and most highly cherished and rationally defensible values and principles. If, as I would hope, the core of Beth's and Clara's overall values and principles include a high degree of trying to see matters from others' points of view, an understanding of the extent to which certain disagreements are rationally irreconcilable, a presumption against settling matters by rank or power, and so on, it would not be surprising if they were to agree that a compromise in this instance were to be more integrity-preserving than the imposition of either of the polar alternatives.

FURTHER CONSIDERATIONS

Although compromise has been neglected by ethical theorists, it has an important role to play in addressing actual issues in health care, including those turning on conflicts of ethical values and principles (Benjamin, 1988, in press; Benjamin & Curtis, 1986, 1987; Weil & Benjamin, 1987). Poole and Anstett (1983) describe 23 cases in which a family physician's response to a patient request for unorthodox or alternative modes of care included an attempt to negotiate some sort of mutually satisfactory agreement or compromise. The results, they conclude, "suggest that certain patients who have requests for alternative health care are willing to negotiate with their physician and to agree on a compromise management plan that may be satisfactory to both the physician and the patient" (p. 772). Moody (1988), in an essay focusing on the nursing home context, emphasizes the role of negotiation in obtaining consent and discusses, among other things, situations involving "negotiating a compromise between a patient's demands and what reality will permit" (p. 66).

As many of the cases in this book suggest, conflicts between residents and between residents and staff are inevitable within a complex social setting like the nursing home, especially when they are a function of limited personal and material resources. In many situations a well-grounded, integrity- preserving compromise may be the best we can do to ameliorate such conflicts. Yet compromise is a complex notion with a number of different, but overlapping meanings (Benjamin, in press). In the health care setting, especially when the needs of staff conflict with those of residents, special attention must be given to compromise *as process* — give-and-take discussion presupposing moral equality and aiming at mutual accommodation. Genuine compromise requires that staff members resist the temptation to exploit their greater power so as to manipulate or coerce residents into the sort of lopsided "compromises" that give the notion a bad name. Compromise, especially on matters of ethics, requires ethics *in* compromise (Benjamin, in press).

Caregivers wanting to improve their skills in negotiating mutually respectful and satisfactory compromises will find Fisher and Ury's *Getting to Yes* (1981) a short and accessible primer drawing on a wealth of empirical research. Institutions interested in facilitating compromise between residents and between residents and staff (and perhaps even between staff members and between administration and staff) might organize in-service training or discussion groups around this book. Like much social scientific work on bargaining and negotiation, however, it gives short shrift to power imbalances (Luban, 1985) and disagreements rooted in opposing ethical convictions (Benjamin, in press).

CONCLUSION

Dress and personal appearance play an important role in preserving integrity and identity in the lives of the elderly and in enabling them to express themselves and assert their own unique individuality. The disabled often need special help in this regard. A caregiver is often required to bridge the gap between a physically disabled person's decisional autonomy ("I'd like to wear my red dress today") and his or her autonomy of execution ("but I can't put it on by myself"). Given the ethical importance of integrity, identity, and autonomy, a caregiver's understandable interest in conversing with "favorite" residents should not come at the expense of the rights of less favorite residents to adequate help with dress and appearance. In some situations, however, limited staffing may not allow a caregiver to spend as much time helping certain residents with dress and appearance as these residents would like. While attempting to remedy such regrettable situations, caregiver and patient should each attempt to appreciate the other's point of view and engage in mutually respectful give-and-take discussion in the hopes of devising a mutually satisfactory, integrity-preserving compromise.

REFERENCES

Benjamin, M. (1988). Rethinking ethical theory: Suggestions from and for the classroom. *Teaching Philosophy, 10,* 285–294.

Benjamin, M. (in press). *Splitting the difference: Integrity-preserving compromise in ethics and politics.* Lawrence, KS: University Press of Kansas.

Benjamin, M., & Curtis, J. (1986). *Ethics in nursing* (2nd ed.). New York: Oxford University Press.

Benjamin, M., & Curtis, J. (1987). Ethical autonomy in nursing. In D. Van De Veer & T. Regan (eds.), *Health care ethics* (pp. 394–427). Philadelphia: Temple University Press.

Collopy, B. J. (1988). Autonomy in long term care: Some crucial distinctions, *The Gerontologist, 28* (Suppl.), 10–17.

Fisher R., & Ury, W. (1981). *Getting to yes: Negotiating agreement without giving in.* Boston: Houghton Mifflin.

Kuflik, A. (1979). Morality and compromise. In J. R. Pennock & J. W. Chapman (eds.), *Compromise in ethics, law, and politics.* New York: New York University Press, 38–65.

Luban, D. (1985). Bargaining and compromise: Recent work on negotiation and informal justice. *Philosophy and Public Affairs, 14,* 397–416.

Moody, H. R. (1988). From informed consent to negotiated consent. *The Gerontologist, 28* (Suppl.), 64–70.

Poole, S. R., & Anstett, R. E. (1988). Patients who request alternative (nonmedical) health care. *Journal of Family Practice, 16,* 767–772.

Rand, A. (1964). *The virtue of selfishness.* New York: Signet.

Weil, W. B., & Benjamin, M. (1987). *Ethical issues at the outset of life.* Boston: Blackwell Scientific Publications.

FOR FURTHER DISCUSSION:
EDITORS' QUESTIONS

1. Should Clara retain control over her wardrobe? In general, how important is autonomy over matters of clothing and dress selection?
2. Whose convenience should be given priority in Clara's case? How flexible ought Vistaview try to be, while maintaining routines that allow for the efficient use of staff time and the safety of the residents?
3. What constitutes a need and what constitutes a luxury? For example, is completion of an outfit with a choice of earrings a need? Is proper adjustment of garments a need? Does a facility have a right to dictate in matters of clothing styles and fasteners for its efficient operation?
4. What efforts should nursing homes make to maintain and enhance the dignity of their residents? Who should define the boundaries of dignity?

5. Did dressing Mrs. McDougal as a clown, for example, violate any boundaries of dignity? Is an adverse reaction from other residents an indicator that Mrs. McDougal was treated inappropriately?

6. If family members came to the home and objected to something they saw, would that be a sign that dignity was inappropriately being violated?

7. If the collective reactions of residents and family members are used to set a standard for decency and dignity, could this end up unreasonably restricting some residents with eccentric appearance and habits? What would be the disadvantage of this kind of standard? How might it affect those residents with diminished cognitive capacities and, with them, a different sense of appropriateness?

8. Returning to the case of Clara, would the obligation of the staff be different if Clara were blind and unable to see her appearance? If she were an Alzheimer's disease resident who didn't care about her appearance? An exhibitionist who *wanted* to look outlandish?

9. Does Clara's dependence on staff for help with dressing lessen her claim to individuality compared to someone who needs no help?

10. Compare and contrast Dr. Benjamin's argument about the obligation to protect the dignity of the resident and those of Dr. Fry in Chapter 16. How does the issue of Clara's dress in this chapter resemble or differ from that of Mrs. Smith's desire for frequent toileting?

11. Apply the ideas about compromise as advanced in this chapter to as many of the other cases as possible. How helpful is this formulation? Why?

Chapter 20

TIPS AND FAVORS

MRS. JONES'S DELICATE WASH

Mrs. Jones has a particularly attractive and varied wardrobe. Shortly after she was admitted to the nursing home, one of the nurse's aides heard her complaining about the poor job that the laundry did on one of her sweaters and the wrinkles that remained in her blouses. The aide offered to take her favorite dress to her own home to launder. Mrs. Jones was so pleased with the results that she proposed a regular arrangement: Mrs. Jones offered to pay the aide for laundering her clothes on a routine basis. Since that time Mrs. Jones has given many articles of laundry to the aide and is delighted with the care that her delicate items now receive. Although not well-to-do, Mrs. Jones has a comfortable income and is pleased to pay the modest charge that the aide makes for this laundry service. Otherwise, she says, her things "either get destroyed or lost, whichever comes first." Both Mrs. Jones and the aide are aware that the nursing home forbids tipping, but they view the laundry arrangement as a mutually beneficial matter that falls outside the tipping prohibition.

In this facility, 60% of the residents receive support from the Medicaid program, the public financing provision for the poor. This means that they have exhausted their resources and that their income is insufficient to meet all or part of their nursing home bill. In this state the Medicaid program allows all residents on Medicaid a monthly income of $40—called a comfort allowance—from which they must meet all of their incidental expenses, including stamps, toiletries, clothing, entertainment, phone bills, greeting cards and gifts, and even some medical supplies. Nursing home staffs are aware that the 60% with incomes that cannot easily be extended to buy a pair of shoes in a month cannot afford to commission even an inexpensive laundry service.

MR. BROWN'S DAILY NEWSPAPER

Mr. Brown, a resident in another facility with a similarly high proportion of Medicaid residents, likes a morning paper. There is a newspaper vending box almost directly in front of the door of this urban nursing home. Mr. Brown has struck up an arrangement with an aide on the morning shift to bring him the paper as she comes to work each morning. (When she is off duty, another aide does this task.) The aides simply put coins in the vending box as they pass and drop the paper off with Mr. Brown as they clock in for their shift. They know that Mr. Brown will pay $1.00 for the daily paper and $2.50 for the Sunday edition. This practice came to the attention of the nursing supervisor, who has now put a stop to what she considers "tipping," a practice forbidden here as well. The nurse reminds the aides that their job is to be helpful generally and to do extra tasks to improve residents' quality of life as they have time. Therefore, if they have time, they should get the correct change from Mr. Brown and buy the paper at the usual retail price. Mr. Brown says he doesn't want any special favors. He wants to read the paper before breakfast, as he has done all his life, and is willing to pay to make it possible. If he doesn't pay, he will not be able to expect the service.

CASE COMMENTARY

Private Contracts Between Residents and Staff

David J. Mayo

I take autonomy to be the capacity for self-rule, that is, the capacity to determine and then to pursue one's own projects, to be the author of one's own actions and life-plan. Of course a person might have this *capacity* but be prevented or prohibited from exercising it. When contemporary ethicists speak of "respect for autonomy," what is usually meant is respect for an individual's liberty in the exercise of his or her autonomy.

According to the liberal conception at the heart of our political heritage, respect for liberty in the exercise of autonomy is a fundamental value. I must *embrace* projects before they can give my life meaning, and I am more apt to embrace projects that I author than projects that are imposed on me from without. Moreover, I define and express who I am, both for myself and for others, by the projects I embrace. It is because autonomy is important to each of us in this way that we all have a prima facie or basic duty to respect each other's liberty.

Since we are social creatures, most of our projects involve others— sometimes as co-authors (e.g., marriage and intentional parenting) but more often when we enlist others for help in our individual projects in accord with some agreement that is mutually attractive. Thus, freedom to exercise our autonomy by entering into contracts with others enhances our opportunities to define and express ourselves and give our lives meaning. Many of our projects would be cut short if we were unable to negotiate or contract with others for goods and services.

The freedom of nursing home residents is characteristically restricted in several ways. First, the conditions that require living in an institution usually impose mental or physical limitations on what a person *can* do. In addition, further restrictions are imposed in the name of institutional convenience and efficiency. Nursing home residents are typically not even free to eat, drink, bathe, or get up and go to bed when they please.

The freedom of nursing home residents is severely attenuated, and, therefore, one of the objectives of nursing home care (and indeed of any nursing care) is to enhance the self-determination of individuals who are unable to meet their own needs unassisted. (Indeed some argue that the ultimate function of medicine itself should be that of enhancing autonomy rather than health.) Because freedom is a fundamental value, any policy limiting the freedom of nursing home residents by restricting the private contracts into they may freely enter stands in need of justification.

The cases of Mrs. Jones and Mr. Brown involve such contracts. Are there considerations that might justify restrictions on these and similar private contractual arrangements between nursing home residents and nurse's aides and other nursing home staff? I will approach this question by first suggesting four possible reasons for restricting such contracts. Then I will assess the force of these reasons and offer some recommendations about what kinds of restrictions these considerations would seem to justify. I will conclude with some reasons why tipping should never be allowed in nursing homes.

Resident competence is a consideration that cuts across most of these reasons, and that I will address shortly. Initially, however, let us presume both residents in question are competent.

FAIRNESS

The first and most prominent of these considerations involves fairness in the sense of distributive justice. It arises because nursing home residents typically live in a world of scarcity of the assistance from staff, which is a good that can enhance their opportunities for self-determination as well as improve their quality of life in other ways. There are obvious economic constraints on the amount of time and attention the staff can give to any one resident.

At the same time there may be almost no upper limit on the amount a resident could benefit from more attention and assistance in pursuing his or her own projects. Some obvious examples: residents suffering mobility problems could benefit from the constant attention of aides who could be their arms and legs and move them or fetch things for them; residents with bad eyesight might benefit from persons always available to read to them materials of their own choosing, help them play cards, and the like. Prompt assistance in fetching a magazine, or attending to a broken pencil, a dropped handkerchief, a soiled blouse, or a full bladder could obviously contribute to the realization of a resident's immediate objectives. Moreover, as an elderly person abandons earlier life projects, these previously minor concerns come to assume a new and major importance.

In short, any reasonably attainable standards of care and assistance in a nursing home are obviously going to fall short of what would be optimal for enhancing residents' opportunities to exercise their autonomy. From the point of view of residents, the amount of one-to-one attention they receive will be one of the limits on their ability to direct their own lives. From the point of view of staff, it will nearly always be true that even a small amount of additional help would yield a tremendous additional benefit in some residents' ability to pursue projects important to them. Thus, the staff stands on the edge of a sort of utilitarian black hole; their situation is rather like that of the person who lives near an icy corner on a country road at which many people regularly slide into the ditch each winter. (Woe to him if he is a dutiful practicing utilitarian, for if so, he may spend most of his waking winter hours helping people get their cars out of the ditch.)

This world in which assistance is scarce sets the stage for unfairness but does not by itself bring it about. With care, a nursing home staff may be able to achieve a just distribution of their assistance even if it is scarce. Concern to avoid "playing favorites" is very real among staff. Quite apart from the problem of determining what is a just distribution in the face of disparate needs, however, is the fact that staff members are only human, and so they probably are disposed to be more attentive to the needs of pleasant and agreeable residents than to those of unpleasant and ungrateful ones. Moreover, general pleasantness aside, some residents will simply be more passive and less apt to ask for help even when they need it.

All of these problems of fairness exist quite apart from private contracts between residents and people who happen also to be their caregivers. What reason is there to think that private contracts would either aggravate or be tainted by them? I believe that there is no *logical* connection here. It *might* be that private arrangements between individual residents and caregivers would have no adverse impact on the problem of distributive justice within the caregivers-residents relationships and would also be free of internal injustices. In fact, if residents were able to get some of their wants and needs (e.g., delivery of the morning paper) met through private arrangements, they might be correspondingly less demanding of scarce staff assistance.

However, I fear a more subtle, empirical connection between private contracts and unfairness in nursing homes. Given that fair treatment of residents is already difficult enough for staff, it seems likely that a private contract between a particular resident and a staff member could create a special sympathy between them that in turn could lead to unfair favoritism in the treatment of that resident within the more general context of staff-resident interaction. Thus, the acute dependence of residents on staff, combined with the scarcity mentioned above, renders the original resident-staff relationship particularly susceptible to "pollution" by feelings of concern or loyalty that could easily be generated or aggravated by a second, independent relationship arising out of a private contract. I speak of these feelings as pollution because I believe they would increase the likelihood that the staff member will give unfair extra attention within the original staff-resident context.

Compare: A ski instructor who has regularly provided each of his sons with a weekly group ski lesson is now approached by his 16-year-old son, who wants to use some of his part-time job earnings to hire his father to give him private lessons in addition to the weekly group lesson with his siblings. I believe such an arrangement would be morally suspect, and I believe it would have to do with fairness. If it doesn't have to do with actual fairness, it may have to do with the appearance of unfairness, which I address next.

THE APPEARANCE OF UNFAIRNESS

Apart from whether a private contractual agreement between a staff member and a resident *actually* led to unfair favoritism within the original staff-resident context, it might very well *create the impression* of unfair favoritism among other residents, a second and independent evil. It is independent both in the sense that either evil can occur in the absence of the other and in the sense that either is an evil whenever it does occur. Thus, there are three troublesome cases: (1) unjust favoritism might exist but go undetected by other residents; (2) it might exist and cause distress when it is detected; or (3) simple jealousy might lead some residents to suffer the genuine unpleasantness of believing that they were being treated unfairly when in fact they were not. (Even parents who manage to treat all of their children fairly sometimes hear complaints from some of them that they show favoritism.) Incompetent and/or childlike residents in particular could feel there was unjust favoritism when they saw that some other resident was provided a daily paper or particularly well-ironed clothes, while they themselves were not. The perception of favoritism could, of course, occur only if those who were not contracting for special services were aware that others were receiving such services, and this in turn will vary with the visibility of those services. Thus, for instance, special arrangements for immaculately ironed blouses to be worn by a resident in public areas would obviously have a greater potential for creating the appearance of unfairness than the delivery of the morning paper to a patient who receives and reads it in a private room.

At this point the libertarian may insist that if all residents are equally free to enter into private contracts with staff, there will be no need for such jealousy or feelings of unfairness. This is true, but in practice some patients will either be too poor or too incompetent (or both) to do so, so the genuine evil of bad feelings may persist.

EXPLOITATION OF RESIDENTS

Except in some very rigorous, libertarian notion of exploitation, even competent nursing home residents are particularly vulnerable to victimization in the form of exploitation—that is, to being taken advantage of unfairly. They are utterly dependent on their caregivers, isolated from the "marketplace," and rarely free to choose or change who those caregivers are to be. They may value (and be willing to pay for) extra assistance out of all proportion to the value it might have to most of us, including persons on the staff who might be in a position to contract with them to provide it. Moreover, they may be reluctant to "shop around for the best deal" (even within the limited community of aides available to approach) for some service in which they are interested, lest they alienate an aide on whom they know they may become increasingly dependent. Instead, they may feel obliged to pay whatever price is demanded by the first aide they approach about some matter.

The potential for exploitation is particularly grave when (as is often the case) a resident suffers some degree of mental impairment and may be incompetent. (Indeed, Minnesota law defines a special category of "vulnerable adults," which includes all nursing home residents, and seeks to protect them from neglect and abuse, including economic abuse. The sort of exploitation that might take place in the context of a private contract between a resident and staff member might qualify as economic abuse of this sort.) Probably the primary reason for restricting private contracts between mentally impaired or marginally competent residents and staff involves the danger of exploitation. However, if mechanisms can be found to control the problem of exploitation adequately, perhaps they will enable even marginally competent patients to participate in some form of "private" contracting for extra services.

EXPLOITATION OF STAFF

A final possible danger with private contracts between residents and staff is the potential for staff exploitation. In a home in which private contracts for extra services are permitted and occur frequently between residents and staff, staff members might feel pressured to "take on their share" of extra work, much as workers elsewhere sometimes feel unjustly pressured (by either their employers or their peers) to take on extra projects or causes.

PRIVATE STAFF-RESIDENT CONTRACTS IN SUMMARY

Are any of these considerations sufficient to justify restricting private staff-resident contracts, and if so, when and how? To a large extent my conclusions here involve "judgment calls" on empirical questions, some of which might be made better by those with more firsthand experience. They are correspondingly tentative.

First, considerations of fairness (real and perceived) will be greater in situations in which different residents have dramatically different sums at their disposal for privately contracting with staff for extra services. In settings in which there are both private patients and also a significant number of Medicaid patients with very limited disposable income, they strike me as decisive. (No more special laundry for Mrs. Jones, at least not from her present laundress.) In nursing homes accepting only private-pay residents, in which most patients have the funds necessary for contracting for special services, considerations of fairness will figure less prominently.

Second, considerations of exploitation of residents strike me as a serious concern but decisive probably (if at all) only where patients who are incompetent are involved. I see no insuperable difficulties to an administrative review of private contracts between staff and competent patients in private nursing homes to assure that they are not exploitative—that is, to see that residents are not being gouged. Admittedly, this makes such contracts correspondingly less private, but I find this unproblematic. In fact, policies requiring that such contracts be reported to and cleared with nursing home administration would probably make it easier to keep tabs on all of the evils we are discussing and to hold them to a minimum. Administrative review of private contracts might even make it possible for some less than fully competent patients to engage in such contracts in private nursing homes.

Third, all of these considerations are addressed to private contracts between residents and *staff*. I see no reason why any of them would preclude private contracts between residents and service providers who are not staff members. Mrs. Jones might arrange to have her laundry done by a commercial laundry firm. Although many of the services residents would like may be so trivial that commercial services are not available, creative solutions might be found in some of these situations. One can imagine, for instance, students seeking part-time work who routinely stop by a home and offer shopping or other services to residents. Mr. Brown might be able to arrange with the local paper (or a local carrier) to deliver the paper to his door.

TIPPING

I believe that tipping should never be allowed in nursing homes because of the potential for each of the first three evils discussed above in connection with private contracts.

In its "cleanest" and most theoretical form, tipping differs from payment for services for which one has contracted in five respects: (1) it involves a reward that is not due the recipient, which is (2) determined unilaterally and (3) after the fact, (4) for performance "above and beyond the call of duty" (5) in ways and areas that are not exactly specified. When tipping occurs in the context of ongoing relationships (as it would if it were to occur between a nursing home resident and a staff member), the most obvious motivation for the tipper would be to encourage futurn acts of supererogation by the person receiving the tip, again in ways or areas that remain unspecified.

Unfortunately the very concept of tipping—and certainly the concept of routine tipping—is morally problematic. Anyone who tips in order to secure better than average service in the future flirts with a violation of the categorical imperative. Moreover, if everyone does this, everyone will fail to secure above-average service (by definition). The supererogatory act of tipping will soon come to be expected and hence will deteriorate into something closely resembling payment for services. At that point the key differences between straightforward payment and tipping will all involve ways in which the tipping arrangement will remain indeterminate. It will be understood that one is to tip, but it will become less clear what one is entitled to expect either with or without the tip, and also what one is expected to tip. Obviously, such indetermination can fuel the three problems, discussed above, of real and perceived unfairness and exploitation.

An arrangement whereby a resident routinely tipped a staff member could easily create unfairness in two ways. First, it could generate expectations on the part of the resident that future (indeterminate) special considerations (remember—in an environment of scarcity of staff assistance) are owed to (or at least can reasonably be expected by) the resident. In addition it could prompt the staff member to show favoritism (again of an indeterminate sort) in the expectation that it would prompt further reward. The same vagaries of tipping would also magnify problems with the perception of unfairness that might arise from an explicit private contract between residents and staff. Finally, the dangers of exploitation would also be magnified. Because no particular payment was being agreed to for services, it would be even more difficult than in the case of private contracts to be sure that tips provided and expected, were not unreasonably high.

At this point it should be clear that I do not believe Mrs. Jones and Mr. Brown were engaged in tipping arrangements with staff. If what begins as a succession of tips between two parties comes eventually to be understood by both as a standard reward due for some very specific task, it ceases to be a tip and becomes a simple payment. This seems to be the case with both Mrs. Jones's laundry services and Mr. Brown's paper delivery. Mr. Brown's arrangement surely passed from tipping to payment at the point that he made known just what he was willing to pay for delivery of his daily paper and that he was willing to pay it to whoever arranged to bring it. Thus, although I have serious reservations about the advisability of the arrangements Mrs. Jones and Mr. Brown have with staff—especially in light of the fact that other Medicaid residents in the home cannot afford similar services—I do not believe these arrangements should be forbidden on the grounds that they involve tipping.

REFERENCES

Cassel, E.J. (1983). What is the function of medicine? In Gorovitz et al., (Eds.), *Moral problems in medicine* (2nd ed.,) Englewood Cliffs, NJ: Prentice Hall.

FOR FURTHER DISCUSSION: EDITORS' QUESTIONS

1. What can we say ethically about these two instances of payment to nurse's aides? Do Mrs. Jones's laundry and Mr. Brown's newspaper raise identical issues?
2. What is the ethical basis for prohibiting or permitting gratuities in nursing homes, and how do these questions relate to resident autonomy?
3. If it is acceptable for persons on the outside—say, in an apartment building—to tip employees or strike up special arrangements, can such arrangements properly be prohibited in nursing homes?
4. Does the ethical point depend on the income of the resident (for example, whether the resident is on Medicaid) or the amount charged for the service, or are these details irrelevant?
5. Is it more appropriate for a resident with means to arrange to purchase service from someone not employed by the nursing home rather than supplement the income of the nurse's aides?
6. Would it be better or worse if the facility organized these efforts and presented residents and aides with an allowable price list for special services?
7. What might be the good and bad outcomes for the entire community of residents associated with allowing these extra-payment practices?
8. What constitutes a kind or generous act and what is exploitative in the kind of resident-staff relationships illustrated here? Would it be any different if one of the professionals—a nurse, a social worker, the administrator—received remuneration for washing the clothes or bringing in the paper?

Chapter 21

FINDING A HOME

PROMISES, PROMISES

Mr. and Mrs. James had been searching for a nursing home for Mrs. James' mother almost since the mother first was admitted to the hospital with a stroke. They were relieved to identify a facility that they liked a lot and that promised them admission. However, the day before the patient was to enter the nursing home, the facility withdrew its offer of a bed.

Apparently, the whole arrangement was contingent on the willingness of a resident already in the facility to move to a room with another man rather than remain in his present double room, where the other bed was currently unoccupied. The resident was unwilling to move, and the home decided to respect his wish. That meant, however, that there was currently no vacancy for a woman.

Mrs. James was outraged. When her mother left the hospital, she was forced to move into a different facility, recommended by the hospital social worker. Mrs. James was "hoping for the best," but she thought it was wrong for the home to restrict access to someone who needed care just to humor another resident.

LONG DISTANCE

Mr. Fielding was helping his aunt find a nursing home for his uncle, who was scheduled to leave the hospital within the week. The uncle was severely demented and had a history of violence in a previous nursing home admission. With the help of the hospital social worker, Mr. Fielding made applications at three facilities, all of which turned them down.

The reasoning of all three facilities was that they were not equipped to give adequate care to a very disturbed resident. One of them told the social worker more informally over the phone that it was not fair to their existing residents to have to cope with disturbing behavior, and there was no room in the locked ward. The social worker was not sanguine about finding a placement unless she were to conceal the patient's history, and she did not think this would be fair to the facility.

A day before the expected discharge, the social worker located a bed at Happytime, a facility in a community about 70 miles away. Mr. Fielding thought this was an unsatisfactory solution because his aunt would be anxious about her husband unless she could see him often, and she did not drive a car. Mr. Fielding also wondered out loud if his uncle was being sent to a place of lower quality. The social worker assured him that she knew of no quality problems at Happytime. In some of the more rural areas there were simply more vacancies, and homes were therefore more open to taking "difficult" residents. Mr. Fielding said he realized his uncle was difficult, but his behavior wasn't his fault. "Doesn't he have rights, and doesn't my aunt have rights? It seems like they are being discriminated against just because they are most helpless." Mr. Fielding suggested that beds should be made available on a "first come, first served" basis.

EQUAL OPPORTUNITY

Mrs. Poluski asked the home care nurse for information about a nursing home for her stepmother, who was living alone. "Her apartment manager is getting worried and says she needs to leave." Mrs. Poluski thinks that her stepmother would like a small facility with emphasis on Catholicism. Also, since her stepmother is Polish-speaking, she would prefer a facility with other residents of Polish ancestry. The nurse said that homes were not allowed to discriminate on the basis of religion or ethnicity. There was, thus, no easy way to find out where Polish-speaking residents might congregate. The nurse suggested that St. Margaret's, a small facility adjacent to a parish church, would meet the requirement for size, location, and religious ambience, but it had a substantial waiting list.

Mrs. Poluski went to visit St. Margaret's and found it very much to her liking. She was sure her stepmother would find the program and the religious artifacts comforting. There even was a substantial group of Polish-speaking ladies in residence. When she found that some people who "weren't even Catholic" were on the waiting list, she asked if she could be given some priority because a place like St. Margaret's would mean so much to her stepmother. The administrator was sympathetic but unable to help. At the end of the month, when the lease was up, her stepmother moved into a large chain facility. She wait-listed herself for St. Margaret's but without much hope. When people are waiting in the community or in a hospital, facilities seldom give preference to those who already have a place. Besides, Mrs. Poluski didn't like the idea that her stepmother would need a whole new adjustment. She thought that St. Margaret's really should have given their space to her stepmother in the first place. "First come, first served is a stupid way to decide who enters a nursing home—that way, nobody can find the place that's right for them."

CASE COMMENTARY

SOME PRINCIPLES GOVERNING
EQUITABLE NURSING HOME ACCESS

Harry R. Moody

Below I offer a tentative list of principles that might be thought to legitimately govern access or admission to nursing homes when there is a scarcity of available beds in the facility.

1. *First come, first served.* This is the principle of pure equality, which refuses to consider such factors as individual needs, desert, or consequences for the institution. Instead, a waiting list is established, and admission is strictly according to the list.
2. *Select the neediest first.* This principle would favor those who are sickest, those with the worst prognosis, those least able to care for themselves at home or those with the shortest life expectancy.
3. *Pick those with best prospects for rehabilitation.* This principle reflects a view of the nursing home as a transitional institution whose highest goal is rehabilitation and discharge. Those with the best prospects for rehabilitation would be given preference

because such a policy creates the best outcomes for individuals and for society.

4. *Recognition for previous contributions.* Voluntary nursing homes can exist only because of contributions made by private citizens to those facilities. A principle of desert would honor by preferential admission those who have made contributions to the institution over the years in the form of either money or volunteer time, or both.

5. *Honoring ties of family and kinship.* The integrity of the family would support preferential admission for the spouse of a current resident or for those with community-residing family caregivers who can maintain ties after admission, for example, because of proximity to the facility.

6. *Select the "kin-wrecked" first.* A substantial percentage of the oldest old have survived all close family members. According to one principle, the nursing home would be viewed as a social or residential institution that should give admissions preference to the socially isolated in order to provide support for daily living.

7. *Maintain the qualitative integrity of the institution.* Under this principle we could legitimately take account of an applicant's ethnicity, religion, affiliation with sponsoring voluntary organizations, or similar attributes as a legitimate criterion for admission, insofar as these attributes help sustain the social character and historical integrity of the facility.

8. *Social responsibility to the local community.* Under this principle a nursing home should give preference in admissions to those from the local surrounding neighborhood, even if applicants do not share the ethnicity or cultural background of current residents of the facility.

9. *Eligibility for public reimbursement.* Under a principle of public reimbursement, the admissions policies of a private facility, whether proprietary or nonprofit, would giver preference to those who are eligible (or are presumed soon to become eligible) for coverage under Medicaid or Medicare reimbursement.

10. *Cash payment.* For proprietary and voluntary facilities, preference could be given to those who make cash contributions at the point of admission. Under this principle, individuals offering high cash payments might be admitted early, and individuals failing to make sufficient payment might not be admitted at all.

11. *Private-pay priority.* To maintain their fiscal viability, proprietary and voluntary facilities may need a certain proportion of patients paying for their care privately (not under public

reimbursement). Under this principle, priority would be given to private-pay patients.

12. *Maintaining ongoing interinstitutional relationships.* Admissions and discharge of residents requires maintaining ongoing ties with an affiliated hospital that may need to discharge patients or receive transfers. It is appropriate to give preferential admission to patients from affiliated organizations where ongoing interorganizational relationships are vital to the welfare of the nursing home.

13. *Select those most suitable for the facility.* Preference should be given to those patients who can best be cared for with the services and staff currently available at the facility. Those needing a higher or lower level of care should be directed elsewhere, a principle increasingly enforced by state reimbursement policies for long-term care (e.g., RUGs).

14. *Quality of life of the residency.* Beyond a certain minimal number (perhaps zero), patients who would seriously disrupt the public quality of life of the facility (e.g., "screamers," violently acting out patients) should be excluded from admission (but not necessarily expelled once admitted). More compliant patients should be given preference at admissions.

15. *Autonomy (noncoercion).* According to the principle of autonomy, patients who resist placement in a nursing home should not be placed there against their will, regardless of family wishes or institutional agreement, unless an appropriate legal authority (e.g., conservatorship) legitimately overrides the patient's preferences. Under this principle, a nursing home should not be occupied by patients who by their own choice do not seek to be there.

Many of these principles reflect familiar ethical concepts, such as (1) egalitarianism, (2) priority for the least advantaged, (3) utility, (4) worthiness, (5) family responsibility, (6) institutional integrity, (7) community obligation, (8) public financing, (9) the free market, (10) economic viability, (11) interinstitutional reciprocity, (12) efficiency, (13) quality of life, and (14) autonomy.

All except the last principle (autonomy) refer to claims of social ethics and organizational or collective obligations. Autonomy, as defined here, is not a principle to apply to admissions, but simply a side constraint on applying the other principles in deciding on admissions.

The principles enumerated here are prima facie principles commonly invoked by those involved with nursing home admissions. There may, of course, be other "good reasons" that motivate decision makers, such as (1) profit (another way of saying that the free market or economic viability should be all-determining), (2) publicity (maintaining the facility's public reputation or avoiding scandal,) or (3) nepotism (securing preferential admission on grounds of family ties, friendship, or "who you know").

However, these "good reasons" fall into the category a diplomat might call "reasons of state." They describe how institutions *do* behave, but they do not furnish principles that can publicly be advocated as to how institutions *ought* to behave—that is, they do not concern the equity or fairness of nursing home admissions. Improving profits, avoiding scandal, or scratching the backs of friends, colleagues, or kin are perfectly familiar, even quite "rational" forms of behavior. But no one comes forward to defend these reasons on grounds of equity or justice. On the contrary, great efforts are made to conceal these criteria, which, of course, does not by itself prove that they are wrong. But for the moment, I will simply assume that these actions not susceptible to public justification are wrong and leave the matter there.

Of course, it could be said, "Well, what about cash payments (bribes?) upon admission? Aren't these also kept covert?" The answer is yes, but the nature of the transaction is different.

Cash payments, even those coerced out of patients' families at the point of admission, could perhaps be defended as contributing to the overall welfare of the institution and therefore to the well-being of all of the residents. If a so-called bribe (like a tip) exists as a well-understood social practice, at what point does the practice become simply part of the price of admission? Is there really a difference between a person who makes substantial gifts over a series of years—as, say, an "insurance policy" guaranteeing preferential admission—and a simply situated person who makes a comparable gift at the point when a relative suddenly needs a place in the nursing home? It could well be that *both* kinds of action are wrong. I leave that question aside for the moment.

The point here is not to justify or to condemn these practices. The point is rather that gift giving and other forms of reciprocity are transactions between applicants and the *institution* as such, not between applicants and individual officeholders (social workers, administrators, etc.). Giving gifts to individual officeholders as a condition of admission is an instance of bribery and would not normally be defensible. Giving gifts to an institution and expecting favorable treatment might well be defensible (but also might not be). A similar analysis could be made regarding preferential treatment for private-pay patients, a practice that facilities may be reluctant to publicize.

Even when a facility cannot defend a practice because of public embarrassment, that fact does not in itself prove that the practice is inequitable or unethical; there is simply a strong presumption in that direction. To put it differently, an institution bears a burden of proof to show *why* preferential admission on grounds of contributions, either as a sustained policy or as an individual act, is acceptable and fair. The facility bears no such burden of proof in the case of, say, a first-come-first-served policy or a policy favoring the neediest first. But once again, in a particular instance it could well be that the latter policies would be the wrong policies to adopt.

The point of this analysis is not to suggest that all of the reasons offered as prima facie principles for equity are on the same level or are justified in the same way. They are not. The point is simply that these principles are all publicly defensible principles in a way that fear of scandal, nepotism, or unrestrained profit making are not. An institution and its managers, like a nation state, may make decisions for "reasons of state" either to defend its existence or to advance its goals, and institutions are properly subject to ethical scrutiny around those decisions. Whether in the case of nation states or institutions, these judgments are rarely easy. But individual officeholders who violate their office by bribery or personal favoritism simply engage in acts of injustice, not defensible forms of compromise.

My general line in analyzing equity in nursing home admissions here is somewhat the same as the framework of Michael Walzer in *Spheres of Justice* (1983). That is, I reject the idea of *simple equality* as a criterion of equity and favor instead concepts of justice that depend on the distinctive features of the institution in question. For example, a long-term-care institution has a qualitative character as a *residential* institution that is different in kind from an acute-care hospital, where patient stays are only temporary. Therefore, long-term-care facilities, I would argue, can properly be given much more scope to "discriminate" in their admissions criteria: for example, to take account of the public quality of life of the facility or of the historical institutional integrity, which may be reflected in factors such as ethnicity and culture. In a more fully public institution, such as hospitals, an "ethics of strangers" should prevail, and acts of discrimination on ethnic or cultural grounds are properly forbidden. But a residential facility is different.

The implication is *not* that long-term-care facilities have an unlimited license to discriminate but rather that a principle of institutional integrity has some proper place in equity judgments there in a fashion it cannot have for an acute-care hospital, a school, or a park. As a private residential facility, a nursing home deserves some discretion in its admissions practices. But as recent legal disputes about whether private clubs can discriminate have demonstrated, the whole question turns on just how "private" a facility can be said to be. When a nursing home accepts public reimbursement, as most private facilities do, then it is arguable that the burden of proof shifts against discrimination. But then, which forms of discrimination (or preferential admissions) are ruled out? The question has no simple answer. But Walzer's concept of "spheres of justice" at least suggests why the analysis that applies to a hospital is likely to be different from that which applies to a nursing home.

Based on this brief discussion of prima facie principles, it is possible to turn now to the questions raised by the case studies. Let me consider the general questions first, then turn back to the specific cases put forward here.

In answer to the first question, I believe there is *no simple answer*, no clear-cut "fair way" to decide who gets vacancies in a particular nursing home. *All* of the prima facie principles can conceivably come into play for any particular admissions case. There is no "rank order" among the criteria mentioned here: disability level, behavior, patient's wishes, convenience of family, date of application (first come, first served), ethnicity and religion, and so on. True, "patient wishes" in terms of noncoercion or respect for autonomy does count as the side constraint, but this doesn't carry us very far. The opposite point—the intensity of a patient's wish for admission—would not appear to weigh much for considerations of access, any more than it would, say, for college admissions or admission to an ICU.

Should each facility be permitted to develop its own admissions criteria? Basically, the answer is yes but subject to the constraints of public policy. There may be ethical constraints as well. Take the law of contracts, for instance. Do patients who apply for admission to a particular facility have some sort of implicit contract that "first come, first served" will apply? If an applicant presumes that, then other opportunities may be forgone, and the applicant will be harmed. Thus, on grounds of ethics, if not of strict law, a facility should be obliged to publish its criteria for admission or at least to make known that a "first come, first served" (or any other presumptive principle) is, in fact, *not* the operative if that is the case.

Are there any prima facie principles that would be ruled out by public policy criteria; that is, principles that are discriminatory in the pejorative sense of the term? I believe that use of racial, religious, and ethnic criteria might fall into that category. That would imply that facilities cannot publish or make use of admissions criteria that say, for example, "Only Catholics are eligible" or "Blacks not considered." But that does not mean that a facility cannot informally *use* these discriminatory criteria to encourage or discourage admissions if the results would contribute to maintaining the social character or historical integrity of the institution. As a *residential* institution, a nursing home should have the right to determine its own character in ways that a school or a hospital does not.

For example, a discharge planner or a nursing home admissions staffer might well point out to an applicant that a facility is 99% Jewish, that it serves kosher meals, and so on, and then make sure the applicant understands what kind of facility it is. The same would hold true for a "Black" or

"Polish" or any other kind of facility. One can argue that it would be a matter of negligence or breach of duty *not* to point out such facts to individual applicants or families, who may not always be aware of the social implications of the distinctive ethnic configuration in a facility. But of course, if an applicant knows and understands the facts and still seeks admission, then it is forbidden to exclude an individual on these grounds.

Do current residents have any standing in deciding who should be admitted? In general, they do not. A nursing home is not a private social club electing individuals to membership. It is an institution existing in the wider social and public world and subject to constraints. But one of those constraints is the need to maintain the quality and character of the facility as it has historically evolved. Therefore, administrators may have the authority to reject applicants—for example, certain disruptive patients—who would also be rejected by the current residents. But the reason has to do with the long-range character of the institution, not the preferences of those who happen to be the residents at one moment in time. Certainly, in arriving at such judgments an administrator would want to take account of the views of current residents but only as one factor. The administrator's basic duty is to the institution. In general, current residents lack standing in such decisions.

Is a facility justified in relocating current residents to make room for new applicants? Yes, under some circumstances. But the administration bears a very heavy burden of proof because, once admitted, an individual acquires certain rights to remain in a room if that room has become tantamount to "home." Admittedly, there is no absolute dividing line here, but the general point is clear enough: A resident who has been living in a room for many years, or even months, has a strong presumptive right to remain there, much more so than a resident who has been in a room (even a very desirable one) for only a few days.

There could be good reasons for forcing a resident to relocate from a room that counts as home. But these would have to be very strong reasons, comparable to the eminent domain power by the government to condemn a private home for important public purposes. Mere interpersonal utility comparisons will not do. The eminent domain analogy makes a serious point: A nursing home resident's room should be regarded with all of the dignity, respect, privacy, and rights accorded ownership of one's own home. Violating those rights just because someone else could make better use of the space is unacceptable except on the highest policy grounds.

Is there a reason to impose uniform standards on nursing homes? Of course there is—for example, in areas such as residents' rights or admissions agreements upon entry into a facility. But there is much *less* ground for imposing such uniform standards in criteria for admissions to nonpublic facilities except where the grounds are those of public policy considerations such as nondiscrimination or levels of efficiency and appropriate reimbursement. The reasons for this lesser stringency in admissions is that persons not yet living in a facility have a much lower standing in terms of mutual rights and obligations than do residents already living there.

In short, applicants and residents are not on the same level. Once having admitted a resident, the facility cannot discharge a person under the same standards it might have used to reject that person from admission in the first place. New rights and obligations arise because of differences in vulnerability and expectations about continuing treatment. Residents living in a nursing home have few options; they cannot easily go elsewhere if conditions are unfavorable. Therefore, patients' rights and the standards for their care must be very strong indeed.

On the other hand, persons seeking admission to a facility have, in principle, much more leeway. Their rights are best protected by policies favoring maximum disclosure and maximum choice, although choices are ultimately shaped by the power and money of those seeking admissions. Furthermore, families at the point of admission are subject to coercive pressure sometimes arising not from arbitrary institutional power but from the very nature of the situation itself: A placement *must* be found very quickly—for hospital discharge, because of deterioration in a patient's state, and so on. There *are* inequalities at this point that deserve redress. But these are best redressed by improving the bargaining position of applicants; for example, by changing reimbursement rates or improving the applicant's ability to make choices.

An analogy may make the point clear. In higher education we have a system with vast inequalities among colleges. Some of these inequalities are tolerable, some not. Yet few people would urge abolishing private higher education or insisting that all states adopt equal standards. The solution to excessive inequalities in college admissions lies in more equal incomes of families (or, what comes to the same thing, more financial aid for the less advantaged), not to mention better preparation of students, affirmative action, and so on. Simply imposing uniform standards of admission on colleges would have a damaging effect on institutions and would by no means necessarily result in greater equality of educational opportunity.

There is, of course, a good case for open admissions, at least among some large segment of public institutions. But that analogy fails for nursing homes; we cannot intentionally take in double the number of applicants expecting to "flunk out" half after the first year, as open-admissions institutions have routinely done.

The point of this analogy is to underscore that the concept of "admissions" or "equality" must have very different meanings depending on the

institutions we are discussing—what Walzer would call "complex equality" and what I am advocating here.

With regard to admissions standards, there are limits to the discretion
of nursing homes to admit whoever they wish. Admissions policy is not
arbitrary but should be determined by the application of the prima facie
principles, which, of course, can conflict among themselves. Then too,
there are cases in which public policy can and should intervene to limit
—for example, coerced gifts as a price of admission or the use of racial
discrimination as a criterion. There may be other prima facie principles
invoked that are subject to argument or may be found unacceptable. But
even after ruling out some criteria, we will be left with a very large list
and with the inevitable conflicts that arise.

Let me turn briefly to some of the specific cases cited for analysis.

Promises, Promises

In this case, the nursing home was correct to deny admission to Mrs.
James. It was proper for the home to restrict access to someone who
needed care for the sake of honoring a resident who was unwilling to
move from a room. (Obviously, the man unwilling to move had been in
his room for a while.) However, the nursing home was wrong in making
the initial offer of the bed and in particular was wrong in not disclosing
that the offer was contingent upon another resident's moving. If the
contingency had been disclosed, the offer might have been acceptable.
Again, the point is that current residents have much stronger rights and
claims than persons seeking admission to a facility.

Long Distance

In the case of Mr. Fielding's uncle, we have three facilities turning down
a disruptive resident. Both the overt reason (inability to care for a very
disturbed resident) and the covert reason (fairness to current residents)
are acceptable prima facie reasons. Thus, the uncle is left in an unhappy
position. Is his position, then, simply "unfortunate but not unfair"? Not
quite. Admission to the one available facility, Happytime, would create
serious disruption of family integrity, and this counts as a strong reason
against that choice. But it's obvious that there aren't any good choices.
The solution does not necessarily lie in forcing the other three facilities
to take disruptive patients, unless this were done according to a collective allocation formula, something like an "assigned risk" pool in car
insurance. Barring that, the real solution lies in creating new institutions

or instituting reimbursement reforms that would make disruptive patients more attractive.

Equal Opportunity

In the case of Mrs. Poluski, we see the important factor of religion and ethnicity. The first point to be made here is that the nurse is simply mistaken (or disingenuous) in saying that, because homes are not allowed to discriminate, there is "no easy way to find out where Polish-speaking residents might congregate." If a discharge planner can't find that out, he or she shouldn't be working in that job. The "informal network" can certainly furnish the answer, and perhaps that's what the nurse's "hint" at St. Margaret's was really all about. The trouble is that St. Margaret's has a waiting list. Mrs. Poluski wants the nursing home to give her stepmother first priority "because it would mean so much to her." But this reason can't count for much in admissions criteria; there are plenty of other applicants who are also eagerly seeking a place.

If Mrs. Poluski has a gripe that St. Margaret's is letting in too many people who "aren't even Catholic," maybe she has a legitimate complaint. Perhaps the institution has strayed from its historical mission and character. If so, it's too bad for Mrs. Poluski's stepmother. The solution would have been for St. Margaret's to discourage (but not forbid) non-Catholics or perhaps non-Poles from applying or getting in in the first place. But once the facility has gone down the road of heterogeneity, there's no turning back. We can't simply move Mrs. Poluski's stepmother up on the waiting list because of her ethnic background. It's too bad that the stepmother now faces the prospect of having to move twice, but no obvious alternative suggests itself.

Incidentally, Mrs. Poluski is quite right to complain that "first come, first served is a stupid way to decide who enters a nursing home—that way, nobody can find the place that's right for them." In her own way, Mrs. Poluski is making a point that Bernard Williams once made in saying that the necessary and sufficient condition for distributing health care is *need* (not simple equality, as the "first come, first served" rule suggests). The trouble is that "need" is not a simple or clear concept. There are many kinds of needs among patients, and there are many legitimate competing concerns that facilities must consider in maintaining an ongoing institution to serve those needs. These are the prima facie principles that are so difficult to reconcile in particular cases. The question of what counts as an acceptable compromise, in this as in other domains, is not one often addressed by applied ethics. In developing ethical guidance for nursing home admissions we will need to think carefully about the nature of compromise among competing principles and about the kind of prudential judgment by practitioners that is required to reach these decisions.

REFERENCE

Walzer, M. (1983). Sphere of Justice: A Defense of Pluralism and Equality. NY: Basic Books.

FOR FURTHER DISCUSSION:
EDITORS' QUESTIONS

1. What is a fair way to decide who gets vacancies in a particular nursing home? What considerations should be given to disability level or behavior of the prospective resident, the wishes of the prospective resident, the wishes or convenience of the family, the date of application, the ethnicity or religion of the applicant compared to the ethnicity or religion of the residents in the proposed facility?
2. Should each facility be permitted to develop its own admissions criteria, and what considerations are legitimate from a facility perspective? Is there any reason to impose uniform standards? If so, who should do it? If not, why not?
3. How can one distinguish between legitimate efforts of a facility to create a congenial grouping of residents and discriminatory practices?
4. What sorts of "discrimination" in admission policies, if any, are justified?
5. Do current residents have any standing in deciding who should be admitted?
6. Is a facility justified in relocating current residents within a facility to make room for new applicants?
7. How do ideas of equality of opportunity and equality of outcome influence allocation of vacancies? In what way is access to nursing home beds similar to or different from access to schools, housing, or other services?
8. What is the obligation of those who make nursing home referrals to disclose information about the prospective resident to the nursing homes? What kind of information should be held confidential? What does a nursing home have a right to know?

Chapter **22**

LETTER OF THE LAW:
Eviction from Homes

"You know, it's funny," Violet whispered. "I used to cry about coming here to die, and now I can't stand that they are making me go." At first Violet thought the stories were gossip, stories about the home being sold and the new owner making the home private pay only. "After all, you can never believe what Mimi has to say, and Lucy has nothing better to do than listen when the girls are on coffee break. You know how those stories get started.

"Then the letters came. At least some people got letters. Mostly, the families got the letters. The girls working here never said anything about it one way or another, but something was going on. You could tell.

"Now I don't know what I'm going to do. I've been here four years. My money's all used up. That's why I went on the Medicaid program two years ago. I went on, but now the home is going off. They can do that all right, but then people like me have to go someplace else.

"My daughter is so angry she could spit. After all the trouble it took to find this place, now what? She says all the decent places that take Medicaid are all filled up. We could wait a year. I have to be out in a month.

"It's not fair, but that's the law, no matter how long we've been here. There isn't any choice about that. But to have to go to someplace

258

like . . . well, you know where. . . . It's like being thrown out in the street.

"I worry about Mimi. It's going to kill her to go. She's been here since before her husband died. She thinks he still lives upstairs. She goes up to say good night every night.

"And Lucy, well, I'll just bet her family will find a way out of it. Her son knows the mayor. They probably have money. Sometimes I think it's people like Lucy who spoil it for all of us. She applied for the program six months ago because she ran out of her money, but then she refused to sell her house. She said she always planned to leave it to her son, who is living there now. She said she hadn't realized you had to sell your house before you could qualify for Medicaid. Lucy had the nursing home over a barrel for months. She just calmly said that she understood the choice, and though she doesn't want to leave the nursing home, she'd rather spend her last few months back at home with her son, 'even though he can't manage the care,' rather than let the house pass out of the family. Someone told me that the nursing home hasn't been paid at all for Lucy since March. The home didn't want the responsibility of putting a sick lady out while she was battling with Medicaid. But now the home has decided not to deal with Medicaid at all. We'll see how Lucy gets out of this one.

"The letter said that the home finds it impossible to run a decent place and count on the Medicaid program for money. There isn't enough money, there's too much paperwork, and sometimes the program decides a resident isn't eligible and then nobody pays for the care. This could be true—I never liked government programs much myself—but is it our fault? I really thought I had paid my share. Lord knows, I gave them all the money I planned to leave for my daughter, and they are still making me leave the nursing home."

CASE COMMENTARY

Loren E. Lomasky

Loss of one's home, even if only a bed in a nursing home, is a misfortune. To be wrenched away from familiar acquaintances and surroundings that provide the stability on which a life is built is disorienting for almost anyone. The perception of loss will be especially severe for an elderly woman for whom almost no prospect is less welcome than the necessity to start over again. So we can easily conclude that the eviction letter is a genuine blow to Violet. Although she once cried about entering the home, now it is indeed *home,* and its impending loss is palpable. Ownership changes and the convolutions of a Medicaid bureaucracy are distant from Violet's ken and yet more distant from her control. So she appears to herself and to us as an innocent victim of decisions in which she has a considerable stake but no part whatsoever. "Is it our fault?" she asks on behalf of her fellow residents, and the answer evidently is no. The circumstances are unfortunate, but are they, as Violet claims, *unfair*?

Perhaps, but who then is the perpetrator of the unfairness? Although Violet is not entirely explicit, she leaves no doubt that she faults the current owners of the nursing home for its shift to a "private payment only" policy. It is tempting to begin and end the suspects list there. That, though, is too abrupt. "I never liked government programs much myself," Violet confesses. She may simply be expressing an instinctive dislike of the distant and impersonal bureaucratic machinery on which she finds herself dependent. However, she may have put her finger on a more specific link to her current misfortune. If the rigidities and insufficiencies of the Medicaid program provide a strong inducement for nursing homes to file for divorce, then the proximate cause of Violet's distress may not be the party on whom the lion's share of culpability should rest.

Lucy's situation may afford a clue. Lucy intends to have it all, and if her resolve and wit hold out, she may well get it. Violet, though, seems likely to end up with nothing or at least not what she most wants at this point of her life. But what makes this illustration of chutzpah-in-action apposite? I may be reading too much into the episode, but it appears to present the nursing home owner as something other than a victimizer. Lucy is playing the Medicaid game with dispatch, and the owner has been either unable or unwilling to call her bluff. General humanitarian concern may be part of the explanation, but if so, why should such concern be extended to a conniving Lucy but not to the obliging Violet? More likely, the home finds itself frustrated and impotent in trying to navigate the labyrinth that is Medicaid. How would it play in the newspapers if it evicts from her surrogate home a sick woman who is fighting to save her "real home"? More to the point, how would it play in front of a jury? Given those circumstances—and other mini-dramas that, for all we know, are simultaneously playing themselves out—it does not appear a piece of unwarranted insensitivity for the owners to wish to rid themselves of the whole bureaucratic tangle in which Violet and Lucy are tokens.

If the current owner is not the villain of this set piece, who then is? The previous owner could have—but did not—insert as a condition of sale that no home occupant be evicted. The Lucys of this world who know how to snatch what they want thereby impose costs on those who are less talented or lucky. Were the Medicaid paperwork gauntlet less fearful, nursing homes would not have so strong an incentive to absent themselves from public welfare programs. The bureaucracy has not, however, imposed on its own volition the requirement that individuals spend themselves into indigence before public provision is afforded; that is a *political* determination. If we, as a society, resolved to show more generosity to aged recipients, that would obviate many of the difficulties in which they find themselves. Finally, is it clear that Violet and her daughter are entirely innocent parties to this dilemma? Although they seem to have *assumed* that lifetime occupancy in the home was assured, they apparently neglected to insist on contractual arrangements to guarantee that result. Most homes that commit themselves to the provision of lifetime care require transfer of substantial assets as a quid pro quo. If Violet and the prospective beneficiary of her estate had not been willing or able to accede to that condition, are they justified in subsequently protesting an eviction notice?

These speculations are both interesting and murky. They also, I believe, tend to divert attention from more salient aspects of the case presented. The search for a *personal* culprit may obscure identification of *systemic* factors that generate results such as this one. Even if each individual acts in a reasonable and morally responsible manner, the output they collectively generate will almost certainly be suboptimal if the institutional structure that conditions their choices is malformed. Because we are strongly inclined to assign blame to recognizable parties, the retreat to institutional criticism can present itself as a cop-out, a diffident reluctance to make tough ethical ascriptions: "It's not *me*, not *you*, not *anyone*, it's the *system.*" Nonetheless, because individual actions are played out in within a context that conditions their choice by imposing particular costs and benefits, the structure of that context may be the single most important factor in understanding why unsatisfactory results have obtained.

More troubling still, it is sometimes the case that adverse outcomes can be attributed *neither* to individual malefactors nor to institutional deficiencies. Rather, behavior and structures that generally yield satisfactory outcomes fail to do so in a particular case, and—here is where the moral bite enters—any move to alter the structure would predictably have the consequences of introducing further and worse distortions.

Although the information at hand concerning the present case is insufficient to ground any confident diagnosis, it is likely that some combination of the preceding considerations is more to the point than would be an apportionment of blame to one or several of the individual actors. It does not appear that any of the dramatis personae is morally exceptionable. Violet is not the sort of troublemaker who would bring eviction upon herself. Nor is there any evidence that the home owners are characterized by malice or venality. They evidently have tolerated with considerable patience one Medicaid-related snafu, and their decision to accept only private patients is, for all we know, an ordinary business decision. Therefore, it is to the context we must turn to achieve a better understanding.

In its broadest confines, that context is characterized by a general social policy determination that, in the first instance, individuals are responsible for their own upkeep but that public support is to be afforded to those in exigency. So deeply embedded in the social contract is this policy that we are apt to overlook its contestability. It is, however, challenged by radicals on both the left and right. The former decry means tests as degrading, arguing that the full panoply of welfare benefits should be extended to all as a basic matter of right rather than charity. (Social Security retirement benefits take essentially this form.) Note that were this position in force, Lucy would not be required to sell her house before gaining eligibility for Medicaid support. Indeed, the prescription from the left would seem to entail state provision of the vast bulk of nursing home services, in much the same way that the preponderance of primary education is supplied collectively. Evictions of the sort encountered here would be moot.

Conversely, it is argued from the right that a vast Medicaid authority is inconsistent with a general policy of self-reliance, that it in fact fosters the very dependency it allegedly is designed to meliorate. The alternative recommended is a general policy of payment by recipients for services rendered, with private charity counted on to provide for those who would otherwise fall through the cracks. Again note that neither Violet's nor Lucy's dilemma could emerge under that scenario.

Although I believe that both critiques deserve serious consideration, they will not receive it here. Rather, they serve an illustrative purpose, suggesting that it is the broad social endorsement of a centrist welfare policy that provides a necessary condition for the existence of the moral quandary confronted in this case—necessary but, of course, not sufficient; other arrangements hewing more or less closely to the political center would obviate this particular kind of impasse. None, though, would be free of social cost. It may be instructive to glance at several possibilities.

First and most obviously, eviction of Medicaid-supported residents could simply be forbidden by law. Any institution that ever accepted public funds to care for a resident would be required to afford that person lifetime occupancy. This proposal has the obvious merit of protecting vulnerable individuals such as Violet, though admittedly at the cost of restricting the ownership prerogatives of proprietors. Because, however, theirs are almost certainly the broader shoulders, the trade-off may seem to be morally promising. That, though, is to attend to only part of the story. For if actual and potential nursing home owners know that they will not be allowed to withdraw from Medicaid involvement should that relationship become more of a liability than an asset, they would have a disincentive to accept Medicaid patients in the first place. All else equal, they would elect to admit only fee-paying occupants. The result would be thoroughly disadvantageous to persons receiving public support. Would Violet have been better off had the nursing home chosen to evict her two years previously when she had used up all her own payment means? Not apparently.

All else need not, of course, be equal. Some homes would contract with Medicaid, but because the effective cost of doing so would include a concomitant loss of flexibility in responding to changing economic and political conditions, those homes, in order to achieve an equivalent return on investment, would typically provide a lower standard of care than that offered by those free from entangling Medicaid alliances. And if the proposed legislation were to lower the overall profitability of investment in nursing home facilities, there would be less of it. The genuine victims then would not be potential proprietors, who can easily enough choose instead to place their capital in shopping malls, treasury securities, or oil rigs; it would be the nursing home clientele.

Even setting the preceding considerations aside, would it really be to Violet's benefit if she were rendered unevictable by legislative fiat? It would be no surprise if such unwanted tenants found themselves enjoying lower-quality care, care that distinctly conveyed the message that their patronage was not desired. Further legislation could be enacted to guard against such unsavory practices, but enforcement would be neither easy nor costless, and it would reinforce existing nursing home disinclination to get involved with Medicaid. Just as rent control ordinances lead to gutted neighborhoods and a dearth of new building, so too would benignly intended nursing home legislation work to the disadvantage of those it was framed to protect.

Alternatively, a longer notice period could be required before nursing home tenants are evicted. However, the case at hand provides no indication that Violet's trouble is caused by any abruptness associated with her removal; she does not wish to leave now, next month, next year, ever. Rather, what it does illustrate is that some homes are loath to deal with Medicaid at all in spite of the assured payment thereby afforded them. Piling regulation upon regulation is not likely to make them more eager to brave the Medicaid system.

These considerations suggest that piecemeal reform could easily generate more problems for residents than it would have any hope of ameliorating. One may therefore become more willing to consider a version of what was described above as the proposal from the left: governmental takeover of the nursing home industry, though with fees charged to those able to pay for their own upkeep. How one appraises the value of this suggestion will be a function of one's assessment of the relative efficiency and responsiveness of governmental versus private service providers. There exists, of course, a vast literature on the subject, one impossible to scrutinize here. But even a casual empiricism does not inspire confidence in the general desirability of substituting political for economic decision making. Will we place more confidence in the skill with which our nursing homes are managed if the incumbents are replaced by bureaucratic soulmates of those Pentagon denizens who purchase $300 hammers and $500 toilet seats? When even the People's Republic of China has become convinced that recourse to private enterprise is necessary for emergence from economic torpor and the Soviet Union is afire with *perestroika,* a contrary policy with respect to American nursing homes seems, at the very least, questionable. But even one considerably more positive than I am about the likelihood of efficient and enlightened management emanating from Washington must concede that this represents an extreme shift from current practice, one justifiable only if prospective benefits were deemed to be substantial. There is nothing in this episode that provides so much as a clue that that is so. One can properly sympathize with a woman on the verge of losing her home without thereby concluding that governmental takeover of the nursing home industry is advisable.

Indeed, the case strongly suggests that it is their perception of being enmeshed in a bureaucratic straitjacket that explains why nursing homes desire to extricate themselves from Medicaid involvement. Because it is costly, time-consuming, and frustrating to comply with Medicaid regulations, they have a strong inducement to opt out. That suggests another systemic alternative: lessen or eliminate the regulatory burden, and the Violets and Lucys of the nursing home world will be as welcome as fee-paying residents.

The suggestion is superficially appealing. By their nature, impersonal bureaucracies are not lovely things. Even those of us who have never been involved with Medicaid have our own rueful tales to tell about jarring encounters with governmental or corporate bureaus. If it were to relax its reporting requirements, were not to require patients to spend themselves down to indigence before receiving public support, and would otherwise strip off its various rigidities, Medicaid would become a more appealing partner of nursing homes and their residents. It would, though, thereby fail to discharge its duty to the citizenry at large. Although it may be estimable for an individual acting in his private capacity to offer assistance without putting the bona fides of the beneficiary under a microscope, a public agency properly enjoys no such discretion. It is not operating with its own resources but with money extracted from taxpayers to whom it owes a fiduciary responsibility. Fulfillment of that responsibility is incompatible with regulatory laxity.

Should Lucy be allowed to retain ownership of her house while Medicaid pays for her upkeep at the nursing home? No one is enthusiastic about dispossessing an old woman from her last remaining asset, but the alternative is clearly morally inferior. Although people may have a right against society that their basic needs be provided, no one needs to leave a considerable estate to his or her heir. It would be highly improper to extract funds from others so that Lucy will be able to provide her son a real estate bonanza. If she elects to leave the nursing home rather than sell the house, that is her decision. Respect for the autonomy of persons does not entail shielding them from the consequences of hard choices; just the reverse. Protracted dithering over eviction in such cases invites both policy confusion and continued bluffing by those intent on beating the system.

Similarly, although the paperwork burden placed on nursing homes by Medicaid is onerous, allowing public money to be dispensed without close scrutiny to determine eligibility would be to fail in a public trust. Bureaucracy is not simply a plague inflicted on us by a malevolent deity; it is, as Max Weber explained, a rationalizing device through which projects that exceed the capacity of any one person to carry through become achievable. No, the Medicaid apparatus may not be lovely, but it nonetheless is a tolerably efficient and humane means for achieving socially approved ends.

That is not, however, to place it above criticism. Like individuals, bureaucracies differ in their sensitivity, flexibility, and responsiveness. We can detect indications in the case under attention suggesting that Medicaid's dealings with nursing homes may be more calcified and unyielding than need be. Violet and her daughter understandably find any move threatening but are especially worried that those homes accepting Medicaid patients fail to provide decent care. Their perception may be clouded by personal involvement, but suppose it is not. That is cause for concern. By law, Medicaid payments are to be adequate to provide fair reimbursement for services provided. If, nonetheless, facilities are unwilling to accept Medicaid recipients, that is evidence that the burden placed on them is excessive. At the very least, eligibility determinations should be made straightforward so that nursing homes do not have to guess whether reimbursement will be forthcoming. Such uncertainty ultimately imposes costs on all residents and unnecessarily stigmatizes legitimate Medicaid clients. The program possesses, as stated above, a fiduciary responsibility to taxpayers, but at least as central to its charge is fulfillment of its responsibility to beneficiaries. If the tentacles of the system have become so threatening that service providers flee its embrace, that latter responsibility is not being fulfilled.

It does not follow, however, that a social obligation is shirked if Medicaid reimbursement levels are below the rates generally paid by patients in private care facilities. To maintain that publicly supported residents are entitled to a decent level of care is one thing; to hold that they must receive the best care that money can buy is quite another. There are theories of social justice that endorse the latter proposition, but these are not the theories that inform American welfare policy. Nor, I believe, should they; but that is a contentious issue best examined elsewhere. Here it is enough to observe that a policy of funding nursing home care at a level of basic adequacy is consistent with other social determinations that enjoy wide support.

One danger of a case study approach to moral problems is that focusing on the particular will lead one to endorse an approach that, if generalized, would have deleterious consequences. That danger certainly looms as one evaluates Violet's situation. That she should be required to move from what has now become her home is regrettable. We are all inclined to empathize with her plight, and that empathy prompts the search for a remedy. Unfortunately, compassion does not guarantee efficacy. Policies intended to shield vulnerable individuals may have the effect of placing yet other people in jeopardy; the impulse to help may instead generate harm. Anecdotal evidence is not sufficient justification for radical restructuring of the Medicaid program of support for nursing home occupants. We can hope that owners of homes, their occupants, and bureaucratic functionaries will all act responsibly. In particular, nursing homes should make it clear to prospective residents whether they guarantee lifetime occupancy. That way there will be no room for a lingering suspicion that the "rules of the game" have been changed midway. If such a guarantee is not part of the package, they should stipulate their willingness to allow a reasonable amount of time for evicted occupants to secure alternative housing and also indicate the measures they will undertake to assist in the search. Contractual specificity is no panacea, but it both protects the legitimate business interests of the home and affords concrete protection to vulnerable residents.

But even if all concerned parties act in a morally responsible fashion, and even if institutional structures are generally fair and efficient, that does not ensure the absence of personal ordeals. Despite our best efforts, some, like Violet, will be afflicted; and others, like Lucy, will gain an edge by ferreting out uncertainties and loopholes within the system. The perfectly frictionless surface is an ideal beyond our attainment in either physical or social system design. We cannot achieve all that we would like. What we can do, however, is to refrain from acting in ways that predictably will multiply misfortune.

FOR FURTHER DISCUSSION:
EDITORS' QUESTIONS

1. What ethical duties do facilities undertake when they accept public subsidies?
2. If a nursing home withdraws from the Medicaid program, what is its obligation to relocate people who no longer qualify for their care? Do the residents and families need to be satisfied with the relocations?
3. What is the obligation of the Medicaid program in such a situation; should it be required to pay the higher private rate for residents caught in the transition?
4. In this situation, the nursing home converted to a private-pay-only status. Would the obligation of the nursing home have been any different if Violet had been fairly warned when she entered 4 years ago that the home did not participate in the Medicaid program?
5. Would the situation be different if the home did accept Medicaid but tried to limit the proportion of its beds at the Medicaid rate? Many homes claim, with some accuracy, that they use the higher rates charged to private-pay residents to subsidize care for all. Overt Medicaid discrimination is illegal, but if Violet were admitted to the hospital from such a home, the facility might not have space for her to return after the hospitalization. Would it be within its ethical rights to take this position?
6. How should one evaluate ethics of the general policy that requires citizens to "spenddown" before becoming eligible for Medicaid? The policy that requires a family home? The morality of a two-tier system?
7. In all of these situations, does a home have greater responsibility to someone who has been with them a longer time? To someone who has already paid out a large sum of money?
8. How should resident autonomy, preferences, and wishes be factored into transfer decisions? What weight should be given to maximizing residents' autonomy? What procedures need to be put in place?
9. What, if anything, is a nursing home's obligation toward a resident who is not paying the bill, or to one who has no payment source? If Lucy is locked in a battle with Medicaid over the disposition of her house, can the facility fairly evict her? What steps must a facility take before terminating care?

PART **III**

TOWARD SOLUTIONS

Chapter 23

BUILDING AN EFFECTIVE CAREGIVING STAFF:
Transforming the Nursing Service

Mila Ann Aroskar, Ene Kristi Urv-Wong,
and Rosalie A. Kane

Despite the name, nursing homes are neither homelike nor known for their quality of nursing care. Elderly people sometimes say that they fear life in a nursing home more than their own death. Until recently, the nursing profession seemed to share this aversion. From a professional and technical perspective, chronic care in nursing homes could be seen as unexciting and unglamorous compared to the action of an acute-care facility. (Note that no one has yet produced a television series about a nursing home.) Within the nursing profession, nursing homes are perceived as full of unpleasant sights, unpleasant sounds, and unpleasant smells (Carter, 1987). Those who, like Selby (1988), believe that work in a nursing home calls for a full range of the highest nursing skills are in a decided minority. If nurses who practice in nursing homes internalize the label of belonging to a professional subclass, they can hardly inspire their staffs.

Even now that some leaders in the nursing field have begun to take an increased interest in nursing home care, a great theoretical void exists about how best to organize the nursing service to meet the goals of a frail clientele that may be in permanent or at least long-term residence. There has been virtually no meaningful testing of alternative ways to render nursing care in nursing homes.

At the bottom of the shaky nursing home pyramid are the nurse's aides or nursing assistants, who occupy what Vladeck (1981) refers to as "the worst job in the world." Yet it may also be one of the most important. Any successful strategy that really makes a difference to the lives of nursing home residents must start from recognition that the bulk of the direct care given in nursing homes is provided by parapro-fessional personnel. Therefore, if the nursing home resident enjoys per-sonal autonomy and lives a life that feels meaningful and interesting, the chances are strong that a nursing assistant has been instrumental in making it possible.

Current nursing literature seems convinced that nurse's aides in nursing homes do have a miserable job (Goodwin & Trocchio, 1987). The physically distasteful aspects—cleaning oozing bedsores and sponge-bathing incontinent residents—are emphasized. The work is viewed as dead-end. The pay is often meager. The nurse's aides are criticized for their lack of skills, the facilities for their weak training programs, and governments for their inadequate funding of nursing home care.

These criticisms have a factual basis. Yet it is easy to deplore the lack of training in this work force and the staggering demands of their positions. It is more difficult, but not impossible, to work with the nursing assistant labor force to produce care that is both technically correct and humanely offered. To do so, however, requires reflection about what a nursing home's purpose is, considerable recasting of the proper roles for staff, and dropping the negativism that pervades the long-term-care nursing field.

In this chapter we explore nursing services in nursing homes and particularly the job of the nursing assistant. Our perspectives come not only from the distressingly limited nursing literature on the subject but also from our own interviews with nursing assistants from nursing homes in five states. Our impressions offer a counterpoint to the gener-ally negative image of nursing homes and point out positive features in the way nursing assistants perceive their roles despite obvious stress. The challenge is to harness the energy of nursing assistants through proper job descriptions, appropriate training, and organizational incen-tives. We conclude the chapter with a laundry list of suggestions for how nursing staff, with the support of a home's administration and both state and federal policymakers, can enhance appropriate autonomy for resi-dents. Some are simple and easily carried out, and some call for radical departure from the status quo.

NURSING IN NURSING HOMES: WHO REALLY "CARES"?

Nursing Service

Typically, the nursing staff is composed of a director of nurses (DON) at the helm, a few (perhaps 2 or 3) registered nurses (RNs), somewhat more (perhaps 2 to 4) licensed practical nurses (LPNs), and a host of certified nursing assistants or nurse's aides (these numbers vary from state to state and between rural and urban areas). Taken together, the nursing service constitutes by far the largest proportion of staff in any facility. Moreover, other staff, including the medical director, physical therapists, pharmacists, and dietitians, tend to be part-time consultants rather than full-time participants in the delivery of care. Designated social workers and activity directors often have little background for their roles and tend to come in quantities of one per facility at most. Thus, by sheer weight of numbers and because their involvement is more than casual or episodic, the nursing staff is a primary force in determining the nursing home's culture. Along with the administrator (who may or may not be professionally trained), the DON is a powerful figure, setting the tone for the work force and the mood of the facility. State nursing home inspectors know that a change in DON can make an instant difference for better or worse in the quality of care in a facility. Therefore, any positive change enacted in a home must emanate from and/or be totally supported by both the administrator and the DON and her professional staff.

Professional nursing practice is not well established in nursing homes. According to the 1977 National Nursing Home Survey, only 47% skilled nursing homes in the United States had 24-hour RN coverage, and the coverage in intermediate care facilities was even thinner (Aiken, 1983). More typically, a moderate-size home has one or two RNs on the day shift. LPNs are more plentiful but still limited. Regulations to be implemented in 1989 require that there be a nursing service person at least at the level of LPN on every shift—hardly a stringent requirement. When residents enter a nursing home because they need "24-hour care," neither they nor their families realize how circumscribed that care might well be.

Because nursing home residents are so heterogeneous, because there is a trend for very sick people to be admitted to nursing homes, and because the multidisciplinary team concept is more ideal than reality, the general list of responsibilities for the nursing service (RN, LPN) is all-encompassing and formidable. Responsibilities include writing care plans, administering medication, bathing, dressing, mobility assistance (toileting, transferring, walking, wheeling), incontinence care, feeding assistance, turning and positioning, decubitus care, special skin care, and highly skilled procedures such as intravenous feeding, oxygen therapy, sterile dressings, tracheotomy care, suctioning, inhalation therapy, multiple injections, and irrigations. They include general nursing maintenance and rehabilitation nursing, such as bowel and bladder training. The nursing service is responsible for routine observations and assessment and for taking vital signs; it is responsible for identifying problems and interacting with physicians about changes in treatment. And nursing service is responsible for documenting all of the above, which means charting, charting, and more charting.

Some of the responsibilities on this list clearly reflect the gradual increase of very sick older persons entering nursing homes for care in the past few years. In addition, given the high proportion of nursing home residents with senile dementia or other psychiatric disorders, nursing service is also responsible for providing or arranging an appropriate array of services to meet these needs.

Planning and organizing nursing services is complicated by the mixture of "high tech" and "low tech" contained in this list. The spectrum of nursing care provided in nursing homes now ranges from custodial care to care that was formerly provided only in hospitals. This range of care needs puts new and greater burdens on nursing staff. In some communities it is made even more stressful by the shortage of all types of nursing personnel in hospitals, home care, and outpatient services as well as in nursing homes. In such instances, nursing homes may need to rely on nursing "pools" for their key personnel, with all of the discontinuities this produces.

The nurse's aides are responsible for supporting all of the goals and activities of the nursing service. And although terms like *nurse's aide* and *nursing assistant* imply that the raison d'etre of the paraprofessional begins and ends with helping nurses, the job surely exceeds those limits.

Who Is the Nursing Assistant?

Who, then, are the nurse's aides who care for our fathers and mothers, grandfathers, and grandmothers? They are usually women. They range widely in age from 16-year-old high school students to 60-year-old grandmothers. In our sample of 144 nursing assistants, the typical aide was about 36 years old and had a high school diploma or its equivalent. On the average, she had worked in her present nursing home for about five years and had usually worked in other homes, too. Because triple-digit turnover is customary in nursing homes, it is sometimes not realized that some people work as aides for decades.

The nurse's aide may be contemplating using the nursing home as a stepping-stone to more rewarding or lucrative work, she may be doing the job to earn money while attending school, or she may think of the occupation as her lifetime work (Tellis-Nayak & Tellis-Nayak, 1989). People in the last group often express profound satisfaction, sometimes religiously derived, because they help and feel they give comfort to the old and infirm. For every person who expresses a sense of being trapped in the role, another says that the job provides intrinsic satisfaction. Those who work in the evenings seem more likely to be students or other temporary personnel. Those who work at night are a different group altogether and seem to include many more men.

Although the aide may contemplate using her position in the nursing home as a stepping-stone to higher levels of nursing, this advancement may never happen. How many actually reach their goals is unknown, and the career lines are not well articulated. Nurse's aides tend to be paid poorly. In some states the aide can work for years and retire at the minimum wage. In other states some aides work themselves up to about $10 an hour. Even at the higher figure, and certainly at the lower figure, nurse's aides may have little financial reserve with which to embark on any new ventures.

Minority group members are proportionately overrepresented in the nurse's aide work force compared to the minority population in the geographic area. Given that nursing home residents are overwhelmingly white and non-Hispanic, the aide may differ from the residents in culture, social class, and even language. The aide may be a recent immigrant to the country or the community, struggling with her own problems of acculturation even as the nursing home resident struggles with acculturation to the facility.

What Do Nursing Assistants Do?

Nursing assistants, or nurse's aides, along with dietary aides, are the home's main labor force. It is the nurse's aides who spend the most time with the residents. They are the home's cadre of bathers, feeders, dressers, toileters, letter readers and writers, comforters, self-appointed disciplinarians, and resident confidantes. They may apply physical restraints, but they also offer the comforting hand. They are often incorrectly viewed as merely the ones who clean up incontinent residents, clean up vomit, and generally just clean up. Certainly, this type of dirty work *is* part of the job description. But much more is involved in being a nurse's aide.

The nursing assistant is given much responsibility but little actual authority to act. She is responsible for getting a resident up, bathed, dressed, to meals, to the bathroom, and conversely, bathed, undressed, and to bed. She applies physical restraints as ordered. Though she is responsible for completing tasks, she has little authority to change a task's timing or operational procedure or to skip a task on any particular day. If she listens, she hears the residents' concerns. She is not expected to act in contradiction to orders, yet she may bear the responsibility and emotional burden of being the only one who hears what the resident thinks. She observes how the resident is either negatively or positively affected by the orders she carries out. She answers to administration, RNs, LPNs, physicians, social workers, and activity coordinators. She is rarely asked to contribute to care plans and, in fact, sometimes hasn't even seen a resident's care plan. She may be terrified that she will witness the death of a resident, or worse, need to attend to a dead body. She may, as so many nurse's aides told us, feel responsible for a resident's peace of mind in his or her last hours, yet she does not have authority even to change her own daily routines (see Wetle, this volume).

The physical tasks of the nurse's aide—the lifting, turning, dressing, feeding, waking, putting to bed, providing pericare, or fixing a resident's hairdo—are demanding and tiring, but they are only one dimension of the work. Clearer insight into the nurse's aide's function is gained by examining the social and psychological functions she may or may not perform. She takes the resident to activities, she talks to the resident, she listens to the resident, she motivates the resident to make efforts toward rehabilitation, she helps the resident make telephone calls, she smiles at the resident, and she makes the resident feel safe. This is sometimes referred to as "high-touch" technology, contrasted to high-tech.

Missing from the usual litany of list of tasks and activities for which nursing personnel are responsible is the entire realm of care for residents' psychological and social needs. Diamond (1986) describes this as "caring work." Caring work, primarily carried out by nursing assistants, is not charted, and is not paid for as a separate service item; therefore, it does not "officially" exist in a nursing home bureaucracy. The special knowledge and skills required in high-touch or caring work are unmentioned in training and reports and hence invisible. Diamond's ethnography of everyday life in nursing homes emerges from his research in several nursing homes where he worked as an observer/participant. His study is a rich analysis of the daily life of nursing assistants and residents. It is one of the few places in the literature where the voices of the nursing assistants are heard. He contends that although the work of nursing assistants is often portrayed as either menial or unskilled (and the tasks sometimes actually are), the overall work can be construed this way only if nursing aides are considered to be subordinates in a world dominated by the hierarchies of medical care and if the deeper caring work is discounted.

According to Diamond (1986), caring work begins with being in touch with someone else's body and its need for constant, intimate tending. It includes mental work and special thought, much of which is obvious only when it is not done, such as when a resident turns up poorly dressed or becomes incontinent when it was the nursing assistant's job to ensure against it. It includes emotional work: holding, cuddling, calming, grieving. Construed this way, the job calls for a great deal of thought, but unfortunately, often the aide must tend to one resident while thinking of another.

Training

Training for aides emphasizes the physical tasks, tends to be perfunctory, and is concentrated on the initial stages of the job. Administrators are reluctant to invest in training nurse's aides because of the high turnover (Kaster, Ford, White, & Carruth, 1979). They worry about investing in education for aides who will "just up and leave." Because administration discourages investing time and money for aide training, in turn the DON will not encourage, if not actually discourage, her supervisory staff (RNs and LPNs) from a similar investment.

Ironically, however, a possible explanation for high nursing aide turnover is that the aides are unequipped to cope with the diversity and intensity of both the physical and emotional demands of their jobs. Picture a high school graduate with high motivation to help old people. She becomes a nurse's aide. After two days of observing a fellow aide on her shift and one day of being observed herself, she is left to fend for herself on an evening shift with 15 assigned residents. She is asked to apply restraints. She notices that a resident is slowly starving herself and wonders what to do. She rarely sees a supervisor. Nurse's aides like her lack adequate education, preparation, and support. Lacking the necessary understanding or training to perform a job competently and confidently could truly create conditions for "the worst job in the world."

The lack of front-end training for nurse's aides will be addressed through the mandates of the federal Nursing Home Reform Act in the Omnibus Budget Reconciliation Act (OBRA) of 1987. The Act stipulates that all aides must receive at least 75 hours of training in programs that address nursing, psychosocial, physical, and environmental needs of residents as well as medical needs. Nurse's aides must be competent to perform the tasks they are assigned. These training goals include inculcation of a more realistic and holistic approach to caring work. Yet even now, as states are struggling to come into compliance with the mandate, many recognize that a few weeks of training prior to assuming the job is a slim bulwark against a difficult and compromising job.

RELATIONSHIP BETWEEN
AIDE AND RESIDENT

A nursing home is the context for a set of relationships between staff and residents. The character of those relationships is influenced by the constraints under which both residents and staff labor: shortages of money, space, and time. Opportunities for conflict and misunderstanding are rampant. Nevertheless, meaningful relationships do emerge between residents and the staff who care for them. And given the intimate nature of the care required, it is hard to believe that personal care could be rendered happily or received comfortably in the absence of some relationship of mutual respect. After all, the tasks that a nurse's aide performs for the resident are the kinds of tasks usually performed for each other by close family members.

In our study, nursing assistants told us about their specific work assignments in minute detail when they were questioned about their job descriptions. But when asked what was most satisfying or memorable in their work, they talked about their special relationships with the residents. Despite differences in background, despite the resident's relative lack of power in the nursing home and perhaps the aide's own general lack of power in both the home and the medical community, and despite the aide's constant work pressure, meaningful relationships do get forged.

Nursing home residents who are cognitively intact seem to strive for these relationships. They often express appreciation of the nurse's aides. They recognize how hard their work is and try not to make excessive demands. They value courteous and affectionate treatment. Conversely, they are distressed when they are treated impersonally, like objects to be processed, when they are patronized as if they were children, or when they are treated rudely. A seminal study by the National Citizens' Coalition for Nursing Home Reform (1985) gathered the opinions of more than 400 residents in 10 states to glean residents' views of quality care. Attitudes and performance of staff ranked first as the prime determinant of quality life and care. Participants cited characteristics such as "being nice and kind to residents." Residents wanted personnel to be affectionate, as well as qualified, well-trained, skilled, and knowledgeable. Residents also valued continuity of care. If they liked an aide, they preferred that aide remain assigned to them and were saddened if these aides were reassigned or left the facility.

Staff members also seem to strive for relationships with residents to give meaning to their world. It would be a mistake to assume that aides are cogs in the nursing home machine that can be interchanged and assigned with impunity. In a study of what contributes to the satisfaction of nurse's aides in nursing homes, Holtz (1982) found that 100% of the respondents cited interpersonal relationships as extremely or very important in influencing them to stay with their work. This was the most important predictor of job satisfaction, followed by quality of supervision. Interpersonal relationships included relationships with patients, supervisors, and co-workers. In other words, most nurse's aides also like continuity and resent being switched.

In our discussions with nurse's aides we learned that many carry out extra tasks for residents gladly because it gives them a good feeling. "Feeling needed" or "feeling good" about their work is one of the intrinsic benefits of nursing aide life. Aides often spend their breaks with residents, help them purchase special products, and often keep a "special eye" on residents, noting unfamiliar or odd behavior. They enjoy their stories, bring them things from home, sometimes introduce them to their children, and sometimes, if the home's rules permit, even take them on outings. Our study also showed that many residents also make special efforts to please the aides. Some efface themselves, determined not to be a burden to the overworked "girls" (a behavior that has its own problems.)

Inevitably, residents have their favorite aides, and aides freely indicated that they had their favorites among the residents. This very human tendency may play out in favors for the favorites, who become the beneficiaries of the extra time and help (see Mayo, this volume). Indeed, many facilities have one or two residents who achieve special status and privileges because they are universal favorites. Feelings are, of course, impossible to standardize and special relationships are inevitable—and perhaps not undesirable. One must guard against the drawbacks, however: Some residents may be favored by nobody, and an aide may unconsciously be lavishing attention and affection on a few residents.

The relationships described here are remarkable because they persist despite, not because of, the structure of the job. The aide is undoubtedly the nursing home workhorse. An aide's life is fixated on physical tasks: tasks that can be quantified, tasks that can be recorded in a medical record, tasks that can be used for reimbursement purposes. "If it's not charted, it didn't happen" (Diamond, 1986). A nursing aide is judged and rewarded for how much she can accomplish physically. Quantity first, quality if there is time left over. As noted before, nursing care directed toward psychological or social well-being is ignored or overlooked in favor of the physical tasks. The very tasks that could help an aide identify more closely with a resident, the very tasks capable of building both residents' and aides' self-esteem such as talking with residents, getting to know their preferences and their feelings, getting to know about their early life—are discouraged. Aides are not rewarded for so-called idle chatter.

Misunderstandings

The potential for relationships is high, but so too is the potential for misunderstandings and insensitivity. As all the case studies illustrate, the nursing home environment compresses a resident's ability to make choices. In that limited world the resident will tend to focus on those areas where he or she can still exercise control. Unfortunately, the areas in which a resident may express a preference are often limited to what might be considered unimportant or even mundane to an outside observer. And these areas are the realm of the nurse's aide. Haphazardly, nurse's aides and residents come together around the small matters of daily life—those mundane choices that, to some residents, are all of the choices that remain.

Furthermore, either because of disability or facility policy, residents may have few areas in which to enact their preferences. If so, a resident may fiercely guard the few opportunities for choice and control that remain. For example, one articulate resident who needed to be spoon-fed told us that the pace at which she was fed was extremely important. She exercised control by refusing to open her mouth, though the staff member could exercise ultimate control by prematurely taking away the tray. The staff member could well interpret this behavior as stubborn and uncooperative, whereas the resident interprets the effort to hurry the meal as the height of hostility and she distinguishes clearly between staff members who let her set the pace and those who do not.

It is the very ordinariness of the residents' choices that can lead to misunderstandings and miscommunication. As Caplan (this volume) has pointed out, the few areas of remaining choice for nursing home residents may be things that others take for granted. Employees seldom give much thought to which day they will take a bath because most can bathe or shower whenever they choose. Therefore, they may not understand why a nursing home resident may make such a fuss over a change in her bath day. It may be difficult to understand until we realize that, given the communal nature of nursing homes, a shortage of nurse's aides to assist, and limited number of bath facilities in a home, a resident gets only one bath per week in many homes. Waiting even one additional day for a bath may be intolerable for a resident accustomed to a daily bath. Being forced to bathe in the morning when the resident prefers the evening may represent impotence to the resident, whereas it is a mere matter of work scheduling to the aide.

Nurse's aides delivering care to residents are not always aware of the compression of autonomy that occurs when a resident moves into a nursing home. A nurse's aide does not have to depend on someone else to bathe her on a strict schedule. Most aides do not even have the luxury of time to consider the fact. When an aide gives Mrs. X her weekly bath, most likely the primary realization is that Mrs. X has to be bathed, as does Mrs. B, Miss C, and Mr. D, E, and F. Secondary is whether or not she can get some help from her co-workers if, for example, she waits and begins her task a half hour from now. The aide has a specific amount of time available to complete her work and little or no time to think about the task (see Fry, this volume).

The aide and the resident approach the realities of the nursing home world from radically different perspectives. The aide leaves the facility each day and leads an independent life outside the nursing home. In contrast, the resident must function within the limited-choice world of the nursing home facility. Both aides and residents have personal sets of values and expectations. The aide may believe that attending daily activities is the most important aspect of a resident's day and therefore stress attendance and make accommodations that allow a resident to participate in a home's various activities. The aide's behavior is reflective of her own priorities (she is unlikely even to ask the resident about hers). A primary focus of the aide's life may be her own leisure time activities, such as bowling or going to movies, and she may assume that the resident finds the home's planned activities pleasant as well.

Unfortunately, then, the aide often overlooks the desires of the resident. In direct contrast to the aide's belief in the importance of the home's activity program to residents, a resident may have personal priorities that include using part of her day to read the newspaper or a new library book. In her belief that the home's activities are a priority to residents, the aide may view the resident's actions as signaling withdrawal, depression, or rebellion. Even though Mrs. X has always enjoyed reading as a hobby, in the context of the nursing home and through the eyes of the aide, Mrs. X is exhibiting antisocial behavior. This type of scenario lends itself to potentially unlimited misunderstandings and miscommunications in spite of the best intentions. If there is little time or expectation that these matters are discussed, the complexities multiply.

Abuse

The growth of nursing homes in the United States has been punctuated by scandals concerning the physical and emotional abuse of residents by aides. Less attention has been given to the fact that residents sometimes "dish out" the abuse, either wittingly or unwittingly. Despite the rosy picture just painted of relationships that work well, the opposite can also be true.

Nurse's aides are exploited in many ways, some more serious than others. Arguably, the more task-oriented the nursing home, the more potential for abuse in either direction. If aides are relegated to the status of routinized robots and residents to passive recipients, the climate for dehumanization is created.

Not everything that an aide calls abusive is necessarily so. Because an aide's job description is so precise, she may be tempted to define anything out of the ordinary as beyond her job. (On the other hand, if her job description encompasses tending to the psychological and social well-being of the resident, there are no limits.) It is unfortunate if the aide's task orientation leads her to view individualization as extra work. "Some residents want us to do our work all over again," said an aide about a resident who wanted to be taken to the toilet twice within a short period of time (see Fry, this volume).

On the other hand, some residents may take advantage of their situation. They may make shrill demands. They may treat aides as subhumans, omitting even the social niceties of "please" and "thank you." They may manipulate an aide through evoking feelings of guilt ("I can't get out of this place like you can") or through blackmail ("If you don't get me a pack of cigarettes, I'll tell the supervisor what you did yesterday" or "what you forgot to do yesterday").

The abuse of aides is not limited to subtle exploitation but can sometimes involve severe verbal abuse (such as profanity and racial slurs) or even physical abuse. Although physical abuse is usually meted out by the mentally incompetent, aides report being subjected to yelling, swearing, and a particularly colorful assortment of name-calling even by residents who are mentally alert. In rarer instances, aides have been struck by canes, hands, and available objects. Residents, both male and female, sometimes pinch and attempt to fondle aides, both male and female.

Abusive residents fall into four groups: (1) those who are manipulative by nature, (2) those who detest being in a nursing home and are taking it out on the aide, (3) those who dehumanize an aide to regain control of their living environment, and (4) those who are demented and not responsible for their acts. Many aides do not allow anything that they consider exploitation or abuse to continue. They report instances to their floor nurse or supervisor, who intercedes; they take a position in a different home; or they go into a new field of work. Unfortunately, aides are rarely prepared in advance for the situations they encounter.

CHANGE STRATEGIES

It is impossible for a creative DON or administrator to eliminate all of the systemic problems that keep the nursing home residents and the aides at cross-purposes and that ultimately compromise the autonomy and dignity of the residents. Some change strategies are long-range and require coalitions and political action. On the other hand, some directions can be taken unilaterally within a home. Anecdotal evidence suggests that they can make a difference in the well-being of residents without adversely affecting nursing home profits. In fact, some approaches can even improve the "bottom line" by reducing turnover of staff, by making the job more efficacious in the long run, or by improving staff morale.

Many of these strategies cost virtually no money and could be implemented immediately. Others require long-term implementation, challenge professional orthodoxy, and perhaps even cost money.

Develop Meaningful Training for Aides

The lack of nurse's aide training has already been deplored, but insufficient thought has been given to optimal training. Training must be practical and continuing. It not only should include the necessary concrete nursing skills but also human relations skills, which include sensitivity training. Nurse's aides have to be helped to discover their own values and prejudices. Such discoveries would help them realize that what they do is valuable and, more important, that why and how they perform their job is crucial. Nurse's aides need to be taught the reasons they make the observations they do and the kind of actions that should follow from observing changes in functioning. Functional assessment skills should not be limited to the professional staff alone. First, the aide is more likely to be present to make the observations; and second, if a person knows why she is collecting information, she is more likely to collect it accurately.

Training should also include attention to matters of personal autonomy. Aides can be encouraged to enter empathetically into the experience of entering a nursing home. On-the-job training should go beyond pedestrian "staff development meetings" to actual monitored assignments. For instance, if staff members are educated in understanding the issues a new resident confronts as he or she moves to a facility, they can be assigned to observe and assist a new resident, and the collective experiences can be the subject of a debriefing. There are countless imaginative ways that training could be integrated into the everyday work because the nursing home itself is available as a laboratory.

Involve Aides in Care Planning

Because aides associate with the residents more than do other staff members, their input could prove invaluable when designing resident care plans, but too often their opinions are ignored, or worse, never even solicited. So the ideas of the people most involved in care—that is, the aides and the residents themselves—are often missing from the resident's care plan. Also, it cannot automatically be assumed that nursing care plans for individual residents are even shared with the aides. We talked to nurse's aides who indicated that they were not supposed to see the medical records, but they found out as much as they could about the resident's condition anyway. This is of import not only because nurse's aides could give valuable input into care planning but because they are hardly likely to implement a plan well if they don't understand its purpose. In an ideal facility every concerned staff member has the opportunity to contribute to a resident care plan. In addition, the resident and a family member should be consulted so that all parties understand which care activities are expected and, most important, why.

Model Behavior for the Aides

Although it sounds obvious, it is often forgotten that actions speak louder than words, especially regarding desired social behavior. Senior professional staff in a nursing home cannot expect aides to follow their advice if they themselves seem to ignore residents, spend little time with them, ridicule them, and fail to attend to their needs. In a truly therapeutic climate it is not beneath anyone's dignity to show a lost resident to her room or attend to someone in distress. If professional staff (RNs and LPNs) do not support efforts at change, implementation becomes counterproductive.

Create Primary Assignments

The concept of primary nursing as developed in the hospital refers to the practice of assigning one staff nurse to one or more patients to be general case manager and advocate. It is also possible to create primary assignments in nursing homes, assigning each day and evening shift aide to one or more residents. Although the aide would have her regular assignments on each shift, her ongoing assignment would be to become the facility expert on her resident or residents—medically, psychologically, and socially—and to represent the resident's interests with other staff. Anecdotal reports suggest that this practice works extremely well as aides become more invested in their work. In at least one home, which has boasted an anthropologist in residence, primary nursing care floors were developed that employed this kind of model (Nicholson & Nicholson, 1982). Turnover of nurse's aides dwindled, and morale improved, compared to other floors.

Primary assignments can take advantage of the natural variation in the skills of the nurse's aide cadre. In any facility some staff will be well educated and psychologically sophisticated, whereas others will have a wealth of practical nursing experience. Staff can be encouraged to consult either formally, through in-service, or on an informal basis with each other to improve understanding of their residents and to learn how to help them better.

Change the Name

A name change can be more than a cosmetic issue. Nurse's aide or nursing assistant may be the wrong term for the paraprofessional in the nursing home. If the term "care assistant" were substituted, it would be at least clear that the nurse's aide tries to implement a wide range of objectives and support the work of the entire professional staff. Better yet, if the term "resident assistant" were substituted, the primacy of the resident's interests over those of the staff would be emphasized. In a model assisted-living program in Oregon, where residents who are all nursing home-eligible, enjoy small private apartments, the staff of the facility are known as home care workers. Although they are employed by the facility, it is conceptualized that they are providing services in the resident's home (Wilson, 1989). Similarly, in many analogous European facilities the caregiving staff, other than those who are literally nurses, are called by terms such as "elder care assistants".

In a more speculative vein, perhaps it would be feasible for staff members *actually* to take their direction from residents, at least for a range of tasks defined beforehand. This would allow residents the ability to make choices in necessary care routines, and aides would know that the resident actually wanted or needed these. One wonders how patterns of care for cognitively intact residents would change if each aide were assigned her residents and told to respond to their requests, dividing their time equitably. This might lead to the same type of difficulty as that of the secretary assigned to five "bosses," all of whom want something immediately. But it would certainly change the balance of power.

Find Business Reasons to Encourage Autonomy

One cannot always do well and do good at the same time, but sometimes it is possible. All staff members should be encouraged to develop techniques and practices that improve autonomy. More important, these procedures should be implemented. Implementation should include education at all levels of nursing home personnel, with everyone understanding the short-term and long-range impact of new procedures. For example, in response to a class assignment to bring about institutional change, an administrator decided that residents at his facility could choose their own bedtimes. Encouraged by initial results, he evaluated the effort more formally (Klanderman, 1983). It seemed that when residents chose their bedtimes, they used fewer sleeping medications, they slept better, there was less incontinence, and both residents and staff were pleased. The administrator concluded that the innovation saved money. Often, the simplest, yet most creatively innovative and effective idea can be found by questioning nurse's aides and asking them what they think could be done to remedy a situation. Nursing aides are too often ignored to the detriment of a home's quality of care.

Models of Excellence

One would be naive to ignore the growing acuity levels in nursing homes and the many special needs for care. In addition to development of nurse's aide programs, improved professional and technical nursing must be encouraged. At a minimum, the nurses also need skills to marshal an enthusiastic work force and create the environment in which autonomy is possible. Without the support of supervisory nursing, personnel change is not possible.

Much needs to be done to improve the practice and image of nursing in nursing homes and to achieve the goals of care found in the unexceptional and ringing phrases of the gerontological nursing standards promulgated by the American Nurses' Association (1987). In order to work on these goals, the nursing profession is planning a study to identify magnet nursing homes, an approach already tried successfully in the hospital sector. The magnet hospital study identified those hospitals and their characteristics that were able to maintain a stable nursing staff. Identification of excellent nursing homes and their characteristics is one objective for such a study.

The National Teaching Nursing Homes Project, funded by the Robert Wood Johnson Foundation, reflects another effort to provide new organizational and service models in nursing homes (Aiken, 1981; Mezey, 1988). The project directly addresses the perceived low status of nursing homes by affiliating with perceived "credible" institutions like schools of nursing and community hospitals. It stresses the importance of assessment of nursing home residents for purposes of preventive early intervention and actively enlists the collaboration of attending physicians and nursing staff in the hospital and nursing home. Liaison activities between the nursing home and the hospital may lessen the relocation trauma that residents so often experience. This liaison certainly lessens the isolation from the medical mainstream for nursing home staff.

No Physical Restraints

It seems axiomatic that nursing home staffs will have trouble respecting autonomy of residents while they continue the general practice of tying residents up, confining them to Geri-chairs, and the like. To those who think elimination of restraints is a romantic and naive notion, we can point out that apparently no other country finds it necessary to use physical or chemical restraints in its nursing homes except as a rare exception (Evans & Strumpf, 1989). In the early days of geriatric medicine in Great Britain, the idea of the drug holiday was invented. Physicians simply took their patients off all of their medications and then, if necessary, started over again. Without drugs, patients began to function better. It seems that in the United States nursing homes might institute both drug holidays and restraint holidays.

Make Ethical Issues a General Concern

Although oddly unrecognized, all nursing personnel in nursing homes, including paraprofessionals, are moral agents. That is, they are responsible for their actions, which can have, after all, profound consequences for the welfare of residents and others in the work environment. Though few would deny that a nurse is a moral agent, the nurse's aide too often is considered a functionary who merely follows orders.

As we repeatedly insist, however, nurse's aides provide most of the care and are therefore closest to the residents. Nursing home administrators must perceive them as responsible and accountable for enhancement or negation of residents' rights. Furthermore, in actuality they have large areas of discretion about whether residents' choices will be respected. As was shown in the chapter by Kjervik (this volume), the nurse's aide may have limited actions available when she sees a problem, but she is bound to work through the hierarchy toward solution. She cannot be justified in ignoring issues.

Professional nursing organizations already recognize a wide array of ethical issues that should concern nurses in nursing homes. These include decisions about emergency treatment, informed consent, confidentiality, surrogate decision making, terminal care, nontraditional treatment modalities, administration of artificial forms of nutrition and hydration, use of restraints, and fair distribution of human and material resources (American Nurses' Association, 1987). To this list we would add the many ordinary matters of daily life cited by the residents we interviewed and reflected in these cases studies.

Thus, we add to the list of matters for ethical scrutiny the selection of roommates and tablemates, policies for separating and mainstreaming persons with dementia, handling of interresident disputes, handling of residents' money, dealing with disagreements between residents and their family members, deciding how often to answer a call button and criteria for ignoring it, defining acceptable risks that residents may take, refining admission and discharge policies, and, of course, determining when, if ever, physical or chemical restraints are justified.

Sometimes the facility can develop a policy that seems fair and workable for the allocation of scarce resources, such as single rooms. (Well-understood queuing policies, for example, were suggested by Miles and Sachs, this volume.) Often what is needed is not a policy—there is a tendency toward too many hard and fast policies anyway—but rather a process for dealing with difficult questions. This legitimates the effort and makes sure the questions are not ignored.

Too often ethical issues and dilemmas arise as crisis situations. A home having appropriate mechanisms in place for dealing with such issues may prevent or eliminate or at least mitigate crises. Nursing home ethics committees should be developed and asked to deal with the questions of living in nursing homes as well as dying in nursing homes. Some nursing homes already have such committees. Trends will become apparent to illustrate problem types. Gradually, problem-solving options will be developed. Ethics committees should include residents, family members, and aides.

CONCLUSION

We would prefer to have federal and state policies and regulators that reward creative efforts to individualize care in nursing homes. We would prefer to have nursing home administrators who understand the importance of supporting management's efforts at offering "high-touch" technology training; who manage staff as investments, not expenses; and who balance risk management with resident autonomy. We would prefer to have more effectively trained professional nurses in nursing homes, nurses who encourage and support innovative care delivery, and nurses who willingly challenge the status quo. We would prefer to have nurse's aides trained in both the physical and social aspects of caring, who are seen as valued members of a caring team, who contribute to and understand both the short-term and long-range consequences of the care they deliver, and who are invested in the work they do. We would prefer to pay nurse's aides better.

Both staff and residents generally bring goodwill to the effort, and if nursing staff are encouraged to care, the personal rewards of the work can be great.

REFERENCES

Aiken, L. H. (1981). Nursing priorities for the 1980's: Hospitals and nursing homes. *American Journal of Nursing, 81,* 324–331.

Aiken, L. H. (1983). Nurses. In D. Mechanic (Ed.), *Handbook of Health, Health Care and the Health Professions,* New York, The Free Press, 407–431.

American Nurses' Association. (1987). *Standards and scope of gerontological nursing practice* Kansas City, MO: Author.

Carter, M. A. (1987). Professional nursing in the nursing home. *Journal of Professional Nursing, 3,* 325.

Diamond, T. (1986). Social policy and everyday life in nursing homes: A critical ethnography. *Social Science and Medicine, 23,* 1287–1295.

Evans, L. K., & Strumpf, N. E. (1989). Tying down the elderly: A review of literature on physical restraints. *Journal of the American Geriatrics Society, 37,* 65–74.

Goodwin, M., & Trocchio, J. (1987). Cultivation of positive attitudes in nursing home staff. *Geriatric Nursing,* January/February, 32–34.

Holtz, G. A. (1982). Nurses' aides in nursing homes: Why are they satisfied? *Journal of Gerontological Nursing, 8,* 265–271.

Kaster, J. M., Ford, M. H., White, M. A., & Carruth, M. L. (1979). Personnel turn-over: A major problem for nursing homes. *Nursing Homes, 28,* 20–25.

Klanderman, D. (1983). *Bedrest—bedtime determinants of long-term care residents.* Masters thesis submitted to the University of Minnesota School of Public Health.

Mezey, M., Lynaugh, J. E., & Cartier, M. (Eds). (1989). *Nursing homes and nursing care: Lessons from the teaching nursing home,* New York: Springer Publishing Co.

National Citizens' Coalition for Nursing Home Reform. (1985). *A consumer perspective on quality care: The residents' point of view.* Washington, DC: Author.

Nicholson, C. K., & Nicholson, J. L. (1982). *Personalized care model for the elderly.* Chittenango, NY: Author.

Selby, T. L. (1988). Long-term care poses challenge for nurses. *The American Nurse, 20,* 1, 26.

Tellis-Nayak, V., & Tellis-Nayak, M. (1989). Quality of care and the burden of two cultures. *The Gerontologist, 29,* 307–313.

Vladeck, B. C. (1980). *Unloving care: The nursing home tragedy.* New York: Basic Books.

Waxman, H. M., Carner, E. A., & Berkenstock, G. (1984). Job turnover and job satisfaction among nursing home aides. *The Gerontologist, 24,* 503–509.

Wilson, K. B. (1989). *Beyond loving care: Developing a social model of care.* Paper prepared for the Oregon Gerontological Society, 1989. (Available from Concepts in Community Living, 3530 SE 84th, 109, Portland, OR 97266).

Chapter 24

DEVELOPING SYSTEMS THAT PROMOTE AUTONOMY: Policy Considerations

Iris C. Freeman

Developing systems that promote autonomy in nursing homes is a mission against formidable odds. Autonomy, by whatever one's chosen definition, connotes some positive level of power, capacity, authority, and prerogative. Nursing home admission, by contrast, brings to mind a constellation of negatives that both trigger and accompany the event. The sequence that goes with admission almost axiomatically reflects deteriorating physical health, mental decline, a farewell to the collected possessions of adulthood, the evaporation of savings, and the severing of connections with people and perhaps pets. It is the time until the end and, by some accounts, a none too dignified environment to complete a life.

Some observe that nursing home applicants' dignity is at risk in the very language of admission, where nursing home "placement" is the commonplace euphemism for "being put." No one wants to be put, because objects are put, not people. Consequently, one characteristically encounters an individual resisting nursing home admission for fear of losing control, for fear of losing authority and prerogative, for fear of metamorphosis from personhood to an object that can, because it is only an object, be "put." Certainly, there are other reasons that people resist admission, from an apprehension that nursing homes are categorically neglectful to a belief that care of an elder is a family matter; however, by and large, the paramount facet is the perceived loss of autonomy.

Set against those perceptions that nursing home residents must overcome a significant probability that living in a nursing home will, intrinsically, reduce their autonomy is a growing body of literature asserting that having a realm of control correlates with improved physical and mental health. The clear message of the "learned helplessness" literature (Teitleman & Priddy, 1988) is that progressive practitioners can and ought to develop practical means for resident to think, to deliberate, to make choices, and to have some, even limited, areas of responsibility. The results of these opportunities and practices are seen to have positive ramifications for residents' self-image, mental status, friendliness, compliance with otherwise unpleasant medical regimens, perceptions of well-being, and, in fact, recovery from illness. Today facilities that have won the respect of their peers, consumers, and regulators are those whose philosophy and programs successfully address the challenge of caring for people who entered the nursing home because they legitimately need both medical help and assistance with activities of daily living without translating a legitimate basis for admission into license for infantilizing the individual altogether.

Arguments are made and refuted that a majority of nursing home residents lack the mental capacity to exercise autonomy in a meaningful way. For this discussion it is sufficient to recognize that there are now and for the foreseeable future will be residents who are fully capable of autonomy that is denied them and that there are several systemic changes (changes in industry behavior as a whole and in public regulation of nursing homes) that will improve the nursing home environment with respect to autonomy.

Principles aside, what does practical autonomy mean for a nursing home resident? As for anyone else, it means having the information necessary for some action or decision and the opportunity to exercise choice and live with the results of decisions. A resident who knows what day her doctor will visit is better able to organize a list of questions about her medication. A resident who knows what her state law provides about goods or services not included in the per diem can decide whether to rent her wheelchair from the supplier recommended by the facility or from some other. A resident who participates in her care conference and can express preferences without restraint or coercion is more likely to have a plan of care that is acceptable to both her and her caregivers. Residents whose council meetings provide a forum to discuss the many sides of a facility problem have the opportunity to play a role in reaching a solution. Even what may seem to the outsider a pitifully insignificant domain of choice, like having the certainty that a substitute dinner will be available when liver is served or choosing an evening bath over a morning shower, can be the objective event that satisfies a goal of enhancing autonomy.

BARRIERS

As we consider means to foster systems that promote resident autonomy, we must be mindful that some barriers to resident autonomy are initiated by neither the facility nor the regulatory agency. These barriers, although not amenable to systems intervention, are more naturally assessed and/or assailed by ombudsmen, legal service offices, and adult protective services.

Some are the beneficent limitations imposed by loved ones—for example, the plight of the resident whose worried daughter pressures the physician and nursing staff to apply physical restraints to an unwilling man who does not want to be bothered using a walker because he perceives the appliance as childish. She does not want him to fall and hurt himself.

Others are not so beneficent. Consider the case of the resident whose English has never been fluent and who months after placement in an urban facility near her nephew's house wants nothing more than to move to a rural facility 90 miles away, where many of the residents and staff speak her native tongue. Someone from her church has volunteered to help with the discharge and readmission requirements; staff members at both facilities are sympathetic and amenable. Nevertheless, the resident's nephew is unyielding in his position that if the renegade gets her way, he will cease paying for her care, rendering her medically indigent and subject to the restrictions of the Medicaid program.

Although community awareness and preadmission screening programs have effectively reduced the problem of people being hoodwinked into nursing homes, one still encounters an example such as the following. An unwilling resident, in the early stages of a dementing illness, has been told by her son that they are going on a shopping expedition. The destination is a nursing home where her application has been signed and sealed. Her sister calls the ombudsman for help in arguing for the resident's desired discharge and for intervention to preserve the resident's property. Whatever the extent of the resident's incapacity, and on that matter convictions diverge vividly, the facts that emerge reflect that her son has systematically been lying to her about her location, her savings, and her possessions.

These examples are somewhat aside from the barriers to the resident's (or applicant's) autonomy inherent in the long-term-care system. It is the latter that this chapter will address. The systems barriers to be explored are (1) failure of nursing homes to meet existing standards; (2) the ironic other side of the coin, slavish adherence to existing standards; and (3) lack of effective in-house problem-solving methods. Improvements will be suggested in each of these areas. The chapter concludes with consideration of the impact of scarcity in creating and deepening autonomy losses for nursing home residents.

Failure of Nursing Homes to Meet Existing Standards

Attention to respect for nursing home residents' autonomy is by no means an issue that has newly entered the nursing home reform agenda. Since the early 1970s, enactment of state and federal bills of rights has been the means to establish standards by which providers have a duty to encourage and honor residents' self-determination. Although overall, practice has improved (Institute of Medicine, 1986), it must be said that a salient threat to resident autonomy is that some nursing homes ignore the standards.

As an example, on the third of the month residents are lined up outside the facility's business office, their Social Security checks taken from the envelopes and turned facedown for endorsement. One by one the residents sign their checks and move on. The administrator asserts that this process ensures timely payment and compliance with Medicaid spend-down procedure. The residents, meanwhile, are deprived of privacy and information in the handling of their financial affairs because their public aid status is very public while the actual amount of their income is simultaneously hidden from them.

In another example, a resident is scheduled for involuntary transfer to a dementia unit in the facility in response to her agitation, vocalizing, and other antisocial behaviors. Intervention by an ombudsman is required to assert her rights to a psychological assessment and review of her medications before imposing a unilateral decision to move the resident's belongings.

In some cases, the facility's action is harder to pin down, most notably when residents' rights to express a grievance are cold-shouldered and quashed with the implication that people who make a fuss may soon find themselves "upstairs" or with the threat that if the situation at hand is so unbearable, perhaps another home might be in order.

This is not to say that residents should have unfettered latitude to assert themselves or that facilities are never entitled to take adverse action against an intransigent troublemaker. Facilities do, however, have an obligation to have orientation and in-service programs aimed at preventing violations of residents' rights due solely to the ignorance or insensitivity of nursing home staff. As a related matter, supervision is required to assure that residents' rights are consistently observed and that conflicts are satisfactorily resolved. Further, a management committed to efficiency above all is more than likely to impose policies that compromise resident autonomy and to encourage staff to stretch laws related to resident involvement in the decisions that affect them. Examples include the willy-nilly shuffling of residents among rooms, as if room assignment were nothing more personal than an ongoing jigsaw puzzle, and the inflexible scheduling of care routines and activities. System changes to challenge these practices should occur in the regulatory and ombudsman sectors.

One of the tenets of consumer advocacy for the regulatory changes passed in the Omnibus Budget Reconciliation Act (1987) was that health officials should view violations of residents' rights as being serious violations, indeed, as serious as infractions related to residents' physical safety. Traditionally, rights violations have been viewed as lapses of a lesser order. In Minnesota, where a schedule of eight levels of fines denotes the severity of infractions, at least six rights related to resident autonomy are violations in the next-to-lowest category. These are rights related to responsive service, the ability to voice grievances without restraint or coercion, telephone privacy, the safety of personal property, the right to establish advisory councils, and the access to protection and advocacy services.

Given that some of the state's sanctions are based on accumulations of violations in the four highest fine categories, the system's implicit message is that even recurrent refusal to comply will not lead to significant trouble. On reflection, experience in most jurisdictions is that when agencies impose their sternest actions against nursing homes, (i.e., revocation, suspension of license, or failure to renew), the core of their basis is more likely to be grounds of safety. The tacit messages are that autonomy is not as important as nursing care and that, besides, the courts would never uphold actions based on rights violations alone.

The Older Americans Act ombudsman program can be seen as a more immediate buffer against facilities' violations of residents' rights and as a means to prod the regulatory system for relief when the informal intervention is fruitless. Fulfillment of the ombudsman mandate, however, will entail two areas of change. First, access to an ombudsman requires knowledge that the program and their personnel exist. For many nursing home residents and their families, the miniature print revealing the ombudsman's whereabouts on the printed materials dealt out at admission and the unobtrusive sign in the hallway are simply ineffective means for alerting people to a source of help. At the same time, ombudsman program directors have an eternal fear of how the world will look on the day that all residents and their families are aware of how to file a complaint. Ombudsman offices are almost universally operating at capacity, and although the Institute of Medicine Committee on Nursing Home Regulation (1986) called for significant changes in the program's funding formula and level, Congress saw fit to make less than a cost of living increase in its most recent appropriation. Glass, (1988) and other sympathetic critics view the expansion of the ombudsman as essential to reinforcing the progress we make in the drafting of appropriate regulatory standards and the improved effectiveness of nursing home inspections.

Playing by the Rules

Many considerate people who work in nursing homes, from administrators to nursing assistants, have nagging second thoughts about the negative effects of decisions they make or the prohibitions they impose on resident autonomy. If it were only up to them, they allow, unwilling residents would not be bullied into breakfast or manipulated into other presumed therapeutic activities. But the matter, they remind us, is not only up to them. Lining the edges of the background are their own fears of reprisal for letting even a competent resident effect a competent choice.

Malpractice lawsuits and regulatory liability are the perceived threats. And although one can reply that by comparison with acute-care facilities, the record of malpractice actions against nursing homes, particularly where adverse events followed from acceding to a resident's rightful self-determination, are rare, most caregivers would rather be safe than sorry. This attitude is prevalent, despite the solid standards of proof that would have to be met that the provider flouted both the duty to protect and common standards or parameters of practice and that the resulting harm to the resident was directly caused by the provider's failure. "It can be stated with certainty," writes Marshall Kapp, (1987) an expert on the issue, "that a health care provider is not held legally liable for every mistake or error in judgment, or for every unfortunate patient outcome, but only for patient injuries that are directly caused by the provision of care that falls below the due or reasonable range" (p.5).

More pressing, it may appear, is the concern that deviating from the "rules" will incur the wrath of regulators. Not only may health department inspectors second-guess a decision to honor the resident's preferences, but one is reminded that the trend in federal and state regulation of nursing homes is to strengthen the sanctions for violations and to hasten the calendar for license revocation and decertification. We begin with the narrow issue of a resident's demurrer and slide precipitously into the specter of a fast-track decertification.

The mindset would be fully laughable were it not for the equally darkly humorous examples of regulatory standards and events that, applied by the hand of one or another surveyor or agency, do inhibit resident autonomy. Consider the resident who has stored liquid shoe polish and a small box of detergent in her nightstand so that she can fulfill a value of personal responsibility to maintain shiny shoes and laundered underwear. This matter, uncontroversial in the privacy of one's own home or apartment, can draw quite another scenario in a licensed, certified nursing home. Surveyors may view the storage as a safety violation; to wit, the storage of poisonous substances in a location where, even if no risk exists for the owner of the contraband, others with dimmer mental capacity may wander in, open the bottle, drink the contents, and be harmed. Conversations among providers and ombudsmen on the topic of "rights and regulations" are now and then a spirited game of one-upmanship, swapping anecdotes of similar regulatory imbroglios.

No nursing home operator welcomes a bad report card, particularly as public policy moves toward full disclosure of surveys to help people make informed decisions about admissions. If the further jeopardy is that the nursing home appears, on the record, to be careless about getting people to breakfast (whether or not they want to go) or to therapeutic reactivities (whether or not the activities are enjoyable, or worse, are inappropriate for the time of day), then the line of thought runs to written orders for correction, reinspections to verify compliance, potentially costly appeals if one means to resist orders, and arguably, a sum total of deficiencies that merits a state decision to seek decertification.

Nonetheless, the history of nursing home regulation is compelling, so even illogical conclusions must be viewed against what has been a stirring need to protect vulnerable individuals from the perils of institutional living. The annals of regulation, to this day, are replete with gruesome experiences of individual and corporate providers whose cynicism and financial incentives overcame their duty to deliver care and protect people from harm. Records of state and federal hearings, reams of documentation, and alarming accounts in the media, not only of neglectful service but of weak-willed inspectors, support the evolution of incrementally stricter standards for the operation of facilities (Institute of Medicine, 1986). Given the unequivocal role of consumers and their organizations in achieving a highly regulated nursing home industry, it becomes difficult, even in the face of a seemingly inappropriate regulatory event, to fault a compliant home (e.g., one whose policies prohibit contraband in a nightstand) or an honorable regulator (e.g., one who imposes a penalty upon discovery of contraband in a nightstand), despite the fact that a resident believes that her rights have been violated more egregiously than anyone's safety. Intuitively, something is amiss.

As we enter what might be termed a second generation of nursing home regulation, the issue is ripe for exploration and offers a salutary context for consumers, providers, and regulators to cooperate on an agenda for improvement. Some pieces of that agenda follow:

1. First, the interested parties have to agree that conflict between resident autonomy and "playing by the rules" is a topic worthy of address. Identification of a few problematic regulations, policies, and case examples can be presented as an impetus for discussion. As likely as not, discussion will yield barrels of additions and a wealth of perspectives that complicate the issue.

2. A singular area for inquiry is whether, in facilities that serve both the cognitively intact and impaired, the short-term rehabilitation client and the long-term residents, all regulations should be applied universally. Questions include the practicality of drafting standards that are individualized to the residents they are supposed to protect, the advisability of combining universal regulations with client-specific exceptions, and the knotty problem of how (in real life) one would deal with the ebb and flow of restrictions upon a resident whose mental capacity wavers or declines. If one of the goals of regulation is to apply clear standards fairly and another is for regulators to demonstrate that their punitive actions are valid and consistent, does reality demand contentment with a certain degree of mechanistic response to any set of facts?

3. Related to this is progress to make in the area of surveyor orientation and training. Distancing ourselves from the pressures of our unique experience as consumers, providers, or regulators, we might all agree that surveyors ought to be able to observe a fact situation that deviates from adherence to a rule and assess whether the salient property is resident autonomy or caregiver neglect. In part, the nursing home's prior record is relevant, as is the current profile of the home as whole. For example, are some residents not getting to breakfast because of dangerous understaffing or because they resist being awakened at 6 A.M.? Looking at the individual resident's record, surveyors should proceed from a principle that residents are entitled to a presumption of competence to make certain decisions about the services they receive. From there, the observer can analyze what documented or observed factors overcome that presumption and what, either for the individual or the society of the home as a whole, are unacceptable levels of risk.

Consumer organization spokespersons suggest that the key to surveyor orientation and training in sorting out such situations is including nursing home residents in their training. Residents are the people who can best describe the critical factors of privacy and autonomy.

Although one hesitates to give surveyors a double message—that is, carry a big stick but be very cautious about applying it—the message may just be realistically complex. The education of regulators calls for sensitive discussion of the differences between regulating the provider and regulating the resident.

4. Another potential system improvement is creating a step in the enforcement process that permits an informal reconsideration process for matters that the facility contends to have been respect for an individual's rights but the agency has recorded as a violation. Typically, once a violation is documented, a facility's only two choices are correction or resistance through some combination of penalty and appeal. Interpreters of the enforcement provisions of the Omnibus Budget Reconciliation Act (1987) suggest that state systems may adopt a fair reconsideration process in which a facility would have 15 business days after notice of penalty to ask for a reconsideration of the order. Their written reconsideration request would detail specific reasons for disagreement with the penalty. For this purpose, general appeals or claiming that the violation no longer exists would not be valid bases for reconsideration. A designated state agency official who did not participate in the initial determination to impose the penalty would review the request and issue a decision within 10 business days. Reconsideration would be based solely on the facility's and agency's documentation. Neither hearings nor oral testimony would be taken (Edelman,). The reconsideration process offers a potentially effective and certainly time-limited option for balancing competing goals of protection and autonomy.

5. Finally, a closer look at some of what has become conventional wisdom in the language of certain nursing home standards reveals implications for the long-term-care research agenda. The broad question is whether some of the regulations that prescribe resident behavior have an adequate empirical basis. Do the socialization goals inherent in group activities and group repasts withstand a fresh evaluation? Are periodic and even more frequent compromises to restrictive diets to be thwarted at all turns?

The challenge of crafting improved standards and processes is substantial; however, the experience of communication about these issues may be productive in its own right. Again, citing Kapp, (1987): "What is needed in health care delivery generally, and in the long-term care setting particularly, is a practical way of balancing the altruistic goals of autonomy and beneficence with the pragmatic needs of facilities to be legally protected within the confines of their staffing and resources" (p. 79). Add to that balancing the vagaries of individual self-determination and the public desire for a coherent regulatory system.

Lack of Effective In-House
Problem-Solving Methods

Improving systems of communication and decision making in nursing homes fosters the autonomy of individual residents. Residents councils are groups that meet regularly in their homes to voice needs and concerns, state preferences, and cooperate with nursing home staff toward change. They are a relatively recent phenomenon, with scattered development in the 1960s and concentrations of intense effort (New York, Washington state, Massachusetts, and Minnesota) in the 1970s. With increasing publicity and growing respect by policymakers and industry trade associations, the 1980s have seen a number of state laws either requiring resident councils in licensed homes (Colorado, Illinois, New York, Oklahoma) or assuring councils the legitimate support of staff liaison, meeting space, and privacy for deliberations (Minnesota). Unfortunately, there remain facility staff who view residents councils as just another activity and minimize the practicality of working with residents to achieve change. Examples of observed events tell us otherwise. Residents at a New York home have a biannual food-tasting event in cooperation with the Food Services Department. Resident food committee members sample new items and rate them as to appearance, taste, and acceptability. High ratings are translated into incorporation in the menu cycle (Grossman & Weiner, 1988). Residents in Minnesota homes have successfully affected telephone access and privacy. In the first, residents took the initiative to contact the telephone company about the cost of lowering the pay phone to wheelchair height. In the second, they persuaded administration to move the public phone to a small private room. Others have achieved changes in their food service, menus, portions, and cutlery. Another council intervened when the Health Department scorned their salad bar. Their petitions convinced the agency that residents liked having choices (Hart, 1988).

Family councils have a similar role in affecting the quality of life and opportunities in a nursing home. Skeptical staff who view a family council as a recreational activity or a support group may be missing a valuable opportunity to address mutual problems in a spirit of cooperation. Again, the principle has been seen at work. A family council in one home persuaded administration to assign nursing assistants to specific residents on a continuing basis. Both residents and their caregivers report that better care resulted from heightened awareness of individuals' needs. Family councils have secured funds for equipment that expands residents' opportunities for self-expression, such as a piano, a stereo, a library of large-print books, and even a van to open opportunities for activities outside the home (Hart, 1988). Family council members can be involved in staff training and are valuable allies in staff recognition. It is little wonder, then, that nursing homes that boast dynamic family councils are exemplars of care and consumer satisfaction.

Comparatively little attention has been given to the role of the nursing home staff member who serves in the role of the council staff advisor. The advisor, or liaison between consumers and administration, is often key to the success or failure of the council. Necessary attributes include objectivity, commitment to the purposes of consumer involvement, enthusiasm, and a capacity to facilitate without imposing. Administrators who are sincere in a goal of fostering effective consumer councils are similarly aware that staff advisors have to be able to devote adequate time to their council duties along with whatever other activities or social service tasks make up the remainder of their job descriptions.

The Omnibus Budget Reconciliation Act (1987), responding to a recommendation of the Institute of Medicine (1986), incorporated for the first time in federal law the right of the "resident to organize and participate in resident groups in the facility and the right of the resident's family to meet with families of other residents." Although the language supports and legitimates the existence of self-help groups, people experienced in the development of effective councils suggest that success requires something more tangible than enabling legislation. Areas of notable council development are by and large areas where an independent community organization or ombudsman program has been involved to a substantial degree in working with residents, family members, and facility staff to define and refine purpose, governance, leadership skills, meeting procedures, ways of increasing active participation, tasks, and problem-solving skills. In 1985 Minnesota was the first state to recognize that the actualization of residents' rights depends in part on the vitality of consumer councils. To promote quality assurance through councils, the state enacted an annual surcharge ($1.73, later amended to $2.75) on the licensing fees of every nursing and boarding care bed. Funds collected are used for the purpose of enabling the statewide nursing home consumer organization to hire educators and develop resources to help resident and family groups throughout the state to improve their capabilities. This model for encouraging consumer self-expression with hands-on help is a promising example of how legislative advocacy can result in a means for enhancing autonomy.

Bioethics committees are newer to nursing homes than to hospitals; however, as they develop, there is reason to consider them as a forum for discussing the ethical perplexities of daily life in the facility. Although bioethics committees are more commonly associated with difficult decisions around withholding and withdrawing medical treatment, the interdisciplinary composition offers a promising means for education, policy development, and consultation on many of the most pressing issues of autonomy and safety, such as the use of restraints, petitions for guardianship, adherence to therapeutic diets, self-medication, and room assignment.

Unlike hospital forums, nursing home bioethics committees can appropriately budget a significant portion of their time to addressing the ethical issues of daily life because so many residents spend hundreds, even thousands, of their days in the facility. Further, their mandate can be structured to address the most timely and provocative issues in their own home, taking cues not only from administration and staff but from resident and family councils.

In all, the lack of effective methods for communication and problem-solving within the confines of the nursing home is a formidable barrier to ensuring attention to residents' autonomy. Although changes in the long-term care regulatory and financing systems are critical to attaining improvement, there are notable benefits to recognizing that the most immediate "system" in a resident's life is that of the home itself.

THE ISSUE OF SCARCITY

As we explore systems interventions that promote autonomy, we unavoidably reach a recurrent theme: so much of what detracts from autonomy in long-term care is a side effect of scarcity. Simply stated, the autonomy problems that confound the daily lives of nursing home residents are also complaints of "not enough." Most of the foregoing case situations reveal illustrations: the rarity of single rooms; the prized chair in the dayroom; the displacement of some residents for others' family events; the regimented mealtime, dressing, grooming, and toileting schedules that are concomitants of limited staff. Access to nursing home care itself—the risk of finding an available space too many miles from home—is an early indicator that resource issues are intrinsic to levels of choice. Categorizing roughly, there are goals that are pipedreams (e.g., every resident having the personal attention necessary to exercise every prerogative and sustain comfort) and conditions that are amenable to improvement. Three examples of the latter follow.

Nursing Home Staffing

Ombudsmen and health department complaint investigators frequently receive reports of unresponsive service, primarily of call lights not being answered fast enough. This is simultaneously an issue of autonomy and safety. How we best can approach the problem demands attention to its proximate cause. If we determine that the nursing home is making a good-faith effort to staff adequately, but the payment system in its jurisdiction is dangerously stingy, then the intervention must aim at the payment system. If, conversely, the management of the home is making decisions to staff at the margin of acceptability—that is, refusing to spend what it can—then the target must be the operator or corporate system, not the laws or overall appropriation under which the state's nursing homes operate. These are difficult and sophisticated assessments to make; however, as in other domains, the fitness of the solution lies in accurate problem definition. Throughout, there are ethical questions for policymakers, consumers, and the industry. What constitutes reasonable expenditures and efforts to fulfill residents' requests? How should adequate ratios of staff to residents be determined for different populations? What principles should govern the allocation of staff time? Should people who express preferences be honored at the risk of slighting others? Discussion on this order will not invent a magic bullet, but it should better inform decisions and agendas for reform.

Space, Privacy, and Autonomy

Autonomy requires privacy, for a call to an ombudsman out of others' earshot, for visits with a mate or friend, to shine a reading lamp without waking a roommate. Privacy to talk with one's physician is rare, although exercise of autonomy would promise that one can receive and weigh information to make a decision. So-called privacy curtains may inhibit view but are never a sound barrier.

Ironically, sometimes the most desirable space in a home is awarded to the least desirable resident. The practical problem is this: Would you assign the only single room on the floor to the most truculent resident or the most cordial? Something is wrong with the incentive, and remedy eludes because many jurisdictions, in a justified quandary to manage nursing home costs, have enacted moratoria on construction and renovation of facilities. Nonetheless, to the degree and in the instances that renovation, replacement, and new construction money is available, attention can be paid to the relationship between the configuration of space and the autonomy of the people who live in it.

Medicare and Medicaid

In 1965 the federal government enacted the health care programs that have come to define much of the long-term care system. The programs were, unquestionably, meant to guarantee life-sustaining care to masses of older persons. Subsequent rules, however, are known to make life miserable for individuals. Two that are notable with respect to autonomy of nursing home residents are the "Medicare bed" and the Medicaid personal needs allowance. Briefly, the Medicare bed is a certified one that the resident must use if the home is to be reimbursed by Medicare. Unless all of the beds in a facility are so certified, a resident returning from hospitalization will rarely return to the familiar space that may have been "home" for a very long time. It is an abrupt and unsettling change, ill-timed and not amenable to negotiation. Further, 1989 changes in Medicare coverage for skilled care have occasioned the transfer of many additional residents (those without acute-care episodes) to new quarters.

The Medicaid personal-needs allowance is the amount of the resident's own income that can be retained for clothing and other needs not supplied by the program. All remaining income must be "spent down" (i.e., paid for care), as a condition of subsidy for the rest of the bill. The federal floor for the allowance is $30 a month. Some state legislatures periodically supplement this amount; however, decisions to increase the allowance are infrequent and do not keep pace with the cost of living. If the personal-needs allowance is a resident's budget for clothing, haircuts, telephone, and nonmedical transportation, the question occurs: how much autonomy can anyone buy for $30 or $40 a month?

Minnesota and Massachusetts are the only states that have enacted an automatic annual cost-of-living increase. Nonetheless, if the spend-down requirements of the Medicaid program will not be fundamentally changed in the short term, then sympathetic attention remains due on the meager base amount and its stifling effect on the daily lives of recipients.

SUMMARY

Developing systems that promote autonomy for nursing home residents tests the commitment, creativity, and patience of those involved. As in individual cases, there is eternal confrontation with the values, needs, and perspectives of the multiple interested parties. It is a process of negotiation, of choosing priorities, of defining standards, testing them and making them accountable.

REFERENCES

Edelman, T.S. State intermediate sanctions under OBRA." Paper prepared for the American Association of Retired Persons.

Glass, A.P. (1988). Improving the quality of care and life in nursing homes," *Journal of Applied Gerontology, 7,* 413.

Grossman, H.D. & A.S. Weiner. (1988). Quality of life: The institutional culture defined by administrative and resident values," *Journal of Applied Gerontology, 7,* 402.

Hart, M. (1988). Report of resident and family council accomplishments—1988. Minneapolis: Minnesota Alliance for Health Care Consumers.

Institute of Medicine, Committee on Nursing Home Regulation (1986). *Improving the Quality of Care in Nursing Homes,* Washington, D.C., National Academy Press.

Kapp, M.B. (1987). *Preventing Malpractice in Long-Term Care: Strategies for risk management.* New York: Springer Publishing Co.

Omnibus Budget Reconciliation Act. (1987). PL 100-203.

Teitleman, J.L. & Priddy, J.M. (1988). From psychological theory to practice: Improving frail elders quality of life through control-enhancing interventions," *Journal of Applied Gerontology, 7,* 298–315.

Chapter 25

AVENUES TO APPROPRIATE AUTONOMY: What Next?

Rosalie A. Kane, Arthur L. Caplan, Iris C. Freeman, Mila Ann Aroskar, and Ene Kristi Urv-Wong

With a focus on nursing home residents, this book has closely scrutinized personal autonomy, a fundamental value in American society and a closely guarded principle for both philosophers and constitutional theorists. Some conclusions about this subject are possible, which, in turn give rise to a multifaceted agenda of practice and policy change and of further inquiry.

PERSONAL AUTONOMY IS UNDULY COMPROMISED

The evidence seems clear. Nursing home residents say they would like more control over many areas of their daily lives and care. They say, too, that currently they have little control. Nursing assistants and other nursing home personnel say, usually with regret, that under present circumstances most residents are assured precious little personal choice and control. Moreover, nursing assistants and other nursing home personnel say that in their view it is important for nursing home residents to exercise control over these mundane matters, even while also saying that it cannot be done under current financial and regulatory constraints.

From an ethicist's standpoint, many of the moral questions are also clear. *We can and ought to arrange nursing home care and other residential care for the elderly in a way that is much more respectful of the personal autonomy of the residents.*

The arguments to justify the status quo are well known and have a realistic basis. Yes, the interests of one resident often compete with those of another; therefore, the expression of autonomy in any residential community cannot be unbridled. And yes, many residents *do* need some protection. Some exercise of beneficence in the interest of their safety and well-being is therefore necessary. Moreover, it is indisputable that many residents have diminished capacity for autonomous decision making and that some are so impaired that respecting autonomy becomes relevant only in the sense of implementing their advance directives. In these cases, many would argue that "respect for persons"—from which the principle of autonomy flows—requires dignified and humane treatment of those who have become hopelessly confused. They might also argue that standard care for persons with cognitive impairment is insufficiently respectful.

We also recognize that autonomy is not a fairy godmother that grants all wishes. Autonomous living necessarily entails negotiation, compromise, getting in line, following procedures. College students, for example, often draw roommates who are incompatible, and we do not say their autonomy is breached. Inevitably, nobody gets everything he or she wants. But although autonomy does not imply a "satisfaction guarantee," autonomous people do require some ability to position themselves to exercise a modicum of choice and control.

Having made obeisance to all of the necessary caveats, consensus remains: No justifications can be found on moral grounds for the extent to which residents' daily lives are compromised. No ethical principle applies that justifies intrusions into the lives of competent people that mandate their rising up and lying down, to use the biblical phrase, and almost everything else that occurs in between. Even nursing home regulations, however heavy-handed, cannot be a scapegoat for such pervasive loss of liberty. That is not what the regulations intend. That is not how they should be applied.

PAYING ATTENTION

The first step toward any social change is paying attention. One cannot work productively on a problem before it is identified and known to exist.

This book was designed to pay systematic attention to matters usually considered too trivial and perhaps also too intractable for ethicists and policymakers to address.

Data from our own studies and those of others illustrate that control over many ordinary matters is important to cognitively intact residents and that such control is often denied them. Our study was an initial effort to pay attention to what residents say and want. At a time when many excellent scholars are preoccupying themselves with studying the functional limitations and acuity levels of nursing home residents, mapping the amount of time needed to care for residents of given disability and acuity, and refining "case-mix adjusted" payment systems, our line of research may seem quixotic and out of step. But we would hope to see more explorations of the preferences and wishes of nursing home residents, weighed against their perceptions of their actual experience. We view this as a form of paying attention.

It would be feasible for nursing home staffs to determine much more about a resident's preferences, both on admission and in an ongoing way. To make such fact finding worthwhile, however, actions must flow from the information. Flexible rising times, bedtimes, and mealtimes; practices that allow some residents to retain use of their checkbooks; ways for residents to consult meaningfully with a physician—all of these would need to be worked out.

Many of those who are cognitively impaired also have the opportunity to express preferences while they are still functioning at higher levels. Part of the tragedy of Alzheimer's disease and other dementias is that the course is so long, and in the early stages persons with the disease are aware of their future fate. This might be the time to learn something about the preferences of the person with Alzheimer's disease. Of course, these preferences would often be elicited long before the older person ever entered a nursing home. Some mechanism would be needed to ensure that the preferences of the demented person followed him or her. Perhaps family members would necessarily become the translators.

ENVIRONMENT

Some features of typical nursing homes interfere enormously with the prospect of personal autonomy for the residents. We would argue that it is time to reconsider them.

Double Rooms

Roommate problems are rampant in nursing homes. Even with compatible roommates, each is limited by the presence of the other. They are limited in their use of the lights and the television, their privacy for visitors, and their privacy for intimate care. Incompatible roommates are sentenced to "doing time" in close quarters, without the escape mechanisms that more mobile people forced to live in close spaces enjoy. Given the heterogeneity of nursing home residents, the mathematics of room assignment cannot ever work out well. Except for married couples, most residents told us they would prefer a single room if they could afford it. Otherwise, they preferred an unobtrusive roommate who blended into the background. We suggest the time has come to simply stop designing residential facilities for the elderly with double rooms.

Remaining in the Same Room

One's room in a nursing home—even a double room—is one's home. Residents may decide they want to change that home, and they may place their names on a list for a room they perceive as more desirable, but they find it disruptive and disturbing to be moved from room to room to meet the needs of the facility or the payment mechanisms. For example, if all beds are not dually certified for Medicare and Medicaid coverage, a resident who wants to claim her Medicare benefit for short periods of time, say, on return from a hospital, may need to literally move out of her room. When her Medicare benefit elapses, she needs to move again. In some states Medicaid rules have been interpreted to mean that a resident who needs heavier amounts of care (and is receiving reimbursement reflecting that) must move to a section where the staffing levels are higher. Facilities also can achieve efficiencies by grouping residents according to their care needs. Finally, residents may be asked to move to accommodate the changing census; for example, more men being admitted may change the room patterns, or someone needing terminal care may be moved to a single room close to the nurses' station.

We argue that in most instances the care should be brought to the resident's room, rather than moving the resident to the care. An exception would be when a resident becomes so cognitively impaired that he or she would benefit from a special unit for dementia, as discussed below.

Separate Programs for Dementia

Cognitively intact residents were disturbed by the palpable presence of demented residents—residents who made noise, who pried into their possessions, who could not participate in an activity or conversation. Long-term-care facilities have recently begun developing special units for Alzheimer's disease. Although these have initially been marketed to the families of persons with Alzheimer's disease as an improved (and usually more costly) environment for the demented, in fact, the interests of both those with and those without dementia are served by the separation.

Common sense dictates that the same programs cannot ideally serve physically impaired but cognitively intact and cognitively impaired residents. For the former, one tries to create obstacle-free spaces; for the latter, one tries to create mazelike paths where the demented person can safely wander. People with dementia can enjoy brief structured programs; they seem to like music; they seem fascinated by programs that others would consider childish. If they are not in an area where their movements would disturb others, the arguments for physical and chemical restraints almost disappear. Meanwhile, persons who are cognitively intact enjoy a more sensible environment.

We recognize that perfect sorting is unlikely to occur in any nursing home. Single rooms, as already advocated, would solve some of the problems.

RESTRAINTS

Being physically restrained against one's will would seem extremely incompatible with enjoying autonomy. Physical restraints are used widely in nursing homes in the Unites States, although no conscious societal decision has been made that our preferred way of handling the aberrant behavior of our grandparents is to tie them up. Unfortunately, ethicists have largely left the issue of physical restraints in nursing homes unexamined. It is time that they turned to it.

Nursing homes in other countries barely use physical restraints at all, whereas in the United States we use them heavily. Ostensibly, they are used to protect the resident, and they may indeed be a cheaper protection than staff supervision. They are also sometimes used to protect other residents from someone who is dangerous. We interviewed a few cognitively intact residents who were in restraints at the time. Stoically, they report "getting used to it." For the most part, restraints are used for confused residents. Family members often get the last word in disputed cases. If family members want a relative to take the risks, usually the facility agrees. But if family members want the resident protected regardless of the resident's wishes, again the family seems to win.

Physical restraints are an important exemplar of the trade-offs between beneficence and autonomy as they occur in nursing homes. But the restraints may not have the beneficient effect we expect. Several factors must be considered. First, there are numerous examples of residents who struggle to get out of the restraints and who fall over the raised bed rails. Second, the effect on staff may be dehumanizing in ways that lead to belittling the residents in general. It is hard to maintain a respectful relationship to someone whom you can tie up with impunity. We asked nurse's aides about how using restraints affected them, and most told us that though it "bothered" them a little at first, they felt better when they understood the reasons.

DEMENTIA AND ADVANCE DIRECTIVES

Undoubtedly, autonomy in the usual sense of self-rule is impossible for persons with severe or even moderate senile dementia. Many of the contributors to this volume point to the importance of discerning and respecting the authenticity of the person based on their previous identity in these sad situations. We are also reminded that a person officially classified as "demented" may still be capable of expressing current preferences on many matters if only we pay enough attention to elicit them. For other, more complex decisions, autonomy is presumably expressed through duly constituted surrogates with or without advance directives from the resident who is now demented. Both advance directives and surrogacy raise many legitimate questions.

Advance Directives

It is unclear what force advance directives should have on the long-term care of cognitively impaired people. Specifically, one can ask whether all properly executed advance directives must be honored. This practice could exert what might be called a "living dead hand" on care providers and on family members. People no longer able to make a decision and weigh new information about risks and benefits of treatments or about available resources would then be controlling decisions as a result of their previously expressed preferences. Proponents of advance directives have ethusiastically adopted this "decide while you still can" solution for permitting autonomy to the cognitively impaired. But little attention has been given to delineating the areas of decisions for which an advance directive should have force.

So far advance directives have largely been used as a mechanism for a person to limit life-sustaining treatments under various conditions. As such they cost little and may save money. In the United States we have not explored whether advance directives place positive obligations on others to continue life-sustaining care for those in irreversible comas or vegetative states, much less to arrange the caregiving milieu in a certain way. It is interesting to speculate, for example, about whether a competent person should be allowed to issue a directive prohibiting the use of physical restraints in the event of becoming afflicted with Alzheimer's disease, or insisting that they must always be cared for in their own home. There must be two parties to a directive: the one who issues it and the one who agrees to carry it out. The latter could all be citizens under a social agreement that is embodied in government policies and laws. We are, of course, a long way from that kind of well-understood social compact.

An advance directive, one would think, has no more force than an expressed preference. It surely can have no more standing than the stated preferences of those who are mentally intact, and those preferences bind others only in special circumstances. Thus, advance directives as the answer to ensuring appropriate autonomy for residents with cognitive impairment is a complex solution and one that needs further detailing.

Surrogates

Another way for nursing home staff to respect the autonomy of the cognitively impaired is to defer to a surrogate decision maker and consult that person's preferences and decisions on behalf of the resident rather than exercise its independent judgment. The surrogate is a stand-in for the resident herself, is presumed to have her best interest at heart, and may, in fact, have been designated by the resident to act in her behalf.

In the nursing home, residents of varying degrees of incapacity often have no formally appointed surrogate such as a guardian or conservator but may have one or more de facto surrogates, such as a representative payer, a specific family member, or perhaps a number of family members. This leads to a potentially chaotic situation, with a facility uncertain about whom to seek for help with a decision, how to act in the case of disputes among these informal surrogates, and what to do if the resident seems opposed to the view of a family member.

On the other hand, seeking formal conservatorships or guardianship arrangements is no perfect solution. Nursing homes too often notice instances when legally designated surrogates seem to be acting outside the best interests of the resident. Even when the resident retains cognitive capacities, she can have great difficulty reversing a guardianship once it has been filed.

Furthermore, the involvement of surrogates begs the question of the appropriate scope of decision making for a guardian, particularly one who spends little time in the facility. Should it extend to minute decisions about how the resident spends her time? Should a guardian be able to limit a friendship, restrict outside visitors, order physical restraints? Is it always more respectful of autonomy to defer to a distant guardian over and above the opinion of those on the scene? When does respect for autonomy require asking the guardian? All of these are issues requiring more attention, not just in the context of the life-and-death decisions but in the context of everyday life.

RISKS AND RISK TAKING

So many of the issues discussed in this book deal with taking risks. Restrictions on mobility, prohibitions against going outside unaccompanied or showering alone, removal of unsafe substances from the reach of any resident, and even physical restraints—all are designed to keep residents safe in a safe environment.

We are confident that residents would rather take some risks. With the risks, however, will come untoward events. If residents are permitted to move about, more of them will fracture their hips. (Hip fractures occur on the outside, and perhaps some should be expected on the inside in facilities that value autonomy.) Some will wander off and get lost.

This issue poses grave difficulties. On the one hand, few would be prepared to exonerate a nursing home from all responsibility for the safety of the residents. Some accidents and untoward events are a result of bad care. But we will be paying only lip-service to the concept of quality of life if our regulatory and legal systems send strong messages to facilities that safety always comes first. Nursing home staffs cannot settle this question alone. Consumer advocates must consider what they *really* want in a long-term-care facility. Typically, they want pleasant, unrestricted environments that are respectful of residents' preferences, but they are also prepared to "cry foul" when hips are broken and accidents occur. Family members of residents may also be quick to consider a lawsuit if something goes wrong for their parent at a nursing home. Until some consensus is reached on the preferred trade-offs and facilities are given unambiguous messages about what is valued, it is understandable that they err on the side of safety.

RESIDENTS' RIGHTS

Many of the topics touched on in this book could be and have been framed
as a matter of residents' rights. Thus, residents could be argued to have a
right to dignified treatment, competent health care, regular toileting, control over their money, freedom from physical restraints, and a choice of
rising time and bedtime. In this potpourri of potential rights, some are
identical to basic rights guaranteed to every citizen under the Constitu-
tion, whereas others have an odd specificity for something to be couched
in rights language.

There are two issues to consider about rights. First, rights are not ensured by declaration alone, particularly rights of vulnerable, dependent
people. If we are serious about a particular right for nursing home residents, we must inform them and their family members fully of that right,
create opportunities for it to be exercised, apply sanctions to those who
violate rights, and educate personnel to understand the existence and
importance of the rights as well as their role in protecting and promoting
rights of residents.

As important as it is to establish and maintain residents' rights, single-
minded attention to rights may be problematic. It is possible to argue that
the staff should be kind to residents, offer them choices, and give them
control over their lives, not because residents have rights kindness, choice,
and control but because virtuous staff members will take that course.

Orientation to rights is very American, and it seemingly is also very
necessary in the context of the American nursing home, where a history of
abuse has occurred. But rights language has the disadvantage of introducing legalistic formulations into the everyday world of the nursing home
residents. In ordinary living situations, such as families and friendships,
we rarely speak of rights. Rather, we treat each other according to the
claims of affection and our own view of how we, as virtuous people,
should behave. A fixation on rights can seem austere and sterile. On the
other hand, the downside of a virtue approach in a human service is
the danger of an arrogant paternalism on the part of authorities.

RIGHTS OF CAREGIVING STAFF

Care attendants also have both rights and duties, but neither are well
spelled out. Professionals such as nurses and social workers subscribe
to a code of ethics that governs their behavior, and they are expected to
be relatively autonomous in carrying out their mandates. In contrast,

paraprofessional members of the caregiving staff have no defined code of conduct, and there is uncertainty about the amount of discretion and autonomy they should have in initiating actions. Before ideal resident autonomy can be achieved, the scope of the care attendant's rights and responsibilities must also be established.

BEYOND THE MEDICAL MODEL

We have struggled in these pages with imperfect success to determine what kind of place a nursing home is or should be. What seems clear, however, is that modeling a nursing home after a hospital is dysfunctional. This is true even acknowledging that some very sick people live and die in nursing homes.

A hospital is a doctor's workshop. The physician is viewed as having a fiduciary responsibility to the patient, and requests concerning the patient are usually filtered through the physician. For their part, the patients usually have accepted some constraints on their autonomy because they perceive they have put themselves into professional hands for a limited period of time in order to achieve potential benefit.

"Consent of physician" in nursing homes is required for a wide range of matters. Physicians are asked to attest that a single room is necessary or that moving from room to room would be detrimental. In some instances, physicians' orders are requested for residents to self-medicate, to have an alcoholic beverage, or to stay up late at night. It is as if the remainder of the resident's life is to be orchestrated by a physician.

The care plan further medicalizes everyday life, determining what residents may eat, whether they are restrained, whether they are given psychoactive medications to control their behavior, and what kind of ambulation assistance, exercise programs, and other help they will receive.

It is not clear by what authority we have the right to so circumscribe a nursing home resident's life and to turn each decision into a health care decision. Indeed, new housing units for frail older persons are being developed on an opposite set of premises. Sometimes called assisted living, and largely available now for the well-to-do, these housing complexes afford their residents the privacy of small apartments and considerable autonomy. The housekeeping and hotel functions of the nursing home are provided and somehow separated conceptually from the delivery of medical and skilled nursing care. Under this model, it is unlikely that a resident's movements would be so restricted.

Much work is ahead to discover the most desirable way of organizing living situations for the frail elderly who are now in nursing homes. Any solution will need to take into account that some nursing home residents some of the time need hospital-like care, which indeed should be under the direction of health care professionals. But to put the lives of all nursing home residents under constant medical direction is to act out a fiction that restricts individual rights and ignores the importance of independence in small everyday decisions.

DEVELOPING PROCEDURES

Although absolute rules are unlikely to be found to govern many of the choices that must be made in nursing homes, procedures can be developed that at least raise issues in an organized way and militate toward fair solutions. Many of the problems reflected in the cases and commentaries concerned allocation—of a single room or a room with a desirable roommate, of table companions, of staff time to give intimate care, of the limited public space for residents' private purposes.

Questions of allocation lend themselves to procedural approaches. For matters of room and table allocation, for example, there could well be general guidelines that residents help shape and that are known to all new residents in advance. The criteria could be a mixture of queuing tempered by any considerations of health and safety that seemed paramount. Mechanisms for making complaints and requesting exceptions could also be clearly spelled out.

Procedures at the time of admission are particularly important. We were startled to learn how little many residents had participated in the decision to enter the facility and how many had misconceptions about the length of the stay. It would seem reasonable to expect that each cognitively intact resident participate in those decisions. Realistically, some residents come to nursing homes directly from acute-care hospitals; they are still sick, and the hunt for a facility with available space was necessarily undertaken in a hurry. Perhaps it is necessary to explore the legal protections that could be offered so that an older person's household would not be prematurely disbanded and so that the resident would still retain decision-making flexibility once recovered.

CONCLUSIONS

We conclude that nursing home residents want to have, could have, and should have more autonomy in everyday matters. In the first chapter, we pinpointed the three Rs—routine, regulation, and restricted opportunity —as the enemies of autonomy in the nursing home. These add up to a complex situation, but none of the complexities should be allowed to obfuscate the real problems or justify the status quo. Moreover, we believe that many of the issues we have identified apply to those receiving home care as well as those in nursing homes.

We foresee a lengthy process of discovering what can be done—first, what can be done without spending another cent or changing any laws, and second what can be done but requires policy change or more money. Ahead of us lie measurement challenges to accurately determine the preferences of nursing home residents. We also have ahead the work of developing and testing procedures that will result in fairer allocation of resources and more autonomous residents. Our plea is that attention be paid and the work begin.

CONTRIBUTORS

Mila Ann Aroskar, EdD, RN, is a professor in the Division of Health Services Administration at the University of Minnesota School of Public Health, where she formerly directed the program in public health nursing. Her teaching and research are concentrated on ethical issues in public health, nursing, and health care in general.

Martin Benjamin, PhD, is a professor of philosophy at Michigan State University. A prolific writer in bioethics, his newest book *Splitting the Difference: Integrity-Preserving Compromise in Ethics and Politics* will be published by University of Kansas Press in 1990.

Margaret Battin, PhD, a professor of philosophy at the University of Utah, is a bioethicist who has written on end-of-life issues for many years. She is the author of *Ethical Issues in Suicide* and co-author or co-editor of *Suicide: The Ethical Issues, John Donne's Biathanatos: A Modern-Spelling Critical Edition, Suicide and Ethical Theory, Should Medical Care Be Rationed by Age?*, and various papers in medical ethics. She is one of several authors of *Ethical Issues in the Professions* and has just completed a new study in applied professional ethics, tentatively entitled *Ethical Issues in Organized Religion*.

Arthur L. Caplan, PhD, a philosopher, was formerly associate director of the Hastings Center for Biomedical Ethics. He is the founding director of the University of Minnesota's Center for Biomedical Ethics. A prolific writer and commentator who blends ethical analysis with empirical research, Dr. Caplan has authored scores of articles and monographs on subjects such as artificial heart transplantation, harvesting of organs for organ transplantation, distinctions between clinical research and clinical treatment, ethics in genetics and fertility programs, and the emergence of a new ethic guiding health care delivery.

James F. Childress, PhD, is the Edwin B. Kyle Professor of Religious Studies and professor of medical education at the University of Virginia, where he is also chairman of the Department of Religious Studies and principal of the Monroe Hill Residential College. He is the author of numerous articles and several books in biomedical ethics, including *Principles of Biomedical Ethics*, and *Who Should Decide? Paternalism in Health Care*.

Steven S. Foldes, PhD, is an anthropologist who has occupied a variety of positions in health services research and health care administration. At present, he is director of the Medicaid Research Unit in the Minnesota Department of Human Services. He has been keenly interested in allocation of health care and the cultural contexts for health care services.

Iris C. Freeman, MSW, is the executive director of the Minnesota Alliance for Health Care Consumers, an organization that performs legislative advocacy on behalf of long-term care consumers, provides ombudsman services for the seven-county metropolitan Twin Cities area, and does training and development for nursing home resident and family councils. Ms. Freeman has gained national recognition for her work on behalf of nursing home residents. She was a member of the Institute of Medicine's Committee on Nursing Home Regulation, 1983-1985.

Sara T. Fry, PhD, RN, is associate professor at the University of Maryland School of Nursing, Baltimore, where she teaches the philosophy of nursing science and health care ethics. Her research interests include the protection of privacy, the use of prenatal diagnostic technologies, decision making on the termination of life-sustaining treatments, and empirical investigation of the moral phenomena of nursing practice.

Andrew Jameton, PhD, a philosopher, is associate professor and interim chair of the Department of Preventive and Societal Medicine, College of Medicine, University of Nebraska Medical Center. He is author of *Nursing Practice: The Ethical Issues*. He has recently published work on the ethical responsibilities of residents in long-term-care facilities and on research methods in nursing ethics.

Rosalie A. Kane, DSW, is a professor in the School of Social Work and the School of Public Health at the University of Minnesota, where she also directs the Long-Term Care DECISIONS Resource Center. Her prolific works on the organization, financing, and evaluation of long-term care, many coauthored with Robert L. Kane, MD, include *Long-Term Care: Principles, Programs, and Policies,* 1987; *A Will And a Way: What the United States Can Learn from Canada about Caring for the Elderly,* 1985; *Values and Long-Term Care,* 1983; and *Assessing the Elderly: A Practical Guide to Measurement,* 1981.

Diane K. Kjervik, JD, RN, is associate professor and director of Graduate Studies at the University of Minnesota School of Nursing in Minneapolis. She is also affiliated with the Center for Advanced Feminist Studies at the University of Minnesota. She is a member of the Advisory Council of National Center for Nursing Research at the National Institutes of Health. Her research interests include informed consent, power inequities, incompetency criteria, and the legal status of the elderly.

Loren E. Lomasky, PhD, is professor of philosophy at the University of Minnesota, Duluth. His research interests include medical ethics, political philosophy, and the philosophy of religion. He is the author of *Persons, Rights, and the Moral Community,* 1987.

Ruth Macklin, PhD, a philosopher, is professor of bioethics in the Department of Epidemiology and Social Medicine at Albert Einstein College of Medicine, Bronx, New York. Her many articles about ethics and health care have appeared in professional journals and in the popular press. Her most recent book, *Mortal Choices,* was released in paperback in 1988. Dr. Macklin is a member of six institutional ethics committees, including two at nursing homes in the Bronx.

David J. Mayo, PhD, an associate professor of philosophy at the University of Minnesota at Duluth, has been working in biomedical ethics since 1974. He has concentrated on issues involving death and dying, active euthanasia, philosophical issues involved in suicide, and most recently, ethical issues associated with AIDS.

Laurence B. McCullough, PhD, a philosopher, is professor of medicine and community medicine in the Center for Ethics, Medicine and Public Issues in the Baylor College of Medicine in Houston. He has published extensively in geriatric ethics.

Steven H. Miles, MD, is associate director of the Center for Clinical Medical Ethics and assistant professor of medicine at the University of Chicago, Pritzker School of Medicine. He is a geriatrician and a Henry J. Kaiser Family Foundation Faculty Scholar in General Internal Medicine.

Harry R. Moody, PhD, a philosopher, is associate director of the Brookdale Center on Aging at Hunter College in New York City. His interests range widely to include negotiated consent processes, intergenerational equity issues, and other themes relating to ethics and aging. His most recent book is *Abundance of Life: Human Development Policies for an Aging Society.*

Reinhard Priester, JD, is a research fellow at the Center for Biomedical Ethics at the University of Minnesota. Primary areas of interest include the allocation and rationing of limited health care resources, transplantation, termination of treatment, cost containment, and the role of market forces in health care. He was formerly a research associate with the Minnesota Coalition on Health.

Robert L. Schwartz, JD, is professor of law at the University of New Mexico, where he has taught since 1977. He has at times taken leave from his teaching to be a legal research associate at the High Court of American Samoa in Pago Pago, to be a post-doctoral fellow at the Hastings Center, to join the law faculty at Cambridge University and the University of Delhi, and to serve as general counsel to the New Mexico Human Services Department.

Rosemarie Tong, PhD, is John Thatcher Professor of Medical Humanities at Davidson College in North Carolina. Her publications include *Women, Sex, and the Law, Ethics in Policy Analysis,* and *Feminist Thought: A Comprehensive Introduction.* Currently, she is co-authoring a book on reproductive and genetic technology and working toward the establishment of an undergraduate program in medical humanities at Davidson.

Ene Kristi Urv-Wong, MHA, is coordinator of the University of Minnesota's Long-Term Care DECISIONS Resource Center. She holds a masters degree in hospital and health care administration. Previously, as research associate in the School of Public Health's Division of Health Services Research and Policy, she managed the field studies for the project "Practical Autonomy in the Everyday Life of Nursing Home Residents."

Maryellen Waithe, PhD, a philosopher, is assistant professor at the University of Minnesota's School of Nursing, where she is part of the undergraduate Ethics Education Project funded by the Fund for Postgraduate Education. She has published and taught in medical, dental and nursing ethics. She is the director of the project on the history of women in philosophy and editor of a four volume series, *A History of Women Philosophers.*

Terrie Wetle, PhD, is director of research for the Braceland Center for Mental Health and Aging at the Institute of Living and is on the faculty of the Travelers Center on Aging at the University of Connecticut. She is the former associate director of the Division on Aging and an assistant professor of medicine at Harvard Medical School and director of the Program in Long-Term Care Administration at Yale University.

INDEX

Activities director, 12, 72, 273, 276
Activities of Daily Living, 7, 41, 114,
    117, 158
ADLs, see Activities of Daily Living
Administration, 35, 76, 132, 276, 300
Administrators, 15, 21, 47, 73, 125,
    131, 133, 137, 144, 223, 253,
    277, 283, 289, 294
Advance directive, 311–312
Agree, E. A., 127, 131, 135
Aides, see Nursing assistants
Aiken, L. H., 287, 289
Alexander, G., 149, 153
Alzheimer's disease, see Cognitive
    Impairment
Ambrogi, D., 83, 88
American Nurses Association, 286,
    288, 289
Arras, J., 40, 50
Autonomy
    definitions, 5, 32, 44–46, 66–68,
        112–116, 127, 141, 144, 146,
        159, 181, 193, 200–201, 225,
        236, 291, 292

    enhance, see opportunity for moral
        agents, 47, 48, 82, 201–202,
        205, 287
    opportunity for, 33, 34, 38, 40, 45,
        69, 116, 120, 127, 168, 183,
        193, 207, 237, 238, 292, 293,
        300, 304, 314
    restrictions on, 5, 19, 39, 45, 47, 62,
        83–84, 86, 88, 93, 117, 119,
        122, 134, 147, 237, 238, 254,
        293–302, 306–307, 317

Bathing, 7, 8, 16, 38, 79, 85, 178–188,
    237, 273, 275, 280, 302
Beauchamp, T. L., 44, 50, 88, 128,
    134, 135
Bed, transfer (in and out), 7, 8, 274
Beneficence, 23, 54, 55, 76, 83, 88,
    128, 129–130, 133, 135, 206,
    293, 307
Benjamin, M., 81, 88, 231, 232–233
Bennett, C., 15, 19
Bill of Rights, resident, 16, 83, 183

Brody, E. M., 130, 136
Brooks, A., 113, 123
Buchanen, A. E., 156, 163

Callahan, D., 131, 136, 151, 153
Caplan, A. L., 45, 50
Care conference, 203, 204, 205,
    206, 292
Care plans, 16, 17, 83, 119, 202,
    273–274, 282, 284, 289
Care routines, 8, 13, 39, 79–81, 85,
    191, 209, 224, 227, 276, 314
Carter, M. A., 273, 290
Cassel, E. M., 244
Certified Nursing Assistant, see
    Nursing assistant
Chang, B. L., 117, 123
Chairs, 15, 46, 54, 71–78, 302
Childress, J. F., 84, 85, 88, 182, 188
Christianson, D., 128, 136
Chronically mentally ill, 7
Code for Nurses, 63
Code of Professional Responsibility,
    63, 201
Coercive, 49, 68, 73, 82, 88, 116, 118,
    202, 206, 249, 250, 255, 292
Cognitive Impairment, 9, 13, 16, 37,
    38, 40, 59, 62, 104, 109, 134,
    165–166, 241, 293, 308, 309,
    310, 311–312
Collopy, B. J., 44, 50, 112, 123, 141,
    144, 153, 158, 163, 193, 197,
    225, 233
Communication, 125, 126, 132,
    207, 300
Compromise, 81, 228, 230, 283, 307
Conservator, 56, 139
Cooper, K. H., 93, 98
CNA, see nursing assistants, 302
Creek, L. V., 219, 220

Dahl, R., 87, 88
Death, 100, 129, 209–220, 271, 276
Demented, see Cognitive Impairment
Dementia, see Cognitive Impairment

Diamond, T., 105, 107, 276, 277,
    279, 289
Dietician, 12, 273
Dignity, 29, 30, 38, 39, 49, 50, 54, 56,
    83, 158–159, 192, 194, 225,
    229, 284, 291, 314
Director of Nursing, 12, 80, 110, 126,
    137, 273, 277, 283
Disorientation, see Cognitive
    Impairment
DNR, see Do Not Resuscitate
Doctors, see Physicians
DON, see Director of Nursing
Do Not Resuscitate, 211
Dressing, 7, 8, 223–232, 273, 275, 302
DSM III, 113, 123
Dubler, N., 143, 153
Durable Power of Attorney, 151
Duties, 38, 39, 65
Dworkin, G., 44, 50, 84, 89, 114, 123,
    141, 153
Deinstitutionalization, 7

Eating, 7, 8, 19, 22, 38, 40, 55, 59, 79,
    88, 109–122, 142, 237, 274,
    275, 297, 302, 308
Edelman, T. S., 299, 304
Emanuel, E., 37, 50
Equity, 25, 39, 50, 75–76, 78, 185,
    247, 250–251
Evans, L. K., 15, 19, 287, 289

Faden, R., 113, 123
Family
    selection of a nursing home, 10, 11
    support, 12, 26, 27, 43, 77–78
    visiting, 11, 74
Feinberg, J., 87, 89
Fisher, R., 232, 233
Freedom, see Autonomy
Fry, S. T., 195, 197

Geri-chairs, see Restraints
Gibson, J., 148, 153

Gilligan, C., 106, 107, 205, 208
Glass, A. P., 296, 305
Goffman, E., 25, 26, 27, 28, 31, 36
Goodwin, M., 272, 289
Gorlin, R., 203, 208
Greenhouse, L., 105, 107
Griswold, 105, 107
Grossman, H. D., 300, 305
Guardian, 56, 137–153, 313

Hall, E. T., 93, 98
Hart, M., 300, 305
Hassler, J., 4, 19
Haworth, L., 31, 36
Hayduk, L. A., 93, 98
Hing, E., 7, 8, 9, 19
Holtz, G. A., 279, 290
Hospice, 42
Hospital, 42, 60, 245
    discharge from, 10, 249, 316
    discharge to, 6, 249, 254
Hulicka, 117

Incontinence, 8, 178–179, 274, 286
Independence, see Autonomy
Individualized care, see Care plan
Informed consent, 43, 142, 182
Institute of Medicine, 17, 18, 20, 294,
    296, 297, 301, 305
Iris, M., 145, 153

Jameton, A., 82, 89, 157, 163
Justice, 18, 25, 49, 50, 83, 88, 107,
    131, 185, 238–239, 251, 266

Kalish, R. A., 213, 220
Kane, R. A., 95, 98
Kapp, M. B., 296, 299, 305
Kaster, J. M., 277, 290
Keeler, E., 6, 20
Kolata, G., 34, 36
Kjervik, D., 202, 208

Klanderman, D., 286, 290
Kuflik, A., 230, 233

Labor unions, 13
Laird, C., 4, 5, 20
Lange, A., 206, 208
Langer, 117, 123
Lawton, M. P., 48, 50
Licensed Practical Nurse, 12, 13, 165,
    200, 205, 271–289
Long, G. T., 93, 98
LPN, see Licensed practical nurse
Luban, D., 232, 233

Married, 100, 107
May, W. F., 103, 107
McCullough, L. B., 126, 127, 131,
    135, 136
Meals, see Eating
Medicaid, 9, 10, 18, 19, 57, 90, 95,
    138, 235, 236, 242, 244,
    258–259, 260–266, 293, 294,
    303–304, 308
    certified bed, 91
    conditions of participation, 17, 161
Medical director, 12, 273
Medicare, 12, 14, 248, 303–304, 308
    certified bed, 91, 304
    conditions of participation, 17, 161,
    248
Memory impairment, see Cognitive
    Impairment
Mezey, M., 287, 290
Mill, J. S., 118, 123
Miller, B. L., 44, 50, 66, 70, 84, 89,
    181, 188
Mishra, P. K., 93, 98
Model resident, see Resident
    individual adaptation
Moody, H. R., 81, 89, 144, 153,
    231, 232
Morford, T. G., 33, 36

National Citizens' Coalition on
    Nursing Home Reform, 278, 290

National Nursing Home Survey, 6, 7,
     8, 9
National Teaching Nursing Home
     Project, 287
Negligence, 162
Negotiation, 81, 133, 186, 231–232,
     237, 304, 307
Nicholson, C. K., 285, 290
Neibuhr, H. R., 82, 89
Nonmaleficence, 83, 88
Nurses, see Registered Nurses,
     Licensed Practical Nurses
Nurses aide, see Nurses assistant
Nursing assistant, 12, 24, 30, 41, 53,
     56, 72, 79, 85, 166, 169, 187,
     190–197, 199–207, 209,
     271–289
  caring work, 276–277, 289
  tasks, 7, 191, 275–277
  training, 13, 277–289
  turnover, 277, 283
Nursing home
  activities, 9, 14, 18, 30, 60, 69, 281
  admissions to, 3, 4, 6, 11, 12, 28, 75,
     82, 97, 102, 157, 169, 245,
     247–257, 291, 308, 316
  as medical facility, 23, 27, 28,
     41–43, 62, 64, 66, 68, 74,
     165, 173, 315–316
  as residential facility, 23, 41–43, 62,
     64–65, 66, 68, 104, 119, 186,
     251, 307
  culture, 23–28, 32, 107, 216–217,
     247, see also total institution
  discharge from 6, 7
  efficiency, 31, 35, 119, 121, 169,
     183, 185, 226, 227, 237,
     249, 309
  environment, 5, 7, 12, 14, 17, 39,
     41, 43–44, 49, 54, 75, 76, 81,
     83, 104, 133, 168, 170, 188,
     192, 194, 197, 201, 237, 291,
     308–310, 313
  ethics committee, 288, 301–302
  length of stay, 6–7
  liability, 21, 43, 49, 156–163, 205,
     263, 296, 313

  policies, 18, 38, 39, 49, 72, 80, 119,
     218, 254, 260, 280, 289, 297,
     312, see also Autonomy,
     restrictions on
  programs, see Nursing home,
     activities
  regimentation, 16–19, 22, 26–28,
     92, 317, see also Nursing
     home, culture
  regulations, 17, 18, 19, 23, 33, 49,
     54, 81–83, 85–88, 295–296,
     299, 317
  religious, 17
  resources, 23, 31, 33, 34, 56, 75, 94,
     116, 122, 183, 243
    allocation of, 91, 186, 288, 302,
       314, 317
  safety, 17, 33, 35, 48, 87, 117, 161,
     166, 170, 172, 183, 295, 297,
     307, 313, 316
  standards, 294–296, 298, 304
  surveyors, 18, 80, 273, 297, 298, see
     also Nursing home,
     regulations
Nursing Home Reform Act, see
     OBRA

Obligations
  of family, 126, 131, 152
  of nursing home, 39, 78, 87, 132,
     161, 187, 214, 216
  of residents, 38, 62–64, 82
  of staff, 56, 132, 195, 196, 202,
     212, 226
Office of Technology Assessment,
     142, 153
Older Americans Act, 152
Ombudsman, 15, 27, 53, 55, 97, 101,
     106–107, 156, 293, 295–296,
     302–303
Omnibus Budget Reconciliation Act,
     277, 293, 299, 301, 305
Organic brain disease, see Cognitive
     Impairment
Outcome measures, see Quality
     of life

Paraprofessional, *see* Nursing
  assistant
Paternalistic, 49, 60, 62, 84, 85, 113,
  118, 128, 182, 314
Patient Tort Liability of Rest,
  Convalescent, or Nursing
  Home, 83 ALR 3d 871, 161, 163
Pellegrino, E. D., 195, 197
Peschel, R. E., 213, 221
Pharmacist, 12, 273
Physical therapist, 12, 273
Physicians, 10, 12, 33, 34, 41, 43, 160,
  183, 203, 287, 308
Poole, S. R., 231, 233
Possey, *see* Restraints
Presidents Commission for the Study
  of Ethical Problems in Medicine
  and Biomedical and Behavioral
  Research, 142, 153, 193, 194,
  198
Primary caretaker, 206, 209, 284–285
Privacy, *see* Private space
Private pay, 260, 262
Private space, 14, 15, 29, 54, 80, 83,
  86, 92, 93, 103, 104, 106, 214,
  303, 316, *see also* Rooms
Protecting nursing home patients,
  161, 163
Pruchno, R. A., 97–98
Public space, 16, 22, 54, 72, 76, 93

Quality of life, 17, 59, 40, 41, 43–44,
  49, 220, 238, 249, 251
  outcome measures, 17–18, 33, 248

Rand, A., 230, 233
Registered nurses, 12, 27, 41, 80, 152,
  165, 169, 205, 271–289, 276,
  284
Rehabilitation, 6, 55, 95, 115, 247, 298
Reimbursement, 14, 18, 19, 91, 251,
  256, 308
Resident
  assets, *see* Resident, resources
  attitude, *see* individual adaptation

belongings, *see* Resident, personal
  possessions
characteristics of, 6–12
cognitively intact, 10, 14, 16, 28,
  30, 38, 41, 45, 48, 49, 69,
  109, 113, 128, 130, 169, 172,
  238, 278, 285, 298, 308, 310,
  see also Cognitive
  Impairment
competency, *see* Residents,
  cognitively intact
decision making capability, 12, 115,
  144, 182–183, 237, *see also*
  Cognitive Impairment
dehumanization, 76
dependence on staff, 7, 8, 29, 35,
  42, 45, 158, 185, 192, 239
eviction, 56, 258–266
expectations for, 21, 23, 28, 32, 35,
  42, 62, 242, 281
expectations of, 17, 22, 35, 102
frail, 5, 127, 129, 161, 162,
  212–213, 240, 271
functional disability, 7, 9
functional impairment, 7, 8, 12,
  146
incompetent, 50, 141, 146, 241,
  298
individual adaptation, 28–31, 49,
  54, 58, 60–65, 67, 68–69, 81,
  82, 96, 125, 178, 184
level of care, 102, 162
personal identity and integrity, 19,
  47, 54, 75–77, 84, 94, 102,
  114, 159, 194, 224–232, 248,
  251, 291, 292
personal possessions, 11, 12, 15, 16,
  18, 22, 29, 35, 39, 40, 54, 86,
  93, 291, 293
physically disabled, 4, 14, 104, 109,
  112–113, 192
relationships, 41, 54, 55, 74, 75, 78,
  95, 102, 104–106, 131, 195,
  214, 219, 239, 241–242,
  278–280, 291
resources, 9, 10, 11, 56, 95, 291,
  314

Resident *(cont.)*
  risk, willingness to assume, 56,
      313
  self-expression, *see* Resident,
      personal identity and
      integrity
  sensory impairments, 8, 12
  vulnerable, 49, 50, 85, 87, 170, 172,
      195, 241, 266, 314
  wandering, 137, 162, 168, 313
  younger, 7
Resident Council, 64, 69, 72, 73,
      106–107, 110, 178, 184, 204,
      292, 300
Responsibilities
  family, 39, 130–131, 135, 175, 249
  nursing assistant, 56, 171, 201, 207,
      214, 275–277
  nursing home staff, 39, 137, 157,
      171, 173, 185, 259, 274, 288,
      301, 313
  resident, 38, 41, 59, 60–63, 68, 82
Restraints
  chemical, 22, 73, 174, 287, 288
  physical, 11, 15, 16, 22, 29, 30, 47,
      56, 156, 165–176, 275–276,
      287, 288, 292, 293, 310–311,
      314
Retirement Research Foundation, ix
Richards, D. A. J., 104, 108
Robinson, M. A., 218, 221
Roe vs. Wade, 105, 108
Roommates
  assignment, 16, 38, 54, 91, 94–98,
      110, 288, 316
  difficulties with, 14, 22, 25, 29, 55,
      59, 92, 102, 187
Rooms
  single, 14, 55, 58–61, 69, 90–98,
      288, 309, 315, 316
  transfer, interinstitutional, 14–15,
      29, 97, 104, 179, 255, 295,
      309, 315
RN, *see* Registered nurses
Ryden, M., 117, 123

Sarton, M., 4, 20
Sartorius, R., 114, 123
Sekscenski, E., 6, 20
Selby, T. L., 273, 290
Self determination, *see* Autonomy
Senile dementia, *see* Cognitive
      Impairment
Shared decision making, *see*
      Negotiation
Shield, R. R., 27, 28, 36
Side-rails, *see* Restraints
Smith, A., 65, 70
Social security benefits, 262
Social worker, 12, 24, 28, 30, 34, 53,
      54, 55, 60, 62, 91–92, 101, 109,
      110, 112, 115, 120–121,
      137–138, 144, 152, 273, 276
Staff
  convenient for, 47–48, 56, 69, 102,
      103, 166, 169, 218
  resources, 8, 186, 218, 239, 298,
      302
  training, 31, 34, 206, 214–215, 218,
      220, 232
Stanley, B., 142, 154
Surrogate decision maker, 113,
      144–145, 148, 149, 153,
      174–175, 206, 288, 311,
      312–313

Table companions, 109–122, 288,
      316
Teilleman, J. L., 292, 305
Telephone, 7, 10, 19, 22, 38, 39, 40,
      125–135, 186, 300
Television, 15, 16, 42, 49, 54, 186
Tellis-Nayak, V., 275, 290
Thomasma, D., 44, 50, 141, 154
Tipping, 235–244, 250
Toileting, 7, 19, 31, 59, 227, 274, 275,
      282, 302, 314
Tolle, S. W., 219, 221
Total institution
  description of, 25–27, 31, 32, 43

Tulloch, J. C., 4, 5, 13, 20
Tolstoy, L., 213, 221

Uniform Guardianship and Protective
    Proceedings Act 1982,
    139–140, 141, 145, 150
Uniform Probate Code 1969,
    139–140, 141, 143, 145, 150

Veatch, R. M., 128, 136
Vladek, B. L., 272, 290

Waithe, M., 113, 114, 115, 118, 123
Waiver of liability, 162

Walkley, F. H., 93, 98
Walzer, M., 251, 257
Weil, W. B., 231, 233
Weisman, A. D., 213, 221
Welfare benefits, see Medicaid
Wethe, T., 212, 219, 221
Wilson, K. B., 285, 290
Winslow, G. R., 94, 98

Zimmer, J., 15, 20